国际经典内科学教科书

第10版
Cecil Essentials of Medicine
希氏内科学精要
中英双语版

原 著　Edward J. Wing, MD, FACP, FIDSA
Former Dean of Medicine and Biological Sciences
Professor of Medicine
Warren Alpert Medical School of Brown University, Providence, Rhode Island

Fred J. Schiffman, MD, MACP
Sigal Family Professor of Humanistic Medicine
Vice Chair, Department of Medicine
Warren Alpert Medical School of Brown University, Providence, Rhode Island

中英双语版　编辑委员会　主任委员　王　辰

U0197200

=== 第1分册 ===

内科学概论·呼吸与危重症医学·术前和术后照护

主　译　王　辰　代华平　赵　晶　黄　慧

北京大学医学出版社

XISHI NEIKEXUE JINGYAO（DI 10 BAN） DI 1 FENCE NEIKEXUE GAILUN·HUXI YU
WEIZHONGZHENG YIXUE·SHUQIAN HE SHUHOU ZHAOHU（ZHONGYING SHUANGYU BAN）

图书在版编目（CIP）数据

希氏内科学精要：第 10 版. 第 1 分册，内科学概论·呼吸与危重症医学·术前和术后照护：汉、英 /（美）爱德华·温（Edward J. Wing），（美）弗雷德·谢夫曼（Fred J. Schiffman）原著；王辰等主译. -- 北京：北京大学医学出版社，2024. 11. -- ISBN 978-7-5659-3245-8

Ⅰ. R5

中国国家版本馆 CIP 数据核字第 2024BB3806 号

北京市版权局著作权合同登记号：图字：**01-2024-4518**

Elsevier (Singapore) Pte Ltd.
3 Killiney Road, #08-01 Winsland House I, Singapore 239519
Tel: (65) 6349-0200; Fax: (65) 6733-1817

Cecil Essentials of Medicine, Tenth Edition
Copyright © 2022 by Elsevier, Inc. All rights are reserved, including those for text and data mining, AI training, and similar technologies.
Publisher's note: Elsevier takes a neutral position with respect to territorial disputes or jurisdictional claims in its published content, including in maps and institutional affiliations.
Previous editions copyrighted 2016, 2010, 2007, 2004, 2001, 1997, 1993, 1990, and 1986.
ISBN-13: 978-0-323-72271-1

This translation of Cecil Essentials of Medicine, Tenth Edition by Edward J. Wing and Fred J. Schiffman was undertaken by Peking University Medical Press and is published by arrangement with Elsevier (Singapore) Pte Ltd.
Cecil Essentials of Medicine, Tenth Edition by Edward J. Wing and Fred J. Schiffman 由北京大学医学出版社进行翻译，并根据北京大学医学出版社与爱思唯尔（新加坡）私人有限公司的协议约定出版。
《希氏内科学精要（第 10 版） 第 1 分册 内科学概论·呼吸与危重症医学·术前和术后照护（中英双语版）》（王辰 代华平 赵晶 黄慧主译）
ISBN: 978-7-5659-3245-8
Copyright © 2024 by Elsevier (Singapore) Pte Ltd. and Peking University Medical Press.
All rights reserved. No part of this publication may be reproduced or transmitted in any form or by any means, electronic or mechanical, including photocopying, recording, or any information storage and retrieval system, without permission in writing from Elsevier (Singapore) Pte Ltd. and Peking University Medical Press.

注　意

本译本由北京大学医学出版社独立完成。相关从业及研究人员必须凭借其自身经验和知识对文中描述的信息数据、方法策略、搭配组合、实验操作进行评估和使用。由于医学科学发展迅速，临床诊断和给药剂量尤其需要经过独立验证。在法律允许的最大范围内，爱思唯尔、译文的原文作者、原文编辑及原文内容提供者均不对译文或因产品责任、疏忽或其他操作造成的人身及（或）财产伤害及（或）损失承担责任，亦不对由于使用文中提到的方法、产品、说明或思想而导致的人身及（或）财产伤害及（或）损失承担责任。

Published in China by Peking University Medical Press under special arrangement with Elsevier (Singapore) Pte Ltd. This edition is authorized for sale in the People's Republic of China only, excluding Hong Kong SAR, Macau SAR and Taiwan. Unauthorized export of this edition is a violation of the contract.

希氏内科学精要（第 10 版） 第 1 分册　内科学概论·呼吸与危重症医学·术前和术后照护（中英双语版）

主　　译：王　辰　代华平　赵　晶　黄　慧
出版发行：北京大学医学出版社
地　　址：（100191）北京市海淀区学院路 38 号　北京大学医学部院内
电　　话：发行部 010-82802230；图书邮购 010-82802495
网　　址：http://www.pumpress.com.cn
E-mail：booksale@bjmu.edu.cn
印　　刷：北京信彩瑞禾印刷厂
经　　销：新华书店
策划编辑：高　瑾
责任编辑：高　瑾　责任校对：靳新强　责任印制：李　啸
开　　本：889 mm×1194 mm　1/16　印张：14　字数：520 千字
版　　次：2024 年 11 月第 1 版　2024 年 11 月第 1 次印刷
书　　号：ISBN 978-7-5659-3245-8
定　　价：96.00 元

版权所有，违者必究

（凡属质量问题请与本社发行部联系退换）

中英双语版 编辑委员会

主任委员

王　辰

委　员（按姓氏笔画排序）

王　洁　　王伊龙　　王建祥　　巴　一　　代华平　　宁　光　　宁晓红　　朱　兰

任景怡　　刘海鹰　　李小鹰　　李梦涛　　李雪梅　　杨爱明　　张福杰　　郑金刚

房静远　　赵　晶　　赵明辉　　郝　伟　　姜　辉　　栗占国　　贾继东　　夏维波

黄　慧　　黄晓军　　曹　彬　　彭　斌　　潘　慧

第 1 分册　内科学概论·呼吸与危重症医学·术前和术后照护

　　　　　主译　王　辰　代华平　赵　晶　黄　慧

第 2 分册　心血管疾病

　　　　　主译　郑金刚　任景怡

第 3 分册　肾脏疾病

　　　　　主译　李雪梅　赵明辉

第 4 分册　胃肠疾病·肝脏与胆道系统疾病

　　　　　主译　房静远　杨爱明　贾继东

第 5 分册　血液疾病

　　　　　主译　黄晓军　王建祥

第 6 分册　肿瘤疾病

　　　　　主译　王　洁　巴　一

第 7 分册　内分泌疾病与代谢疾病·女性健康·男性健康·骨与骨矿物质代谢疾病

　　　　　主译　宁　光　朱　兰　姜　辉　夏维波　潘　慧

第 8 分册　肌肉骨骼与结缔组织疾病

　　　　　主译　栗占国　李梦涛

第 9 分册　感染性疾病

　　　　　主译　刘海鹰　张福杰　曹　彬

第 10 分册　神经疾病·老年医学·缓和医疗·酒精和物质使用

　　　　　主译　彭　斌　王伊龙　李小鹰　宁晓红　郝　伟

医学名词审定指导

任慧玲　　李晓瑛　　冀玉静　　张燕舞　　李军莲

3

　　让我国医学生与国际医学生站在同一起跑线上的首要之事，是为其提供具有世界先进水平的标准教材。我们应争取使每一位医学生都能接触到内容经典、充分代表现代医学水平的国际权威原文教材并力求准确翻译，提供原文与中文双语对照版本，使医学生和医生在学习中形成双语医学词语、概念、概念间逻辑及由此构成的医学知识体系。在这样的思想驱动下，国际经典内科学教科书《希氏内科学精要（第10版）》中英双语版应运而生。

　　《希氏内科学》原著以其论述严谨准确、系统全面，被誉为"标准的内科学参考书"。自1927年首次出版以来，在内科学领域渐享世界级声誉，成为全球众多优秀医学院校，包括哈佛医学院、斯坦福大学医学院、约翰斯·霍普金斯大学医学院、牛津大学医学部、剑桥大学医学院、墨尔本大学医学院、新加坡国立大学医学院及多伦多大学医学院等普遍采用的内科学参考书。首版《希氏内科学精要》则诞生于1986年，旨在凝炼其全本的精华和要点，以最为简洁明确的方式向以医学生为主体的医学界精辟传达《希氏内科学》的核心信息，包括书中所体现出的人文精神。此后，每版精要本都力求凝炼地反映当时最新医学成果和医疗实践指南，愈来愈成为各国医学生、住院医师、专培医师及教师学习和传授内科学的主要教本，在世界医学教材体系中居引领地位。《希氏内科学》和《希氏内科学精要》两个版本不仅在英语国家被广泛使用，更被翻译为葡萄牙语、西班牙语、希腊语、意大利语、日语、简体中文版，为全球医学界广泛采用。

　　中国的医学生、住院医师、专培医师需要培养国际专业信息获取能力。将精要本原文引进并准确翻译，以中英文对照的形式呈现，便于读者进行双语对照阅读和学习，使之在学习理解国际标准医学内容的同时，学习好中英文医学词语，为国际医学交流打好基础。相信此举对于提高我国的医学教育水平，培养国际型医学人才至为有益。

　　《希氏内科学精要》精练地涵盖了内科学的所有主要领域，包括心血管疾病、呼吸疾病与危重症、消化疾病、肾脏疾病、内分泌和代谢疾病、风湿疾病、血液疾病、肿瘤、感染性疾病、神经与老年疾病等，构建了较为系统的知识体系。在翻译引进过程中，我们遵循将相关内容集中的原则，将原书按系统器官拆分为十个分册，使其更具有专科阅读的对应性，以更加灵活轻便的形式为读者提供多样化的阅读选择。

为确保译文质量，我们在译者遴选上采取了严谨的标准。从《希氏内科学（第 26 版）》翻译团队中择优选取责任心强、译文优质的译者，同时吸纳了临床医学专业"101"计划核心教材的编者团队。每个分册均由主译专家带领各自译者团队完成翻译、审校、交叉互审、通审四级审校工作。这些译者具备扎实的英语与专业能力，他们在翻译过程中，深入理解原文，准确阐述作者思想，并多角度审视译文的准确性、流畅性与风格一致性，确保译文的忠实性、规范性与可读性，在不同的语言和文化间架起坚实的桥梁。尤其值得称赞的是，对原著中疏漏或不够完善之处，译文中以"译者注"的形式加以适当解释和说明，使译文内容在忠实于原著的基础上更为准确。

　　本书读者定位于具有一定学习能力和基础的高等医学院校医学专业 8 年制、5 年制学生以及相关医学专业人员，可作为医务人员的内科学参考书、住院医师规范化培训和专科医师规范化培训辅导教材、研究生入学考试辅导教材、内科学教师参考书、内科学各专科医师复习回顾其他专科知识的重要读本。

呼吸与危重症医学教授
中国医学科学院院长
北京协和医学院校长
2024 年 11 月

对学习者教科书重要。

对学医者内科学重要。

世界上的内科学教科书，

首推《希氏内科学精要》。

中文是中国医生主要执业用语。

英文是国际医学交流的主要文字。

学习医学，当以双语对应阅读为好。

如此，可获纵横国际之效。

本书力求有助于此。

In Memoriam

Thomas E. Andreoli, MD

Dr. Thomas Andreoli, along with Drs. Lloyd Hollingsworth (Holly) Smith, Jr., Fred Plum, and Charles C.J. Carpenter, was one of the four founding editors of *Cecil Essentials of Medicine.* He served as editor for editions one through eight before he passed away on April 14, 2009. Dr. Andreoli was born in the Bronx, New York, in 1935, attended Catholic primary and high schools, and graduated from St. Vincent College and the Georgetown School of Medicine. He trained as a resident at Duke University under legendary Chair of Medicine Dr. Eugene Stead, who recognized him as a brilliant physician and scientist and encouraged his research career. Dr. Andreoli received his research training at the NIH and then in the laboratory of Dr. Tosteson at Duke. His research focused on the biochemical and biophysical properties of renal tubular cell membranes and their role in water and electrolyte transport. He made fundamental discoveries on the normal renal physiology, illuminating the way to subsequent work by many others on renal health and disease. His research was recognized with numerous awards and election to honorific societies both in the United States and in Europe. Dr. Andreoli also served as editor of *The American Journal of Physiology: Renal Physiology* and Editor in Chief of *Kidney International.*

Tom's national prominence and leadership qualities were recognized early in his career when he became head of Nephrology at the University of Alabama in Birmingham. There he helped faculty and trainees develop outstanding research, organized clinical services, and created a hemodialysis program to build one of the outstanding Divisions of Nephrology in the country. In 1979, Dr. Andreoli was appointed Chair of the Department of Internal Medicine at the University of Texas, Houston, where he assembled an outstanding faculty focused on research, clinical care, and teaching. In 1988, he accepted the position as Chairman of Internal Medicine at the University of Arkansas School of Medicine, a position he held until his death. There he again assembled a distinguished faculty who were outstanding researchers but also dedicated to outstanding clinical care and teaching. Morning report and clinical rounds with Dr. Andreoli were rigorous and riveting, focusing on the individual patient, not only their diagnoses and treatment but also on each patient's personal concerns and well-being. Dr. Andreoli was revered by medical students, his house staff, faculty, and colleagues, and I (EJW) personally can attest to what he regarded as his most cherished role—the mentorship and education of the next generation of physicians.

One of Dr. Andreoli's great interests was *Cecil Essentials of Medicine,* for which he was the editor/chief editor for eight of its ten editions, an interest that reflected his commitment to the education of students, house staff, and other physicians in the "essentials" of Internal Medicine.

Dr. Andreoli was devoted to his family. He was married to Elizabeth Berglund Andreoli from 1987 until his death. He was previously married to Dr. Kathleen Gainor Andreoli, mother of his three children and their ten grandchildren. Being of Italian ancestry and from Bronx, New York, it is not surprising that Dr. Andreoli was a passionate fan of the New York Yankees, Italian opera, which he could sing in Italian, and Frank Sinatra.

Dr. Andreoli's legacy lives on in his numerous previous students, house staff, colleagues, and in this book.

缅 怀

托马斯·安德里奥利博士

托马斯·安德里奥利（Thomas E. Andreoli）博士携手李奥德·霍灵斯沃斯·史密斯［Lloyd Hollingsworth（Holly）Smith］博士、弗雷德·普拉姆（Fred Plum）博士和查尔斯·卡彭特（Charles C.J. Carpenter）博士同为《希氏内科学精要》的创始编者。他在 2009 年 4 月 14 日去世前，曾担任该书第 1 至第 8 版的编者。安德里奥利博士于 1935 年出生于美国纽约布朗克斯区，就读于天主教小学和中学，后毕业于圣文森特学院和乔治城大学医学院。他在杜克大学医学院接受住院医师培训期间师从著名内科主任尤金·斯特德（Eugene Stead）博士，后者将其视为杰出的医生和科学家，并鼓励他投身科研事业。安德里奥利博士在美国国立卫生研究院接受科研训练后，前往杜克大学托斯特森（Tosteson）博士的实验室继续深造。他重点研究肾小管细胞膜的生化和生物物理特性及其在水和电解质转运中所发挥的作用。他在正常肾脏生理学方面的重要发现为后续关于肾脏健康和疾病的研究铺平了道路。安德里奥利博士的研究工作荣获多个学术奖项，并入选美国和欧洲的多个荣誉学会。他还担任《美国生理学杂志：肾脏生理学篇》（*The American Journal of Physiology：Renal Physiology*）的编辑以及《国际肾脏杂志》（*Kidney International*）的主编。

安德里奥利博士担任阿拉巴马大学伯明翰分校肾脏病学系主任后不久，即因其杰出领导力而赢得全美业内声誉。他帮助本校师生们取得科研突破，负责临床业务的组织实施，并因开创血液透析业务而使该科跻身全美顶级肾脏内科之列。1979 年，安德里奥利博士被任命为得克萨斯大学休斯敦分校内科学系主任，他在该系组建了一支科研、临床诊疗和教学并重的优秀教职团队。自 1988 年起，他担任阿肯色大学医学院内科学系主任，直至辞世。在这里他再次组建了一支卓越的教职团队，他们不仅科研工作出色，临床诊疗和教学工作也出类拔萃。安德里奥利博士带领的晨会报告和查房非常严谨而引人入胜，不仅尽心竭力于每位患者的诊断和治疗，还关注到他们每个人的个体情况和福祉。安德里奥利博士深受医学生、住院医师、教职人员和同事的崇敬，我（EJW）可以证明，他最珍视的角色当属培养和教育下一代医生。

安德里奥利博士对《希氏内科学精要》倾注了满腔热忱，先后担任了该书 10 版中 8 版的编者／主编，践行他为医学生、住院医师和其他各科医生们传授内科学"精要"的承诺。

安德里奥利博士高度重视家庭。他与第二任妻子伊丽莎白·伯格兰德·安德里奥利（Elizabeth Berglund Andreoli）的婚姻从 1987 年延续到辞世。他与第一任妻子凯瑟琳·盖娜·安德里奥利（Kathleen Gainor Andreoli）博士育有三个子女和十个孙辈。作为意大利裔和纽约布朗克斯人，安德里奥利博士是纽约洋基队、意大利歌剧（他能用意大利语演唱）和美国著名歌手、演员、主持人弗兰克·辛纳屈（Frank Sinatra）的忠实拥趸。安德里奥利博士将永远被他的众多学生、住院医师和同事怀念，并因本书而流芳百世。

Charles C.J. Carpenter, MD

Dr. Charles C.J. Carpenter joined Drs. Thomas Andreoli, Lloyd Hollingsworth Smith, Jr., and Fred Plum as a founder of *Cecil Essentials of Medicine*. He served as editor for seven editions and was followed in that role by Dr. Ivor Benjamin and then Dr. Edward Wing. Sadly, Chuck passed away on March 19, 2020, surrounded by his wife and children. He was Professor Emeritus of Medicine at The Warren Alpert Medical School of Brown University and Physician-in-Chief Emeritus at The Miriam Hospital.

Chuck was born in Savannah, Georgia, on January 5, 1931. He attended college at Princeton and medical school at Johns Hopkins where he also did his house staff training, including chief residency, and then joined the Johns Hopkins faculty. With his young family, he travelled to Calcutta, India, where he carried out landmark studies for the treatment of cholera.

Before coming to Brown in 1986, he was Chair of Medicine at Baltimore City Hospital and Case Western Reserve University.

His contributions to medical science and clinical care were many. While in Calcutta, using basic scientific evidence coupled with practical approaches, Dr. Carpenter developed "oral rehydration therapy" to address the cholera epidemic there. This treatment has saved millions of lives. While at Case, one of his innovations was to develop the nation's first Division of Geographic Medicine because of his strong belief that all physicians should be medical citizens of the world. In 1987, as he became deeply involved in the clinical management of persons living with HIV, he initiated a unique program in which Brown University faculty and trainees assumed responsibility for all HIV care in the Rhode Island State prison system.

Dr. Carpenter served as Chairman of the American Board of Internal Medicine and President of the Association of American Physicians. He has been a member of the NIH AIDS Executive Committee, the National Advisory Allergy and Infectious Diseases Council, and the USPHS AIDS Task Force. He was Chair of the Antiretroviral Treatment Panel of the International AIDS Society-USA and authored their recommendations on antiretroviral treatment. He also served as Chair of the Treatment Committee to evaluate the President's Emergency Plan for HIV/AIDS Relief. He became the director of the Brown University International Health Institute and the director of the Lifespan/Brown Center for AIDS Research with several Boston hospitals.

Throughout his career, Dr. Carpenter was the recipient of many international, national, and regional awards, accepting each with characteristic humility. With both small and large groups of learners, Chuck made certain that every member of his team was well educated, and each felt that they contributed to the well-being of their patients. His ability to sit calmly at the bedside, hold the patient's hand, comfort them, and listen in a genuinely focused way, influenced so many physicians. He was truly grateful for the opportunity to care for those less fortunate than he, and the feeling of being privileged to do so was clearly transmitted to all. Dr. Carpenter was a wonderful blend of profound compassion combined with the adherence to scholarship and teaching. Sir William Osler wrote that physicians should "Do the kind thing and do it first." Chuck lived by this precept. Vigor and insight characterized his approach to clinical and ethical challenges, always with younger colleagues at his side. In a recent tribute to him, many emphasized that Dr. Carpenter dedicated his life to his patients, many of whom were the most vulnerable members of society. We hope that we will have some of his strength and use his example as our compass as we are challenged to reduce suffering and improve the health of all for whom we are responsible.

He is survived by his wife of 61 years, Sally; three sons, Charles, Murray, and Andrew; and seven grandchildren.

查尔斯·卡彭特博士

查尔斯·卡彭特（Charles C.J. Carpenter）博士与 托马斯·安德里奥利（Thomas E. Andreoli）博士、李奥德·霍灵斯沃斯·史密斯（Lloyd Hollingsworth Smith）博士和弗雷德·普拉姆（Fred Plum）博士共同开创了《希氏内科学精要》。他共担任了 7 版的编者，嗣后由艾弗·本杰明（Ivor Benjamin）博士和爱德华·温（Edward Wing）博士接任。查尔斯·卡彭特博士于 2020 年 3 月 19 日在妻子和子女们的陪伴下辞世。他曾担任布朗大学沃伦·阿尔珀特医学院的内科学系名誉教授和米里亚姆医院的名誉主任医师。

查尔斯·卡彭特博士于 1931 年 1 月 5 日出生于美国佐治亚州萨凡纳市。他在普林斯顿大学获得学士学位后进入约翰斯·霍普金斯大学医学院，并完成了包括住院总医师在内的住院医师培训，随后加入了约翰斯·霍普金斯大学的教职团队。他曾携妻子和年幼的孩子前往印度加尔各答，在当地对霍乱的治疗进行了具有里程碑意义的研究工作。

在 1986 年入职布朗大学之前，他曾担任巴尔的摩市医院和凯斯西储大学医学院的内科学主任。

他在医学科学研究和临床诊疗领域建树颇多。在加尔各答期间，基于基础科学证据及临床实践，查尔斯·卡彭特博士开创了"口服补液疗法"以遏制当地的霍乱疫情。这一疗法拯救了数百万人的生命。秉承医生无国界的世界公民理念，他在凯斯西储大学做了一项开创性工作，建立了美国首个地缘医学部（研究地理环境因素对人体健康和疾病影响的学科）。1987 年，他深度参与人类免疫缺陷病毒（HIV）携带者的临床管理，并发起了一个独特的项目——由布朗大学教职团队和医学生们承担罗德岛州监狱系统内所有艾滋病相关诊疗工作。

查尔斯·卡彭特博士曾担任美国内科医师委员会主席和美国医师协会主席。他曾是美国国立卫生研究院艾滋病行政委员会、美国国家过敏与传染病咨询委员会以及公共卫生服务部艾滋病工作组的成员。他还曾担任国际艾滋病学会–美国分会抗逆转录病毒治疗组主席，并撰写了抗逆转录病毒治疗建议。他还担任过艾滋病治疗委员会主席，该委员会负责评估美国总统防治艾滋病紧急救援计划；曾担任布朗大学国际健康研究所所长，以及大学与多家波士顿当地医院合办的生命周期 / 布朗大学艾滋病研究中心主任。

查尔斯·卡彭特博士在职业生涯中获得过诸多国际性、全美和地区性奖项，同时展现其谦逊品格。无论学员人数多寡，查尔斯·卡彭特博士都会确保人人都能受到良好教育，并让他们感到自己也对患者的健康做出了贡献。他能够安静地坐在病床边，握住患者的手，安慰他们，并全神贯注地听取患者倾诉，这一举动深深地感染了许多医生。他十分珍视诊治不幸染病者的机会，并且能够将这种殊荣感传递给所有人。查尔斯·卡彭特博士完美地融汇了对患者的宅心仁厚与对学术和教学的坚守。威廉·奥斯勒（William Osler）爵士曾写道，医生应该"行善事，为人先"，而这正是查尔斯·卡彭特博士一生奉行的信条。他在面对临床和伦理挑战时充满活力和洞察力，始终重视提携年轻同事。许多人的悼词中都重点指出，查尔斯·卡彭特博士将毕生致力于患者福祉，其中许多人属于社会上最弱势群体。我们希望，在我们面临减少患者痛苦及改善其健康状况的挑战时，能够拥有他的力量，并以他为榜样获得指引。

查尔斯·卡彭特博士与妻子萨丽（Sally）共度了 61 年的婚姻时光，育有查尔斯（Charles）、穆雷（Murray）和安德鲁（Andrew）三子以及七个孙辈。

Dr. Edward J. Wing was an editor of *Cecil Essentials of Medicine,* editions 8 and 9, and is the lead editor of edition 10. He graduated from Williams College in 1967 and from the Harvard Medical School in 1971. He was a resident in Internal Medicine at the Peter Bent Brigham and completed an Infectious Diseases Fellowship at Stanford University. Joining the faculty at the University of Pittsburgh in 1975, he focused his NIH-funded research on mechanisms of cell-mediated immunity as well as various clinical aspects of Infectious Diseases. From 1990 to 1998, the University and UPMC appointed him as Physician-in-Chief at Montefiore Hospital, then Chief of Infectious Diseases, and finally Interim Chair of Medicine.

In 1998, Dr. Wing became Chair of Medicine at Brown University (1998–2008) where he consolidated the department across hospitals, practice plans, and training programs. As Dean of Medicine and Biological Sciences at Brown University (2008–2013) he strengthened ties with affiliated hospitals (Lifespan and Care New England), increased research, and oversaw the construction of a new medical school building. International exchange programs with medical schools in Kenya, the Dominican Republic, and Haiti were established during his years as chairman and dean. Dr. Wing has cared for patients with HIV since the beginning of the epidemic in outpatient clinics. He continues to be active in research, clinical care, and teaching.

Dr. Fred J. Schiffman, who along with Dr. Edward Wing is editor of *Cecil Essentials of Medicine,* 10th edition, attended Wagner College and then the New York University School of Medicine, from which he graduated in 1973. He performed his early house staff training at Yale-New Haven Hospital and then spent two years at the National Cancer Institute. He returned to Yale as Chief Medical Resident followed by a hematology fellowship. He became Medical Director of Yale's Primary Care Center before coming to Brown University in 1983, where he has been a leader in the medical residency program as well as Associate Physician-in-Chief at The Miriam Hospital.

Dr. Schiffman holds The Sigal Family Professorship in Humanistic Medicine at The Warren Alpert Medical School of Brown University. His scholarly interests include the structure and function of the human spleen and the intersection of the arts and medical care. He has directed or championed many projects and programs, including those that encourage and reinforce wellness and resilience in patients, families, and caregivers. He began a novel program that places medical students and physicians with other nonmedical professionals as they share in the viewing of works of art in the Museum of the Rhode Island School of Design. Dr. Schiffman recently led a Brown University edX course entitled, "Artful Medicine: Art's Power to Enrich Patient Care," with worldwide participation. Dr. Schiffman has also edited texts on hematologic pathophysiology, consultative hematology, and the anemias.

爱德华·温（Edward J. Wing）博士是《希氏内科学精要》第 8 版和第 9 版的编者，以及第 10 版的主编。他先后于 1967 年和 1971 年毕业于威廉姆斯学院和哈佛医学院。他曾在彼得·本特·布里格姆医院任内科住院医师，后在斯坦福大学完成了传染病学的专科医师（Fellowship）课程。自 1975 年加入匹兹堡大学医学院以来，他通过美国国立卫生研究院资助的研究项目，探索细胞介导免疫的机制以及传染病学各领域的临床诊疗工作。1990—1998 年期间，他先后被匹兹堡大学及其医学中心任命为蒙特菲奥里医院的主任医师、传染病科主任，后担任内科临聘主任。

1998 年起，温博士担任布朗大学医学院的内科主任（1998—2008 年）。在此期间，他在不同医院、实践计划和培训项目间对内科进行整合。在担任布朗大学医学与生物科学院院长（2008—2013 年）期间，他加强了与各附属医院（Lifespan 医院和 Care New England 医院）间的联系，提升了科研工作的水准，并为医学院建成了一座新楼。在担任主任和院长期间，他还建立了与肯尼亚、多米尼加共和国和海地的医学院的国际交流项目。温博士自艾滋病流行初期便在门诊诊治艾滋病患者，并始终工作在科研、临床和教学一线。

弗雷德·谢夫曼（Fred J. Schiffman）博士与爱德华·温（Edward Wing）博士共同担任《希氏内科学精要》第 10 版的主编。他就读于瓦格纳学院，随后进入纽约大学医学院，并于 1973 年毕业。他在耶鲁大学附属纽黑文医院接受早期住院医师培训，随后在美国国家癌症研究所工作了两年。回到耶鲁大学后，他担任住院总医师，然后完成了血液学专科医师课程，随后成为耶鲁初级保健中心医学主任。他于 1983 年入职布朗大学，领导医学住院医师项目并担任米里亚姆医院的副主任医师。

谢夫曼博士担任布朗大学沃伦·阿尔珀特医学院人文医学系的西格尔家庭医学教授。他的学术兴趣涵盖人体脾脏的结构和功能，以及艺术与医疗的交叉融合。他主持或参与了许多项目和计划，其中包括许多旨在鼓励和加强患者、家人和医护人员的福祉与康复能力的项目。他所创办的一个新项目可以让医学生和医生与其他非医学专业人士一起，共同欣赏罗德岛设计学院博物馆的艺术作品。谢夫曼博士近期还主持了布朗大学名为"艺术与医学：艺术赋能患者照护"的 edX 课程，此课程的参与者来自全球多个国家。谢夫曼博士还出版了有关血液病理生理学、血液科会诊和贫血的著作。

原著者名单

Jinnette Dawn Abbott, MD

Rajiv Agarwal, MD

Marwa Al-Badri, MD

Hyeon-Ju Ryoo Ali, MD

Jason M. Aliotta, MD

Khaldoun Almhanna, MD, MPH

Mohanad T. Al-Qaisi, MD

Zuhal Arzomand, MD

Akwi W. Asombang, MD, MPH

Su N. Aung, MD, MPH

Christopher G. Azzoli, MD

Christina Bandera, MD

Debasree Banerjee, MD

Mashal Batheja, MD

Jeffrey J. Bazarian, MD, MPH

Selim R. Benbadis, MD

Ivor J. Benjamin, MD, FAHA, FACC

Eric Benoit, MD

Marcie G. Berger, MD

Clemens Bergwitz, MD

Nancy Berliner, MD

Jeffrey S. Berns, MD

Pooja Bhadbhade, DO

Ratna Bhavaraju-Sanka, MD

Tanmayee Bichile, MD

Ariel E. Birnbaum, MD

Charles M. Bliss, Jr., MD

Andrew S. Blum, MD, PhD

Bryan J. Bonder, MD

Russell Bratman, MD

Glenn D. Braunstein, MD

Alma M. Guerrero Bready, MD

Richard Bungiro, PhD

Anna Marie Burgner, MD, MEHP

Jonathan Cahill, MD

Andrew Canakis, DO

Benedito A. Carneiro, MD, MS

Brian Casserly, MD

Abdullah Chahin, MD, MA, MSc

Philip A. Chan, MD

Kimberle Chapin, MD

William P. Cheshire, Jr., MD

Waihong Chung, MD, PhD

Emma Ciafaloni, MD

Joaquin E. Cigarroa, MD

Michael P. Cinquegrani, MD

Andreea Coca, MD, MPH

Harvey Jay Cohen, MD

Scott Cohen, MD, MPH

Beatrice P. Concepcion, MD, MS

Nathan T. Connell, MD, MPH

Maria Constantinou, MD

Roberto Cortez, MD

Timothy J. Counihan, MD, FRCPI

Anne Haney Cross, MD

Cheston B. Cunha, MD, FACP

Joanne S. Cunha, MD

Susan Cu-Uvin, MD

Noura M. Dabbouseh, MD

Kwame Dapaah-Afriyie, MD, MBA

Erin M. Denney-Koelsch, MD

Andre De Souza, MD

An S. De Vriese, MD, PhD

Neal D. Dharmadhikari, MD

Leah Dickstein, MD

Don Dizon, MD, FACP, FASCO

Robyn T. Domsic, MD, MPH

Kim A. Eagle, MD

Michael G. Earing, MD

Pamela Egan, MD

Wafik S. El-Deiry, MD, PhD, FACP

Mitchell S. V. Elkind, MD, MS

Tarra B. Evans, MD

Michael B. Fallon, MD

Dimitrios Farmakiotis, MD

Francis A. Farraye, MD

Ronan Farrell, MD

Panayotis Fasseas, MD, FACC

Mary Anne Fenton, MD

Fernando C. Fervenza, MD, PhD

Sean Fine, MD

Arkadiy Finn, MD

Timothy Flanigan, MD

Brisas M. Flores, MD

Andrew E. Foderaro, MD

Theodore C. Friedman, MD, PhD

Joseph Metmowlee Garland, MD,
AAHIVM

Eric J. Gartman, MD

Abdallah Geara, MD

Raul Macias Gil, MD

Timothy Gilligan, MD, FASCO

Michael Raymond Goggins, MB BCh
BAO, MRCPI

Geetha Gopalakrishnan, MD

Vidya Gopinath, MD

Susan L. Greenspan, MD, FACP

Osama Hamdy, MD, PhD

Johanna Hamel, MD

Sajeev Handa, MD, SFHM

Mitchell T. Heflin, MD, MHS

Robert G. Holloway, MD, MPH

Christopher S. Huang, MD

Zilla Hussain, MD

T. Alp Ikizler, MD

Iris Isufi, MD

Carlayne E. Jackson, MD

Paul G. Jacob, MD, MPH

Matthew D. Jankowich, MD

Niels V. Johnsen, MD, MPH

Jessica E. Johnson, MD

Rayford R. June, MD

Tareq Kheirbek, MD, ScM, FACS

Alok A. Khorana, MD, FACP, FASCO

Sena Kilic, MD

David Kim, MD

James Kleczka, MD

James R. Klinger, MD

Patrick Koo, MD, ScM

Pooja Koolwal, MD

Mary P. Kotlarczyk, PhD

Nicole M. Kuderer, MD

Awewura Kwara, MD

Jennifer M. Kwon, MD, MPH

Richard A. Lange, MD, MBA

Jerome Larkin, MD

Alfred I. Lee, MD, PhD

Daniel J. Levine, MD

David E. Lewandowski, MD

Kelly V. Liang, MD, MS

Kimberly P. Liang, MD, MS

David R. Lichtenstein, MD

扫描二维码了解更多信息

Douglas W. Lienesch, MD

Geoffrey S.F. Ling, MD, PhD

Ester Little, MD, FACP

Yi Liu, MD

Nicole L. Lohr, MD, PhD

John R. Lonks, MD, FACP, FIDSA,
    FSHEA

Gary H. Lyman, MD, MPH

Jeffrey M. Lyness, MD

Shane Lyons, MD, MRCPI, MRCP(UK)

Diana Maas, MD

Talha A. Malik, MD, MSPH

Sonia Manocha, MD

Susan Manzi, MD, MPH

Frederick J. Marshall, MD

F. Dennis McCool, MD

Russell J. McCulloh, MD

Kelly McGarry, MD, FACP

Eavan Mc Govern, MD, PhD

Robin L. McKinney, MD

Anthony Mega, MD

Shivang Mehta, MD

Douglas F. Milam, MD

Maria D. Mileno, MD

Abhinav Kumar Misra, MBBS, MD

Orson W. Moe, MD

Niveditha Mohan, MBBS

Larry W. Moreland, MD

Alan R. Morrison, MD, PhD

Steven F. Moss, MD

Christopher J. Mullin, MD, MHS

Sinéad M. Murphy, MB, BCh, MD, FRCPI

Sagarika Nallu, MD, FAAP, FAAN,
    FAASM

Javier A. Neyra, MD, MSCS

Ghaith Noaiseh, MD

Thomas A. Ollila, MD

Steven M. Opal, MD

Biff F. Palmer, MD

Jen Jung Pan, MD, PhD

Anna Papazoglou, MD

Aric Parnes, MD

Nayan M. Patel, DO, MPH

Ari Pelcovits, MD

Mark A. Perazella, MD

Michael F. Picco, MD, PhD

Kate E. Powers, DO

Laura A. Previll, MD, MPH

Nilum Rajora, MD

Adolfo Ramirez-Zamora, MD

John Reagan, MD

Rebecca Reece, MD

Harlan Rich, MD, AGAF, FACP

Jennifer H. Richman, MD

Lisa R. Rogers, DO

Ralph Rogers, MD

Michal G. Rose, MD

James A. Roth, MD

Sharon Rounds, MD

Jason C. Rubenstein, MD

Abbas Rupawala, MD

Jenna Sarvaideo, DO

Ramesh Saxena, MD, PhD

Fred J. Schiffman, MD, MACP

Ruth B. Schneider, MD

Kristin A. Seaborg, MD

Anil Seetharam, MD

Stuart Seropian, MD

Jigme Michael Sethi, MD

Sanjeev Sethi, MD, PhD

Elizabeth Shane, MD

Esseim Sharma, MD

Shani Shastri, MD, MPH

Barry S. Shea, MD

Lauren Shevell, MD, MPH

Joseph A. Smith, Jr., MD

Robert J. Smith, MD

Davendra P.S. Sohal, MD, MPH

Christopher Song, MD, FACC

Thomas Sperry, MD

Jeffrey M. Statland, MD

Emily M. Stein, MD

Jennifer L. Strande, MD, PhD

Rochelle Strenger, MD

Thomas R. Talbot, MD, MPH

Christopher G. Tarolli, MD, MSEd

Yael Tarshish, MD

Pushpak Taunk, MD

Philip Tsoukas, MD

Allan R. Tunkel, MD, PhD

Jeffrey M. Turner, MD

Zoe G.S. Vazquez, MD

Stacie A. F. Vela, MD

Paul M. Vespa, MD, FCCM, FAAN,
    FANA, FNCS

Wanpen Vongpatanasin, MD

Marcella D. Walker, MD

Eunice S. Wang, MD

Sharmeel K. Wasan, MD

Thomas J. Weber, MD

Brandon J. Wilcoxson, MD

Edward J. Wing, MD, FACP, FIDSA

Ellice Wong, MD

John J. Wysolmerski, MD

Rayan Yousefzai, MD

Thomas R. Ziegler, MD

Rebecca Zon, MD

ACKNOWLEDGMENTS

Dr. Schiffman and I wish to thank first of all, the authors of the 128 chapters that make up the tenth edition of *Cecil Essentials of Medicine*. They have worked diligently to compose the material for each chapter and apply their mastery as they added the newest information, in clear language, to the text. Their efforts are apparent in the excellence of the book, and we are immensely grateful for their work. We wish to also thank Marybeth Thiel, Jennifer Ehlers, and Dan Fitzgerald from Elsevier who guided and supported our work as editors and whose expertise has made this volume possible. Finally, we are always thankful to our wives, Dr. Rena Wing and Ms. Gerri Schiffman, without whose love, support, and especially humor, this book would not have happened.

致　谢

　　谢夫曼博士和我首先要致谢《希氏内科学精要》第10版全书128章的各位作者。感谢他们精益求精地撰写每一章节，并运用其专业知识，以简明的语言将前沿资讯呈现在书中。正是他们的辛勤努力确保了本书的卓越地位，对他们唯有由衷的感激。我们还要感谢爱思唯尔出版集团的玛丽贝丝·蒂尔（Marybeth Thiel）、詹妮弗·埃勒斯（Jennifer Ehlers）和丹·菲茨杰拉德（Dan Fitzgerald），他们对本书的编辑工作给予了指导和支持，其专业水准保障了本书的完稿。最后，要特别感谢我们的妻子——蕾娜·温（Rena Wing）博士和盖瑞·谢夫曼（Gerri Schiffman）女士，对她们的爱和支持，特别是积极乐观的心态始终心存感激，她们为本书的圆满完成发挥了不可或缺的作用。

总目录

第1分册

内科学概论·呼吸与危重症医学·术前和术后照护

第1分册译者名单

主　译

王　辰　代华平　赵　晶　黄　慧

译　者（按姓氏笔画排序）

王　辰　中国医学科学院北京协和医学院　　陈闽江　中国医学科学院北京协和医院

王　珞　中国医学科学院北京协和医院　　　邵　池　中国医学科学院北京协和医院

王丁一　中日友好医院　　　　　　　　　　赵　晶　中日友好医院

王诗尧　中日友好医院　　　　　　　　　　赵　静　中国医学科学院北京协和医院

王孟昭　中国医学科学院北京协和医院　　　柳　涛　中国医学科学院北京协和医院

王莉芳　中日友好医院　　　　　　　　　　侯　刚　中日友好医院

石　穿　中国医学科学院北京协和医院　　　徐　燕　中国医学科学院北京协和医院

代华平　中日友好医院　　　　　　　　　　徐作军　中国医学科学院北京协和医院

曲木诗玮　中日友好医院　　　　　　　　　黄　慧　中国医学科学院北京协和医院

刘　悦　中日友好医院　　　　　　　　　　童　润　中日友好医院

李卫霞　中日友好医院　　　　　　　　　　詹庆元　中日友好医院

吴小静　中日友好医院　　　　　　　　　　翟振国　中日友好医院

陈茹萱　中国医学科学院北京协和医院

第1分册目录

第 1 篇　内科学概论　Introduction to Medicine

第 2 篇　呼吸与危重症医学　Pulmonary and Critical Care Medicine

第 3 篇　术前和术后照护　Preoperative and Postoperative Care

CECIL ESSENTIALS OF
MEDICINE

Introduction to Medicine

Pulmonary and Critical Care Medicine

Preoperative and Postoperative Care

SECTION I

Introduction to Medicine

内科学概论

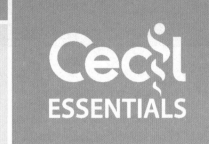

1

Introduction to Medicine

Edward J. Wing, Fred J. Schiffman

Cecil Essentials of Medicine presents a core of internal medicine and neurology information that every physician should know. This book provides an essential framework so physicians can appropriately assemble the key elements of history, physical examination, and laboratory data to understand their patient's illness and develop an appropriate diagnostic and therapeutic strategy. Furthermore, in order to understand advances in medicine, physicians must have a strong background for the acquisition and categorization of new medical knowledge.

Cecil Essentials of Medicine is designed for medical students as well as physicians in training, and we hope it will be an appropriate vehicle for course and examination review. We also believe, however, that physicians at all stages in their careers will find it to be a valuable resource for review and reference. This book also serves as a companion to the 26th edition of *Goldman-Cecil Medicine*, which is more comprehensive in scope and detailed in its content.

Cecil Essentials of Medicine is organized into sections, most often representing organ systems, with introductory and then organ-specific, disease-based chapters. The chapters themselves are subdivided. For example, the cardiovascular disease chapter is divided into Epidemiology, Anatomy, Pathophysiology, Clinical Diagnosis, and Treatment. The Suggested Readings sections at the end of each chapter include selected critical reviews, guidelines, and important randomized controlled trials. They are not meant to be an exhaustive reference list, but rather to highlight the essential information that physicians should know.

We believe that the information in *Cecil Essentials of Medicine* will encourage evidence-based diagnostic and therapeutic decision making. Importantly, the rational approach to medical problem-solving must be interwoven with the attentive presence of the physician at the bedside, clinic or office, undistracted by electronic devices (particularly the computer), displaying mindful humanistic patient care. Humanistic practice includes integrity, compassion, altruism, respect, service, and empathy, but also excellence. Both the art and the science of medicine must be part of the approach to any patient encounter. The editors believe that these concepts have been best expressed by Frances Peabody, who famously stated that "the significance of the intimate personal relationship between physician and patient cannot be too strongly emphasized, for in an extraordinary large number of cases both the diagnosis and treatment directly depend upon it. One of the essential qualities of the clinician is interest in humanity for the secret of the care of the patient is in caring for the patient," and by Sir William Osler, who said, "The practice of medicine is an art not a trade; a calling not a business; a calling in which your heart will be exercised equally with your head."

We believe that the fundamentally important bond between caregiver and patient is the starting point to the care of the patient. This is followed by a thorough history and a directed physical examination, which allow a diagnosis in the great majority of encounters. Laboratory data and imaging are supplementary. The focus of the diagnostic process should be on diseases that are common and treatable. Common presentations of common diseases account for the vast majority of cases; next in frequency are unusual presentations of common diseases; less common are typical presentations of rare diseases. Concentrate on common diseases, but know the rare ones as well.

We sincerely hope that *Cecil Essentials of Medicine* will be used to provide the basic and clinical data that are essential for us to practice medicine in a manner informed by both compassion and evidence, so that we may truly heal those with whose care we are entrusted.

内科学概论

王丁一 译 代华平 王辰 审校

《希氏内科学精要》提供了每一位内科医生应知应会的内科学和神经医学知识。本书为医生提供了包含病史、体格检查、实验室检查在内的核心知识框架，有助于帮助他们了解患者的病情，并制定恰当的诊断和治疗策略。此外，本书也有助于医生们学习掌握获取新知识并进行分类的技能，进而了解医学进展。

《希氏内科学精要》适用于医学生和正在接受培训的住院医师及专科医师。我们也希望本书成为医学课程学习和考试复习过程中的适宜参考书。我们更相信本书对处于各个职业生涯阶段的医生都具有很大的查阅和参考价值。本书也可以与《希氏内科学（第26版）》搭配阅读，后者的内容更加全面，涵盖范围更广，内容也更加翔实。

《希氏内科学精要》分为数个篇章，多按器官系统分类，先进行总论概述，进而按特定器官、疾病进行章节设置。各章节内又细分条目。例如，心血管疾病的章节分为流行病学、解剖、病理生理学、临床诊断和治疗几个部分。每个章节末尾的推荐阅读部分包括了精选的评论综述、指南和重要的随机对照临床试验。其并非详尽的参考文献列表，而是强调医生应该掌握的精华信息。

相信《希氏内科学精要》的内容能够鼓励循证诊断和治疗决策的制定。重要的是，解决医疗问题离不开医生在电子设备（尤其是计算机）之外，在床旁、门诊或办公室的细心工作和用心的人文关怀。人文主义实践包括正义、同情、利他、尊重、服务意识和同理心，也包括卓越性。医学的艺术性和科学性应该有机地融入对患者的照护中。编者们认为，Frances Peabody 的一句名言很好地表达了这一概念——"医患之间亲密的个人关系怎么强调都不为过，因为在非常多的病例中，诊断和治疗都直接依赖于这种关系。临床医生的基本品质之一是有仁爱之心，因为照护患者的秘诀就在于关爱患者。"现代医学之父 William Osler 爵士说过："行医是一门艺术，而不是一场交易，是一项使命而不是一笔生意；是一项需要用心用脑来完成的使命。"

我们认为医疗照护的提供者首先应该建立与患者之间的互信和良好关系，随后进行充分的病史采集和体格检查，这在多数情况下得以对患者进行诊断。实验室检查和影像检查提供补充信息。诊断过程的重点应放在常见和可治疗的疾病上。常见病的常见表现占据接诊的绝大多数病例，其次是常见病的不常见表现，罕见病的典型表现不太常见。我们需要关注常见病，但也要了解罕见病。

我们诚挚地希望《希氏内科学精要》能提供临床实践中必备的疾病原理和临床数据，让我们能够基于悲悯之心和客观证据开展临床实践，这样我们就可以真正地治愈那些托付给我们对其进行照护的患者。

SECTION II

Pulmonary and Critical Care Medicine

呼吸与危重症医学

Lung in Health and Disease

Sharon Rounds, Debasree Banerjee, Eric J. Gartman

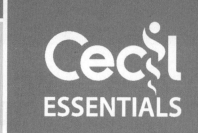

INTRODUCTION

The lung is part of the respiratory system and consists of conducting airways, blood vessels, and gas exchange units with alveolar gas spaces and capillaries (Fig. 2.1). The neural control of the respiratory system includes the brain cortex and medulla, the spinal cord, and peripheral nerves that innervate the skeletal muscles of respiration, airways, and vessels. The airways of the respiratory system include the upper airway—the nose, pharynx, and larynx—where inspired air is humidified and particulate matter is filtered. The intrathoracic airways continue down the trachea to the carina where the mainstem bronchi branch defining the right- and left-sided airways. Bronchi continue to branch into smaller airways (bronchioles) that eventually take on gas exchange capacity and end in alveolar sacs. Both pulmonary arteries and veins and lymphatics follow the branching patterns of the airways. The lung also has systemic circulation via the bronchial arteries. The bony structure of the chest wall protects the heart, lungs, and liver, and the lungs are maintained in an inflated state by mechanical coupling of the chest wall with the lungs. The skeletal muscles of respiration include the

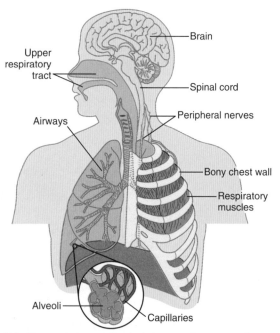

The Respiratory System

Fig. 2.1 The respiratory system includes neural structures that control breathing, the chest wall and skeletal muscles of breathing, the upper airway, and lung parenchyma.

diaphragm and the accessory muscles; the latter are important when disease causes diaphragm fatigue.

The lung is a complex organ with an extensive array of airways and vessels arranged to efficiently transfer the gases necessary for sustaining life. The organ has an immense capacity for gas exchange and can accommodate increased demand during exercise in healthy individuals. In lung disease, however, as exchange becomes compromised, the host's activities and function become increasingly compromised. The most dramatic consequence of acute and chronic abnormalities in lung function is systemic hypoxemia, which causes tissue hypoxia in multiple other organs.

In addition to gas exchange, the lungs have other functions, such as defense against inhaled infectious agents and environmental toxins. The entire cardiac output passes through the pulmonary circulation, which serves as a filter for blood-borne clots and infections. Additionally, the massive surface area of endothelial cells lining the pulmonary circulation has metabolic functions, such as conversion of angiotensin I to angiotensin II.

Lung disorders are common and range from well-known conditions such as asthma and chronic obstructive pulmonary disease (COPD) to rarely encountered disorders such as lymphangioleiomyomatosis. The chapters in Section II discuss the diagnosis, evaluation, and management of pulmonary disorders that develop in direct response to lung injury and those that develop indirectly through injuries to other organs. Section II also addresses critical illness such as acute lung injury, which is frequently managed by pulmonary or critical care specialists.

This chapter reviews the structural-functional relationships of the lung during development, the epidemiology of pulmonary disease, and the classification of pulmonary disorders.

LUNG DEVELOPMENT

The lung begins to develop during the first trimester of pregnancy through complex and overlapping processes that transform the embryonic lung bud into a functioning organ with an extensive airway network, two complete circulatory systems, and millions of alveoli responsible for the transfer of gases to and from the body. Lung development occurs in five consecutive stages: embryonic, pseudoglandular, canalicular or vascular, saccular, and alveolar postnatal (Table 2.1).

During the embryonic stage (between 21 days and 7 weeks' gestation), the rudimentary lung emerges from the foregut as a single epithelial bud surrounded by mesenchymal tissue. This stage is followed by the pseudoglandular stage (between 5 and 17 weeks' gestation), during which repeated extensive branching forms rudimentary airways, a process called *branching morphogenesis* (Fig. 2.2). Coinciding with airway formation, new bronchial arteries arise from the aorta.

肺的健康和疾病状态

王珞 译 赵静 柳涛 审校 黄慧 王辰 通审

引言

肺是呼吸系统的一部分，包括传导气道、血管和肺泡-毛细血管组成的换气单元（图 2.1）。控制呼吸系统的神经包括大脑皮髓质、脊髓和支配呼吸系统骨骼肌、气道及血管的周围神经。呼吸系统的气道包括上呼吸道，即鼻、咽和喉，它们加湿吸入的空气，过滤颗粒物质。胸腔内的气道由气管继续向下延续到隆突，并在此主支气管分为左、右主支气管。支气管继续分支成更小的气道（细支气管）并最终具有气体交换功能，最后终于肺泡囊。双侧肺动脉、静脉和淋巴管都伴随气道而分支。肺也通过支气管动脉进行体循环。

骨性胸壁保护心脏、肺和肝脏，肺通过胸壁与肺之间的机械耦合保持充气状态。参与呼吸的骨骼肌包括膈肌和辅助呼吸肌；当疾病导致膈肌疲劳时，则由辅助呼吸肌发挥重要作用。

肺是一个复杂的器官，广泛分布着气道和血管，能有效转运维持生命所需的气体。该器官具有庞大的气体交换能力，可满足健康人体运动时气体需求的增加。然而在肺病时，随着气体交换功能受损，患者的活动和功能也日益恶化。急慢性肺功能异常最明显的后果是全身性低氧血症，并导致其他器官组织缺氧。

除了气体交换，肺还具有其他功能，如抵御吸入性传染源和环境中的毒素。右心输出的全部血液都要途径肺循环，并通过肺循环过滤血栓和病原体。此外，肺循环的血管内皮细胞表面积巨大，具有代谢功能，如将血管紧张素 I 转化为血管紧张素 II。

肺病很常见，既有熟知的哮喘和慢性阻塞性肺疾病（COPD）等疾病，也有淋巴管肌瘤病等罕见病。本篇各章节将讨论直接肺损伤所致的或其他器官损伤间接导致的各种肺病的诊断、评估和治疗。本篇还将介绍呼吸科或危重症医学科专科医师经常处理的急性肺损伤等危重疾病。

本章回顾了肺在发育过程中结构与功能的关系、肺病的流行病学和分类。

肺的发育

肺在妊娠期前 3 个月开始发育，经过复杂而彼此紧密相接的过程，将胚胎的肺芽转变为具有广泛气道网络、2 个完整血液循环系统和数百万个肺泡的功能器官，负责全身气体的输送与回收。肺的发育分为 5 个连续阶段：胚胎期、假腺期、小管期、囊泡期和出生后肺泡期（表 2.1）。

在胚胎期（妊娠 21 天至 7 周），原始肺自前肠萌生，这是一个被间充质组织包围的单层上皮肺芽。接下来是假腺期（妊娠 5 到 17 周），肺芽重复、连续分支并形成原始气道，这一过程称为分支形态发生（branching morphogenesis）（图 2.2）。在气道形成的同时，新的支气管动脉也从主动脉发出。

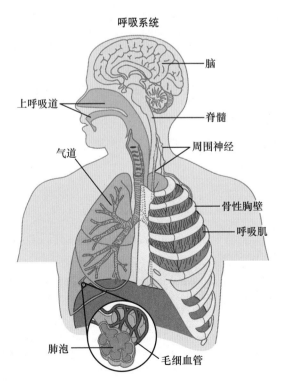

呼吸系统

脑

上呼吸道

脊髓

周围神经

气道

骨性胸壁

呼吸肌

肺泡

毛细血管

图 2.1 呼吸系统包括调控呼吸运动的神经结构、胸壁、参与呼吸运动的骨骼肌、上呼吸道和肺实质

TABLE 2.1	Stages of Lung Development	
Stage	**Period**	**Comments**
Embryonic	3-7 wk	Embryonic lung bud emerges from the foregut.
Pseudoglandular	5-17 wk	Airway tree is formed through a process of extensive branching accompanied by growth.
Canalicular	17-24 wk	Angiogenesis and vasculogenesis form the developing vascular network.
Saccular	24-38 wk	Alveoli begin to form through thinning of the mesenchyme, apposition of vascular structures with the air spaces, and maturation.
Alveolar (postnatal)	36 wk-2 yr	Further alveoli development and maturation occurs.

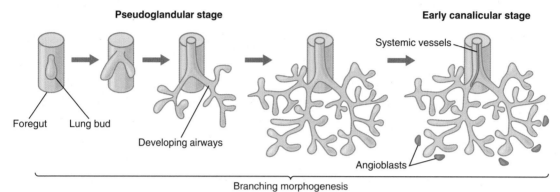

Fig. 2.2 Lung branching morphogenesis occurs during the pseudoglandular stage of lung development. It is the process by which the embryonic lung develops the primitive airway system through extensive branching.

The canalicular stage (between 17 and 24 weeks' gestation) is characterized by the formation of the acinus, differentiation of the acinar epithelium, and development of the distal pulmonary circulation. Through the processes of angiogenesis and vasculogenesis, capillary networks derived from endothelial cell precursors are formed, extend from and around the distal air spaces, and connect with the developing pulmonary arteries and veins. By the end of this stage, the thickness of the alveolar capillary membrane is similar to that in the adult.

During the saccular or prenatal alveolar stage (between 24 and 38 weeks' gestation), vascularized crests emerging from the parenchyma divide the terminal airway structures called *saccules.* Thinning of the interstitium continues, bringing capillaries from adjacent alveolar structures into close apposition and producing a double capillary network. Near birth, capillaries from opposing networks fuse to form a single network, and capillary volume increases with continuing lung growth and expansion.

During the alveolar postnatal stage (between 36 weeks' gestation and 2 years of age), alveolar development continues, and maturation occurs. The lung continues to grow through the first few years of childhood with the creation of more alveoli through septation of the air sacs. By age 2 years, the lung contains double arterial supplies and venous drainage systems, a complex airway system designed to generate progressive decreases in resistance to airflow as the air travels distally, and a vast alveolar network that efficiently transfers gases to and from the blood.

The processes that drive lung development are tightly controlled, but mishaps occur. Congenital lung disorders include cystic adenomatoid malformation of the lung, lung hypoplasia or agenesis, bullous changes in the lung parenchyma, and abnormalities in the vasculature, including aberrant connections between systemic vessels and lung compartments (e.g., lung sequestration) and congenital absence of one or both pulmonary arteries. In children without congenital abnormalities, lung disorders are uncommon, except for those caused by infection and accidents.

Congenital lung disorders are rare compared with the number of infants born annually with abnormal lung function as a result of prematurity. In premature infants, the type II pneumocytes of the lung are underdeveloped and produce insufficient quantities of surfactant, a surface-active substance produced by specific alveolar epithelial cells that helps to decrease surface tension and prevent alveolar collapse. This disorder is called neonatal *respiratory distress syndrome* (RDS). The treatment of neonatal RDS is administration of exogenous surfactant and corticosteroids to enhance lung maturation. To sustain life while allowing maturation, mechanical ventilation and oxygen supplementation are required but may promote the development of bronchopulmonary dysplasia (see Chapter 10 for further discussion).

PULMONARY DISEASE

Epidemiology

Diseases of the adult respiratory system are some of the most common clinical entities confronted by physicians. According to the Centers for Disease Control and Prevention data for 2017, chronic lower respiratory diseases, influenza or pneumonia, and cancer (including lung cancer) are among the top 10 causes of death due to medical illnesses in the United States.

COPD is a leading cause of both death and disability in the United States. At a time when the age-adjusted death rate for other common disorders such as coronary artery disease and stroke is decreasing, the death rate for COPD continues to increase. More than 16 million Americans are estimated to have COPD, but the number is expected to rise because COPD takes years to develop and the incidence of cigarette smoking (the most common etiologic factor for COPD) is staggering. In 2017, more than

表 2.1　肺的发育阶段		
发育阶段	胎龄 / 年龄	描述
胚胎期	孕 3～7 周	胚胎肺芽从前肠萌生。
假腺期	孕 5～17 周	随着胚胎成长，气道广泛分支并形成支气管树。
小管期	孕 17～24 周	血管新生和血管生成形成了发育中的血管网络。
囊泡期	孕 24～38 周	通过间充质变薄、血管结构与气腔贴合和成熟，肺泡开始形成。
出生后肺泡期	孕 36 周至出生后 2 年	肺泡进一步发育和成熟。

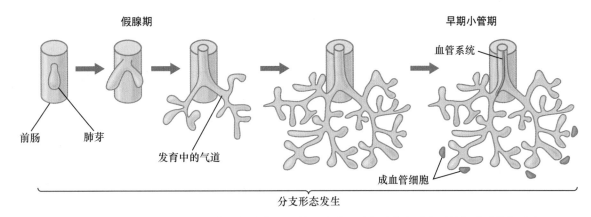

图 2.2　肺分支形态发生在肺发育的假腺期，这是胚胎肺通过广泛分支形成原始气道系统的过程

小管期（妊娠 17 至 24 周）的特点是肺腺泡形成、腺泡上皮分化和远端肺循环发育。通过血管新生和血管生成，由内皮细胞前体细胞衍生的毛细血管网形成，从远端肺泡向四周延伸，并连接发育中的肺动脉和肺静脉。这一阶段结束时，肺泡毛细血管膜的厚度与成人相似。

在囊泡期或出生前肺泡期（妊娠 24 到 38 周之间），起源于实质的血管嵴将称为囊泡（saccules）的终末气道结构分割开来。肺间质继续变薄，使相邻肺泡结构的毛细血管贴合，形成两套毛细血管网。临近出生时，两套毛细血管网会融合成一套，毛细血管的容量会随着肺的不断生长和扩张而增加。

在出生后肺泡期（妊娠 36 周至 2 岁之间），肺泡进一步发育并逐渐成熟。在儿童期的前几年，肺继续生长，并通过分隔更多的肺泡囊，而形成更多的肺泡。到 2 岁时，肺部已包含双重动脉供血和静脉回流系统、一个使得气流阻力随着气体向远端流动逐渐减小的复杂的气道系统，以及可有效地将气体扩散到血液或从血液中排出的庞大的肺泡网络。

肺部发育过程受到严格调控，但也会发生意外。先天性肺病包括肺囊性腺瘤样畸形、肺发育不良或缺失、肺实质的大疱样改变以及血管异常，包括体循环血管与肺部之间的异常相通（如肺隔离症）和先天性一侧或双侧肺动脉缺失。在没有先天畸形的儿童中，肺病并不常见，除非由感染或意外所致。

与每年因早产而导致肺功能异常的婴儿数量相比，先天性肺病并不多见。早产儿肺部的 Ⅱ 型肺泡细胞发育不全，产生的表面活性物质不足。这种表面活性物质由特定的肺泡上皮细胞产生，有助于降低表面张力，防止肺泡塌陷。这种疾病被称为新生儿呼吸窘迫综合征（RDS）。新生儿呼吸窘迫综合征的治疗方法是应用外源性表面活性物质和糖皮质激素来促进肺成熟。为了在促肺成熟时维持新生儿存活，需要进行机械通气和氧疗，但这可能会导致支气管肺发育不良（更多内容见第 10 章）。

肺病

流行病学

成人呼吸疾病是医生最常面对的临床情境。根据 2017 年美国疾病控制预防中心的数据，慢性下呼吸道疾病、流感或肺炎以及癌症（包括肺癌）均为美国十大致死病因。

慢性阻塞性肺疾病是导致美国人死亡和残疾的主要原因。当冠心病和卒中等其他常见疾病的年龄调整死亡率下降时，慢性阻塞性肺疾病的死亡率却在持续上升。据估计，有超过 1600 万美国人患有慢性阻塞性肺疾病，但由于慢性阻塞性肺疾病发病需数年，而且民众吸烟（慢性阻塞性肺疾病最主要的致病因素）率惊人，因此预计这一数字还会上升。2017 年，超过

34.3 million Americans were daily smokers and 16 million Americans had a smoking-related illness. The true disease burden of COPD is much greater than these numbers indicate.

Other pulmonary conditions are also common. Asthma affects 8% of adults and 9.5% of children in the United States. The prevalence, hospitalization rate, and mortality rate related to asthma continue to increase. In 2016, there were 257,000 hospital visits related to pneumonia and almost 50,000 deaths. Sleep-disordered breathing affects an estimated 7 to 18 million people in the United States, and 1.8 to 4 million of them have severe sleep apnea. Interstitial lung diseases are increasingly recognized, and their true incidence appears to have been underestimated. For example, idiopathic pulmonary fibrosis, the most common of the idiopathic interstitial pneumonias, affects 85,000 to 100,000 Americans annually.

These conditions affect males and females of all ages and races. However, a disproportionate increase in the incidence, morbidity, and mortality related to lung diseases exists for minority populations. This finding is true for COPD, asthma, certain interstitial lung disorders, and other diseases. Although these differences point to genetic differences among these populations, they also indicate differences in culture, socioeconomic status, exposure to pollutants (e.g., inner-city living), and access to health care.

Classification

Lung diseases are often classified on the basis of the affected anatomic areas of the lung (e.g., interstitial lung diseases, pleural diseases, airways diseases) and the physiologic abnormalities detected by pulmonary function testing (e.g., obstructive lung diseases, restrictive lung diseases). Classification schemes based exclusively on physiologic factors are inaccurate because distinctly different disorders with different causes, consequences, and responses to therapy have similar physiologic abnormalities (e.g., restriction from pulmonary fibrosis versus restriction from neuromuscular disease) (Fig. 2.3).

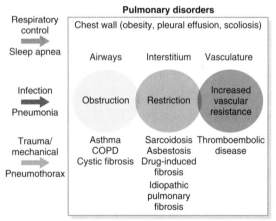

Fig. 2.3 Lung diseases are caused by abnormalities in the lung structure (e.g., airways, interstitium, vasculature) or in the chest wall or by external forces (e.g., infection). Disorders affecting the lung structure cause physiologic derangements (e.g., obstruction to airflow, restricted lung volumes, pulmonary hypertension, hypoxia). These derangements are not necessarily specific to any particular lung diseases, but there is extensive overlap among them, so that different disorders can have similar physiologic abnormalities. *COPD,* Chronic obstructive pulmonary disease.

The obstructive lung diseases have in common a limitation of airflow, called an *obstructive pattern,* as determined by pulmonary function testing. Obstructive lung diseases include COPD, asthma, and bronchiectasis.

The interstitial lung diseases are less common disorders and are more difficult to categorize because they include more than 120 distinct entities, some of which are inherited, but most of which are without an obvious cause. These disorders are characterized by a restrictive physiologic condition due to decreased lung compliance and small lung volumes, which is the reason they are often referred to as *restrictive lung disorders* (e.g., idiopathic pulmonary fibrosis). However, not all interstitial lung diseases exhibit a purely restrictive pattern on pulmonary function testing. They may have airflow limitation as a result of small airway involvement (e.g., sarcoidosis, cryptogenic organizing pneumonia).

In the pulmonary vascular diseases, involvement of the pulmonary vasculature causes increased pulmonary vascular resistance. These diseases range from disorders caused by obstruction to blood flow as a result of blood clots (e.g., pulmonary embolus) to disorders characterized by tissue remodeling and obliteration of blood vessels by vascular remodeling (e.g., pulmonary arterial hypertension).

Disorders of respiratory control include conditions in which extrapulmonary abnormalities cause respiratory system dysfunction and abnormal ventilation. Included are sleep disorders such as obstructive sleep apnea and neuromuscular system disorders such as myasthenia gravis and polymyositis, in which ventilatory abnormalities result from poor excursion of the respiratory muscles.

Disorders of the pleura, chest wall, and mediastinum are classified as such because they affect these structures. Infectious agents, commonly viruses and bacteria, cause infectious diseases of the lung. Neoplastic disorders of the lung include benign (e.g., hamartomas) and malignant (e.g., lung carcinoma) tumors, which can affect the lung parenchyma or its surrounding pleura (e.g., mesothelioma).

PROSPECTUS FOR THE FUTURE

Important questions about lung development remain. What are the primary stimuli for branching morphogenesis? How does gene regulation alter lung development? How is lung airway and blood vessel development coordinated? What are the environment-gene interactions that cause abnormal lung development and subsequent lung diseases? What impact does air pollution and climate change have on our lung health?

There are important fundamental questions about the epidemiology of lung diseases. For example, it is not clear whether or how childhood asthma and adult COPD are related. The role of fine particulate matter air pollution in the pathogenesis of lung diseases is unknown, and the causes and pathogenesis of many lung diseases, such as sarcoidosis, are unclear.

SUGGESTED READINGS

Schraufnagel DE, editor: Breathing in America: diseases, progress, and hope, New York, 2010, American Thoracic Society.

Whitsett JA, Haitchi HM, Maeda Y: Intersections between pulmonary development and disease, Am J Respir Crit Care Med 184:401–406, 2011.

3430 万美国人每天吸烟，1600 万美国人患有吸烟相关的疾病。慢性阻塞性肺疾病的真正疾病负担远比这些数字所显示的要大得多。

其他肺病也很常见。在美国，8% 的成年人和 9.5% 的儿童患有哮喘。与哮喘有关的患病率、住院率和死亡率持续升高。2016 年，有 257 000 人因肺炎到医院就诊，近 50 000 人死亡。据估计，美国有 700 万至 1800 万人受到睡眠呼吸障碍的影响，其中 180 万至 400 万人患有严重的睡眠呼吸暂停。间质性肺疾病正逐渐被认识，其真实发病率可能被低估。例如，特发性肺纤维化是特发性间质性肺炎中最常见的一种，每年累及 8.5 万至 10 万美国人。

这些疾病影响着各年龄段和种族的男性女性。然而，在少数族裔人群中，某些肺病的发病率、患病率和死亡率却出现了不成比例的增长。这个发现在慢性阻塞性肺疾病、哮喘、某些间质性肺疾病和其他疾病中存在。尽管这些差异表明不同人群之间存在遗传差异，但也表明他们在文化、社会经济地位、污染物暴露情况（如市区内生活）和医疗照护可及性方面存在差别。

分类

肺病通常根据受影响的肺部解剖区域（如间质性肺疾病、胸膜疾病、气道疾病）和肺功能检查发现的生理异常（如阻塞性肺疾病、限制性肺疾病）进行分类。但只基于生理学异常的分类方案是不准确的，因为病因不同、预后不同和治疗反应不同的疾病可能表现为相似的生理学异常（例如，肺纤维化引起的限制性通气功能障碍与神经肌肉疾病引起的限制性通气功能障碍）（图 2.3）。

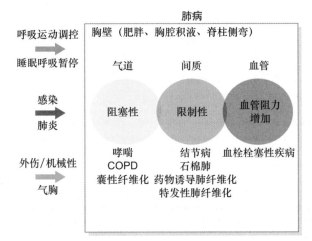

图 2.3　肺病是由肺部结构（如气道、肺间质、血管）或胸壁异常或外部因素（如感染）引起的。影响肺部结构的疾病会导致生理学异常（如气流受限、肺容量受限、肺动脉高压、低氧）。这些异常并不一定是某一种肺病所特有的，它们之间存在广泛的重叠，不同的疾病也有相似的生理异常。COPD：慢性阻塞性肺疾病

阻塞性肺疾病的共同点是气流受限，被称为阻塞性模式，这种生理学异常可通过肺功能检查确定。阻塞性肺疾病包括慢性阻塞性肺疾病、哮喘和支气管扩张症。

间质性肺疾病少见，而且很难分类，因为它们包括 120 多种不同的疾病，其中一些是遗传性的，但大多数病种没有明确病因。这些疾病的特点是由于肺顺应性降低和肺容积变小而导致的限制性障碍，这也是它们通常被称为限制性肺疾病（如特发性肺纤维化）的原因。然而，并非所有的间质性肺疾病在肺功能检测中都表现出纯粹的限制性模式。它们也可能因小气道受累而导致气流受限（如结节病、隐源性机化性肺炎）。

在肺血管疾病中，肺血管受累会导致肺血管阻力增加。这些疾病包括因血凝块导致血流受阻而引起的疾病（如肺栓塞），以及组织和血管重塑导致血管闭塞为特征的疾病（如肺动脉高压）。

呼吸控制障碍包括肺外异常导致呼吸系统功能失调和通气功能障碍，包括阻塞性睡眠呼吸暂停等睡眠障碍和重症肌无力、多发性肌炎等神经肌肉系统疾病，这些疾病的通气功能障碍是由呼吸肌运动减弱造成的。

胸膜、胸壁和纵隔疾病是依照其受累结构进行分类的。传染性病原体，通常是病毒和细菌，会导致肺部感染性疾病。肿瘤性肺病包括良性肿瘤（如错构瘤）和恶性肿瘤（如肺癌），可影响肺实质或其周围的胸膜（如间皮瘤）。

未来展望

有关肺发育的重要问题依然存在。诱发分支形态发生的启动因素是什么？基因调节如何改变肺的发育？肺气道和血管的发育是如何相互协调的？环境与基因之间的相互作用会导致肺发育异常和继发肺病吗？空气污染和气候变化对肺部健康有什么影响？

肺病的流行病学中仍存在一些重要的基础性问题。例如，儿童哮喘和成人慢性阻塞性肺疾病是否相关尚不清楚。空气细颗粒物污染在肺病发病机制中的作用仍不明确。许多肺病（如结节病）的病因和发病机制也未阐明。

推荐阅读

Schraufnagel DE, editor: Breathing in America: diseases, progress, and hope, New York, 2010, American Thoracic Society.

Whitsett JA, Haitchi HM, Maeda Y: Intersections between pulmonary development and disease, Am J Respir Crit Care Med 184:401–406, 2011.

General Approach to Patients With Respiratory Disorders

Michael Raymond Goggins, Brian Casserly, Eric J. Gartman

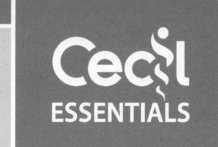

INTRODUCTION

History taking is of paramount significance in the assessment of a patient who may have pulmonary disease. Patients with respiratory disorders often complain of one or more of the following symptoms: dyspnea, fatigue, exercise intolerance, wheeze, cough, sputum production, hemoptysis, and chest pain. Aside from the establishment of a trusting doctor-patient partnership, history taking gives the physician the opportunity to ask critical questions and clarify crucial details that may point towards a specific diagnosis.

Common symptoms of respiratory disease, such as chest pain and fever, frequently occur with diseases of other organ systems (Table 3.1). For example, chest pain is a cardinal symptom of cardiovascular disease. Fever, though it is commonly observed in pneumonia, may also be attributable to a wide array of hematologic and rheumatologic conditions. A thorough assessment of the past medical history, family history, social history, and occupational history combined with a focused physical examination and an understanding of the symptomatology are the pertinent aspects of a systemic approach to patients with respiratory disease. Applying a structured process guides the investigations necessary to determine the underlying respiratory pathology.

❖ For a deeper discussion on this topic, please see Chapter 77, "Approach to the Patient with Respiratory Disease," in *Goldman-Cecil Medicine*, 26th Edition.

CLINICAL PRESENTATION

Dyspnea (i.e., breathlessness) is perhaps the most common presentation of patients with respiratory conditions (Table 3.2). The time of onset (i.e., nocturnal), rate of onset (swift vs. gradual), exacerbating and alleviating factors (i.e., environmental triggers), frequency, and degree of functional impairment are fundamental components of the history. Determining the associated symptoms such as cough, hemoptysis, chest pain, wheeze, orthopnea, stridor, allergic rhinitis, sinusitis, and paroxysmal nocturnal dyspnea is also imperative in developing a differential diagnosis. For example, if dyspnea is of sudden onset and accompanied by chest pain then the list of differential diagnoses should include the following: pneumothorax, pulmonary embolism, myocardial infarction, and flash pulmonary edema. Conversely, long-standing dyspnea indicates that chronic conditions such as chronic obstructive pulmonary disease (COPD), interstitial lung disease, pulmonary arterial hypertension, and neuromuscular disorders are most likely.

The evolution of chronic dyspnea may be insidious, thus questions regarding variations in functional capacity over time are essential. Exertion may precipitate dyspnea or it may occur at rest. Intermittent exertional dyspnea suggests parenchymal lung disease or cardiovascular disease. Dyspnea that is seasonal or provoked by environmental exposure suggests diseases such as asthma and hypersensitivity pneumonitis.

Positional dyspnea can develop in patients with severe obstructive airway disease, diaphragmatic paralysis or neuromuscular weakness.

Orthopnea, dyspnea occurring in the supine position, may result from a reduction in vital capacity caused by abdominal contents applying pressure upon the diaphragm. Paroxysmal nocturnal dyspnea, a sudden onset of shortness of breath transpiring one to several hours after lying flat, is a commonly described symptom of decompensated congestive cardiac failure. This condition is a result of interstitial pulmonary edema secondary to increased venous return to the heart. Nocturnal dyspnea in the setting of asthma has also been frequently documented and is understood to be the consequence of decreased vital capacity in the supine position, decreased production of endogenous agents with bronchodilator functions, and increased exposure to allergens in bedclothes. Exercise-induced asthma causes dyspnea disproportionate to the level of exertion, with symptoms often being most distressing in the 15 to 30 minutes after cessation of exercise.

Wheeze, the continuous whistling noise of air passing through a narrowed tube, while often associated with asthma, may be the result of a variety of conditions. The presence of wheeze does not definitively establish asthma as the diagnosis, nor does the absence of wheeze exclude asthma as a diagnosis. Congestive heart failure, endobronchial obstruction, vocal cord abnormalities, and acute bronchitis are all causes of wheeze.

Cough is often a frustrating symptom because the underlying diagnosis may be surreptitious. The three most common sources of a chronic cough are postnasal drip, asthma, and gastroesophageal reflux disease. Cough may be mild and sporadic. However, it may also be forceful enough to provoke emesis or syncope. Cough may be dry or may generate sputum or blood (i.e., hemoptysis). The symptom may commence months after initiation of a drug (e.g., angiotensin-converting enzyme [ACE] inhibitors), resulting in a dry, hacking cough. *Bordetella pertussis* infection (i.e., whooping cough) and viral lower respiratory tract infections can produce a cough that may last longer than 3 months. Patients with asthma often have a cough, and occasionally it is their only symptom (cough-variant asthma). Nocturnal cough suggests asthma, heart failure, or gastroesophageal reflux disease.

Sputum expectoration occurring more than seldom is atypical and should be characterized with regard to volume, color, timing, frequency, diurnal variation, and presence or absence of blood. Chronic bronchitis is defined as a productive cough for more than 3 months in each of the past 3 years. Asthma patients often have a productive cough due to excess mucus production. Colored sputum may not always represent bacterial infection because the concentration of cellular debris—predominantly white cells in inflammatory processes—affects sputum color. Poorly controlled asthma and the finding of brown plugs or casts of the small bronchi in sputum may indicate allergic bronchopulmonary aspergillosis.

呼吸疾病患者的接诊

邵池 译 柳涛 赵静 审校 黄慧 王辰 通审

引言

病史采集对于评估怀疑肺病的患者意义重大。呼吸疾病的患者常见以下一种或多种症状：呼吸困难、疲劳、活动耐量下降、哮鸣、咳嗽、咳痰、咯血和胸痛。病史采集不仅让医生有机会提出核心问题，理清关键细节，从而指向某一特定诊断，还有助于建立信任的医患关系。

呼吸疾病的常见症状，如胸痛和发热，常常也出现在其他器官系统的疾病中（表3.1）。例如，胸痛是心血管疾病的主要症状。发热虽然常见于肺炎，但也可能由各种血液病和风湿免疫性疾病引起。全面评估既往史、家族史、社会史和职业史，结合有针对性的体格检查和对症状学的分析，是全面处理呼吸疾病患者的重要手段。结构化的流程可以指导我们进行哪些必要检查来确定背后的呼吸系统病症。

❖ 有关此专题的深入讨论，请参阅 *Goldman-Cecil Medicine* 第26版第77章"呼吸疾病患者的接诊"。

临床表现

呼吸困难大概是呼吸疾病患者最常见的症状（表3.2）。该病史采集的基本组成部分包括发病时间（是否为夜间）、起病急缓（迅速还是逐渐）、加重和缓解因素（即环境触发因素）、频率和功能受损程度。对于鉴别诊断来说，确定合并症状（如咳嗽、咯血、胸痛、哮鸣、端坐呼吸、喘鸣、过敏性鼻炎、鼻窦炎和夜间阵发性呼吸困难）也至关重要。例如，如果是突发呼吸困难并伴有胸痛，则鉴别诊断应包含：气胸、肺栓塞、心肌梗死和一过性肺水肿。相反，长期的呼吸困难则提示患者可能患有慢性阻塞性肺疾病（COPD）、间质性肺疾病、肺动脉高压和神经肌肉性疾病这些慢性疾病。

慢性呼吸困难相关疾病往往起病隐匿，此时肺功能随时间变化的相关问题非常重要。呼吸困难可以是劳力性的，也可以是静息性的。间歇性活动后呼吸困难常提示肺实质疾病或心血管疾病。季节性或环境暴露引发的呼吸困难则提示哮喘和过敏性肺炎这样的疾病。重度气道阻塞性疾病、膈肌麻痹或神经肌肉无力的患者则会出现体位性呼吸困难。

端坐呼吸，即仰卧位时发生的呼吸困难，可能是由于腹腔内容物对膈肌施压导致肺活量下降所致。夜间阵发性呼吸困难，即平卧后一至数小时后突发呼吸困难，通常用于描述失代偿性充血性心力衰竭。发病机制是由于静脉回流增加导致间质性肺水肿所致。哮喘患者出现夜间呼吸困难也非常常见。一般认为这是由于平卧时肺活量下降、具有支气管扩张功能的内源性物质产生减少以及床上用品中的过敏原暴露增加所致。运动诱发哮喘会导致与运动程度不成比例的呼吸困难，症状往往在停止运动后 15～30 min 内最为严重。

哮鸣，即空气通过狭窄管道时发出的持续哨声，通常与哮喘有关，但也可能是多种疾病的结果。哮鸣的存在并不能明确诊断哮喘。没有哮鸣也不能排除哮喘的诊断。充血性心力衰竭、支气管内阻塞、声带异常和急性支气管炎都可以引起哮鸣。

咳嗽往往是一种令人困扰的症状，因为背后的原因可以非常隐匿。慢性咳嗽最常见的三个病因分别是鼻后滴漏、哮喘和胃食管反流。咳嗽可以轻微且不规律，但也可能严重到引起呕吐或晕厥。咳嗽可以是干咳，也可伴有咳痰或咯血。咳嗽症状，如干咳可以是在开始服用某种药物（如血管紧张素转换酶抑制剂）数月后才出现。百日咳鲍特菌感染（百日咳）和病毒性下呼吸道感染可导致咳嗽持续时间超过3个月。哮喘患者常有咳嗽，有时甚至是他们的唯一症状（咳嗽变异性哮喘）。夜间咳嗽提示有哮喘、心力衰竭或胃食管反流。

多于平时水平的咳痰往往是非特异症状，应根据痰量、颜色、时间、频率、昼夜变化以及有无血性进行描述。慢性支气管炎的定义为过去3年中每年有超过3个月的咳嗽咳痰。哮喘患者经常因黏液分泌过多而出现咳嗽咳痰。非白色的痰液并不总是代表细菌感染，因为细胞碎片的浓度（炎症过程中主要为白细胞）会影响痰液颜色。哮喘控制不佳且痰液中发现棕色痰栓或小支气管管型可能提示变应性支气管肺曲霉病。

TABLE 3.1	Major Symptoms of Respiratory Disease
Cough	
Sputum	
Hemoptysis	
Dyspnea (acute, progressive, or paroxysmal)	
Wheeze	
Chest pain	
Fever	
Hoarseness	
Night sweats	

Hemoptysis is an alarming symptom. The volume of blood may be scant or considerable enough to cause asphyxiation or exsanguination. Bronchitis is the most common cause of hemoptysis in the United States, whereas pulmonary tuberculosis is the predominant cause worldwide. Hemoptysis is frequently small in volume and self-limited or resolves with treatment of the underlying process. Massive hemoptysis, variably defined as 250 to 500 mL of blood in 24 hours, is a rare medical emergency caused by the following: lung cancer, lung cavities containing mycetomas, cavitary tuberculosis, pulmonary hemorrhage syndromes, pulmonary arteriovenous malformations, and bronchiectasis. Clinicians should distinguish hemoptysis from epistaxis and hematemesis with comprehensive upper airway examination as many patients have difficulty identifying the source of the hemorrhage.

Chest pain attributable to a respiratory cause results from pleural disease, pulmonary vascular disease, or musculoskeletal pain precipitated by coughing as no pain receptors exist in the lung parenchyma. For example, lung cancer does not cause pain until it invades the pleura, chest wall, vertebral bodies, or mediastinal structures. Disease or inflammation of the pleura causes pleuritic chest pain characterized as a sharp or stabbing pain with deep inspiration. Pulmonary emboli, infection, pneumothorax, and collagen vascular disease often cause pleuritic chest pain. Pulmonary hypertension causing right ventricular strain and demand ischemia may produce dull anterior chest pain unrelated to respiration. Additional examples of noncardiac chest pain are esophageal disease, herpetic neuralgia, musculoskeletal pain, and trauma. Thoracic pain secondary to vertebral compression or rib fractures may be seen in elderly patients or those with a history of chronic systemic steroid use.

Adequate analgesic relief, including narcotic use, in patients with chest pain and respiratory disease is essential to prevent a reduction in vital capacity due to splinting of the chest in reaction to the pain. Musculoskeletal chest pain, which is often reproducible with movement or palpation over the affected area, should only be considered as a diagnosis once other causes have been excluded.

HISTORY

The examiner should always inquire about previous respiratory illness, including pneumonia, tuberculosis, or chronic bronchitis, and chest radiograph abnormalities that have been reported to the patient. Acquired immunodeficiency syndrome (AIDS) increases the risk of developing *Pneumocystis jirovecii* pneumonia and other respiratory infections, including tuberculosis. Immunosuppression from chronic steroid use may predispose to tuberculosis and other lung infections.

Many classes of drugs can be linked to lung toxicity. Examples include pulmonary embolism due to the oral contraceptive pill, interstitial lung disease from cytotoxic agents (e.g., methotrexate, cyclophosphamide, bleomycin), bronchospasm from β-adrenergic receptor blockers or

TABLE 3.2	Causes of Dyspnea
Classification	**Examples**
Airways disease	Chronic obstructive pulmonary disease
	Asthma
	Laryngeal disorders
	Epiglottitis, bronchiolitis, and croup in children
	Tracheal stenosis or obstruction (foreign body or tumor)
	Tracheomalacia
	Bronchiectasis (immunodeficiency states, allergic bronchopulmonary aspergillosis, ciliary dyskinesia, cystic fibrosis)
Parenchymal lung disease	Pneumonia
	Interstitial lung diseases
	Obliterative bronchiolitis
	Pulmonary edema due to increased vascular permeability (acute respiratory distress syndrome)
	Infiltrative and metastatic malignancies
Pulmonary circulation disorders	Pulmonary thromboembolism
	Pulmonary arterial hypertension
	Pulmonary arteriovenous malformation
Chest wall and pleural disorders	Pneumothorax
	Pleural effusion or large-volume ascites
	Pleural tumor
	Fractured ribs, flail chest
	Chest wall deformities
	Neuromuscular diseases
	Bilateral diaphragmatic paresis
Cardiac disorders	Pulmonary edema due to left heart failure
	Myocardial infarction
	Pericardial effusion or constrictive pericarditis
	Intracardiac shunt
Hematologic disorders	Anemia
	Methemoglobinemia
	Carbon monoxide poisoning
	Acute chest syndrome (sickle cell disease)
Noncardiorespiratory disorders	Psychogenic diseases (hyperventilation)
	Midbrain lesion
Metabolic or endocrine disorders	Metabolic acidosis (diabetic ketoacidosis, sepsis, severe dehydration, inborn errors of metabolism)
	Hyperthyroidism
	Hypothyroidism
	Hyperammonemia
	Hypocalcemia (laryngospasm)
	Anaphylaxis
	Smoke inhalation
	Chemical agent exposures (phosgene, chlorine, cyanide)
	Drug overdose (salicylates)
Other causes	Biologic and chemical weapons (anthrax, tularemia, phosgene, nitrogen mustard, nerve agents, ricin)
	Submersion injury (near-drowning)

nonsteroidal anti-inflammatory drugs, and cough from ACE inhibitors. Physicians should be conscious that illicit substances known to cause lung disease (e.g., cocaine, heroin) may not be mentioned by the patient.

An accurate history of tobacco use and other toxic and environmental exposures is vital for patients with respiratory symptoms. Tobacco smoke is the primary environmental toxin causing lung disease. It is the physician's obligation to ask about tobacco use and attempt to motivate patients to quit smoking. The risk of smoking-related lung disease is directly correlated to individual genetic susceptibility and the total

表 3.1　呼吸疾病的主要症状

咳嗽
咳痰
咯血
呼吸困难（急性、进行性或阵发性）
哮鸣
胸痛
发热
声嘶
盗汗

　　咯血是一种需要引起警惕的症状。咯血量可以很少，也可以多到导致窒息或出现失血表现。在美国，咯血的最常见病因是支气管炎，而就全球来说，主要病因则是肺结核。咯血量通常很少，且具有自限性，或可通过治疗原发疾病缓解。对大咯血的定义不尽相同，24 h 内出血量可以在 250 ～ 500 ml 之间。大咯血是一种少见的急症，可由以下原因引起：肺癌、包含真菌球的肺空洞、空洞性结核、肺出血综合征、肺动静脉畸形和支气管扩张症。临床医生应通过全面的上呼吸道检查将咯血与鼻出血以及呕血区分开来，因为许多患者自己很难分清出血来源。

　　由于肺实质中不存在痛觉感受器，呼吸系统来源的胸痛是由胸膜疾病、肺血管疾病或咳嗽引发的肌肉骨骼疼痛引起的。例如，肺癌除非侵犯胸膜、胸壁、椎体或纵隔结构，否则不会引起疼痛。胸膜疾病或炎症会引起胸膜性胸痛，其特征是深吸气时出现尖锐性疼痛或刺痛。肺栓塞、感染、气胸和结缔组织病（胶原血管病）常常会引起胸膜性胸痛。肺动脉高压引起右心室负担增加和需氧增高性缺血，可能会产生与呼吸无关的钝性前胸痛。其他非心源性胸痛的病因还包括食管疾病、疱疹性神经痛、肌肉骨骼疼痛和创伤。老年患者或有长期全身使用类固醇激素史的患者可能会出现因脊椎压缩性骨折或肋骨骨折而导致的胸痛。

　　对于患有胸痛和呼吸疾病的患者，充分的镇痛治疗（包括使用麻醉剂）对于防止因疼痛引发胸部活动受限而导致的肺活量下降至关重要。肌肉骨骼性胸痛通常在运动或患处触诊时可诱发，只有在排除其他病因后才可诊断。

病史采集

　　检查者必须询问患者既往的呼吸道疾病史，包括肺炎、肺结核或慢性支气管炎，以及患者既往行胸部 X 线片曾发现的异常结果。获得性免疫缺陷综合征（艾滋病）会增加罹患耶氏肺孢子菌肺炎和其他呼吸道感染（包括结核病）的风险。长期使用类固醇激素导致的免疫抑制可增加结核病和其他肺部感染的概率。

　　多种类型的药物可出现肺毒性。例如口服避孕药可引起肺栓塞，细胞毒性药物（如甲氨蝶呤、环磷酰胺、博来霉素）可引起间质性肺疾病，β- 肾上腺素受

表 3.2　呼吸困难的原因

分类	举例
气道疾病	慢性阻塞性肺疾病
	哮喘
	喉部疾病
	儿童会厌炎、细支气管炎和喉炎
	气管狭窄或阻塞（异物或肿瘤）
	气管软化症
	支气管扩张症（免疫缺陷状态、变应性支气管肺曲霉菌病、纤毛运动障碍、囊性纤维化）
实质性肺疾病	肺炎
	间质性肺疾病
	闭塞性细支气管炎
	血管通透性增加导致肺水肿（急性呼吸窘迫综合征）
	浸润性和转移性恶性肿瘤
肺循环疾病	肺血栓栓塞症
	肺动脉高压
	肺动静脉畸形
胸壁与胸膜疾病	气胸
	胸腔积液或大量腹水
	胸膜肿瘤
	肋骨骨折、连枷胸
	胸壁畸形
	神经肌肉疾病
	双侧膈肌麻痹
心脏疾病	左心衰竭引起的肺水肿
	心肌梗死
	心包积液或缩窄性心包炎
	心内分流
血液系统疾病	贫血
	高铁血红蛋白血症
	一氧化碳中毒
	急性胸部综合征（镰状细胞病）
非心肺疾病	心因性疾病（过度换气）
	中脑损伤
代谢或内分泌疾病	代谢性酸中毒（糖尿病酮症酸中毒、感染中毒症、严重脱水、先天性代谢缺陷）
	甲状腺功能亢进
	甲状腺功能减退
	高血氨
	低钙血症（喉痉挛）
	过敏反应
	吸入烟雾
	化学物质暴露（光气、氯、氰化物）
	药物过量（水杨酸盐）
其他原因	生物和化学武器（炭疽、土拉菌、光气、氮芥、神经毒剂、蓖麻毒素）
	淹没损伤（溺水）

体阻滞剂和非甾体抗炎药可引起支气管痉挛，血管紧张素转换酶（ACE）抑制剂可引起咳嗽。医生还应该意识到，一些会导致肺病的违禁药物（如可卡因、海洛因）可能不会被患者提及。

　　对于有呼吸道症状的患者来说，准确地采集吸烟史和其他毒素和环境暴露史至关重要。烟草烟雾是导致肺病的主要环境毒素。医生有义务询问烟草使用情况并鼓励患者戒烟。吸烟相关肺病的风险与个人遗传易

pack-years history, while it is inversely related to the age at onset of smoking and, in the case of lung cancer, the interval since smoking cessation.

A history of exposure to other inhaled toxins, irritants, or allergens should be elicited. A thorough occupational history can uncover exposure to inorganic dust or fibers such as asbestos, silica, or coal dust. Organic dusts predispose to hypersensitivity pneumonitis and other interstitial lung diseases. Solvents and corrosive gases also induce pulmonary disease. The presence of house pets should be documented. Cats are the most allergenic for asthma while birds may cause hypersensitivity or fungal lung disease.

A travel history is pertinent in evaluating infectious causes of pulmonary disease. For example, histoplasmosis is endemic to the Ohio and Mississippi River valleys whereas coccidioidomycosis is observed in the desert Southwest. Travel to or immigration from developing countries heightens the risk of exposure to tuberculosis. A family history is crucial to establish the risk of genetic lung diseases such as cystic fibrosis and α_1-antitrypsin deficiency and predisposition to asthma, emphysema, or lung cancer.

PHYSICAL EXAMINATION

The physical examination should be comprehensive while also focusing on areas highlighted by the history. Observation and inspection when the patient's chest is bare are the initial steps in the physical examination of the patient with pulmonary disease. The physician should begin by assessing the patient's general appearance with particular attention given to the presence or absence of respiratory distress. This observation points toward the diagnosis and identifies the level of urgency.

Body habitus is relevant because morbid obesity in a patient with exercise intolerance and somnolence suggests a diagnosis of sleep-disordered breathing, whereas dyspnea in a thin, middle-aged individual with pursed lips may indicate emphysema. Race and sex are relevant as specific cohorts have a predisposition for certain conditions. For example, sarcoidosis is frequently encountered in African Americans in the Southeast, whereas lymphangioleiomyomatosis is a rare disorder that principally affects young women of childbearing age. Tachycardia and pulsus paradoxus are essential signs of severe asthma.

The physician should observe the effort required for breathing. Increased respiratory rate, accessory muscles use, pursed-lip breathing, and paradoxical abdominal movement indicate increased work of breathing. Paradoxical abdominal movement signifies diaphragm weakness and imminent respiratory failure. An inability to complete full sentences indicates severe airway obstruction or neuromuscular weakness. The potential presence of a cough should be discerned and the strength of the cough observed because it may signal respiratory muscle weakness or severe obstructive lung disease. The rib cage should expand symmetrically with inspiration. The shape of the thoracic cage should be considered. Increased anteroposterior diameter is appreciated in the setting of hyperinflation secondary to obstructive lung disease. Severe kyphoscoliosis, pectus excavatum, ankylosing spondylitis, and morbid obesity can produce restrictive ventilatory disease due to distortion and restriction of the thoracic cavity volume.

Hand examination may yield significant signs of respiratory pathology. Clubbing is often associated with respiratory disease. An uncommon association with clubbing is hypertrophic pulmonary osteoarthropathy (HPO) characterized by periosteal inflammation, swelling, and tenderness at the distal ends of long bones, the wrists, the ankles, the metacarpals and metatarsals. Rarely, HPO may occur without clubbing. The causes of HPO include pleural mesothelioma, pulmonary fibrosis, and chronic lung infections, such as lung abscess.

Finger staining (caused by tar because nicotine is colorless) is a sign of cigarette smoking. Dorsiflex of the wrists with the arms outstretched

and fingers spread may result in a flapping tremor (i.e., asterixis) seen with severe carbon dioxide retention. Wasting and weakness are signs of cachexia due to malignancy or end-stage emphysema. Peripheral lung tumor compression and infiltration of a lower trunk of the brachial plexus produces wasting of the small muscles of the hand and finger abduction weakness.

Head and neck examination is critical. The eyes are inspected for Horner syndrome (i.e., constricted pupil, partial ptosis, and loss of sweating), which may result from an apical lung tumor compressing the sympathetic nerves in the neck. The voice is evaluated for hoarseness, which may indicate recurrent laryngeal nerve palsy associated with lung carcinoma (usually left-sided) or laryngeal carcinoma. However, the most common cause is laryngitis.

The nose is evaluated for nasal polyps (associated with asthma), engorged turbinates (various allergic conditions), and a deviated septum (nasal obstruction). Sinusitis is indicated by tenderness over the sinuses on palpation.

The tongue is examined for central cyanosis. The mouth may hold evidence of an upper respiratory tract infection (e.g., erythematous pharynx, tonsillar enlargement with or without a coating of pus). A damaged tooth or gingivitis may predispose to lung abscess or pneumonia. Superior vena cava obstruction can cause facial plethora or cyanosis. Obstructive sleep apnea patients may be obese and have a receding chin, a small pharynx, and a short, thick neck.

Chest palpation is performed by first palpating the accessory muscles (i.e., scalene and sternocleidomastoid) of respiration in the neck. Hypertrophy and contraction suggest increased respiratory effort. Tracheal palpation should demonstrate the trachea residing in the midline of the neck. Deviation is suggestive of lung collapse or a mass. Neck masses should be documented.

The physician should place both hands on the lower half of the patient's posterior thorax with thumbs touching and fingers spread; the hands should be kept in place while the patient takes several deep inspirations. The physician's thumbs should separate slightly and the hands should move symmetrically apart during the patient's inspiration. Causes of asymmetry include pain, chest wall abnormalities, consolidation, and tension pneumothorax.

Fremitus is a subtle vibration appreciated best with the edge of the hand against the patient's chest wall while the patient speaks. Increased fremitus occurs in areas with underlying lung consolidation, and decreased fremitus occurs over pleural effusions. Next, the patient's chest should be percussed and the diaphragm level should be determined bilaterally. The percussion note should be compared on each side starting at the apex and moving down, including the posterior, anterior, and lateral aspects. Pleural effusions, consolidation, masses, or elevated diaphragms can produce dullness to percussion and pneumothoraces or hyperinflation can cause hyperresonance.

Lung auscultation is utilized to gauge the quality of the breathing and to detect extra sounds not heard in normal lungs. Normal breath sounds have two qualities, vesicular and bronchial. Bronchial breath sounds are heard over the central airways and are louder and coarser than vesicular breath sounds, which are heard at the lung peripheries and bases. Bronchovesicular sounds are a combination of the two and are heard over medium-sized airways. Bronchial sounds have a longer inspiratory component, whereas vesicular sounds have an elongated expiratory component and are much softer. Bronchial breath sounds and bronchovesicular breath sounds at the lung peripheries are abnormal and may be due to underlying consolidation. In the setting of consolidation, increased vocal sound transmission, called *whispered pectoriloquy,* ensues; *egophony,* in which the spoken letter *e* sounds like an *a* over the area of consolidation, is heard and sometimes likened to the bleating of a goat.

感性及总吸烟包-年数直接相关,而与开始吸烟年龄成反比;对于肺癌来说,还与戒烟时间成反比。

应询问患者是否有接触过其他吸入毒素、刺激物或过敏原的病史。详尽的职业史采集可发现无机粉尘或纤维(如石棉、二氧化硅或煤尘)的接触史。有机粉尘容易引发过敏性肺炎和其他间质性肺疾病。有机溶剂和腐蚀性气体也会引发肺病。应记录家中是否有宠物。猫是最容易引起哮喘的过敏原,而鸟类则可能引起过敏性或真菌性肺疾病。

旅行史对于评估肺病的感染性病因至关重要。例如,组织胞浆菌病是俄亥俄河和密西西比河流域的流行疾病,而球孢子菌病则出现在美国西南部的沙漠地区。前往发展中国家或来自发展中国家的移民结核病暴露的风险增加。家族史对于确定遗传性肺病(如囊性纤维化和 α 1-抗胰蛋白酶缺乏)的风险以及哮喘、肺气肿或肺癌的易感性至关重要。

体格检查

应全面进行体格检查,同时还应重点关注病史采集中有所提示的区域。让患者裸露胸部进行视诊是肺病患者体格检查的起始步骤。医生应首先评估患者的总体外观,特别注意是否存在呼吸窘迫。这一观察结果有助于诊断并确定疾病的紧急程度。

体型评估很重要,对于一个活动耐量下降和嗜睡的患者来说,病态肥胖常提示存在睡眠呼吸障碍;而对于一个身材瘦削、缩唇呼吸的中年人来说,呼吸困难则提示可能存在肺气肿。种族和性别特征也很重要,因为特定人群对某些疾病有易感性。例如,结节病在美国东南部的黑人中很常见,而淋巴管平滑肌瘤病则是一种主要影响育龄期年轻女性的罕见疾病。心动过速和奇脉是严重哮喘的重要症状。

医生应该观察患者呼吸时的用力情况。呼吸频率增加、辅助呼吸肌参与、缩唇呼吸和腹部反常运动意味着呼吸作功增加。腹部反常运动提示膈肌无力,即将出现呼吸衰竭。无法说出完整的句子提示气道严重阻塞或神经肌肉无力。应注意观察患者是否有潜在的咳嗽,以及咳嗽的强度,因为这有助于识别呼吸肌无力或严重阻塞性肺病。胸廓应随着吸气对称扩张。胸廓的形状亦应予以注意。在阻塞性肺病引起肺部过度充气时,可以观察到胸廓前后径的增加。严重的脊柱侧后凸、漏斗胸、强直性脊柱炎和病态肥胖会因胸腔扭曲和容积限制而产生限制性通气问题。

手部检查可发现提示呼吸疾病的有意义征象。杵状指通常与呼吸疾病相关。肥大性肺性骨关节病(HPO)是可出现杵状指的一种少见呼吸疾病,其特征是长骨远端、腕骨、踝骨、掌骨和跖骨的骨膜炎症、肿胀和压痛。在罕见情况下,HPO 可以不出现杵状指。HPO 的病因包括胸膜间皮瘤、肺纤维化和慢性肺部感染,如肺脓肿。

手指染色(由焦油引起,因为尼古丁是无色的)是吸烟的征象。双臂伸展、手腕背屈、手指张开时出现扑翼样震颤,见于严重二氧化碳潴留。消瘦和虚弱是恶性肿瘤或终末期肺气肿导致的恶病质的征兆。外周型肺肿瘤压迫和侵及臂丛神经下干可导致手部小肌肉萎缩和手指外展无力。

头部和颈部检查至关重要。应检查眼睛是否存在霍纳综合征(即瞳孔缩小、部分眼睑下垂和出汗减少)。这可能是由于肺尖肿瘤压迫颈部交感神经所致。检查是否存在声嘶,虽然其最常见原因是喉炎,但也可能提示存在与肺癌(通常为左侧)或喉癌相关的喉返神经麻痹。

检查鼻部是否有鼻息肉(与哮喘有关)、鼻甲充血(各种过敏性疾病)和鼻中隔偏曲(鼻塞)。鼻窦区有压痛则提示鼻窦炎。

检查患者舌头以了解是否存在中心性发绀。口腔检查可提供上呼吸道感染的证据(如咽部发红、伴或不伴脓苔覆盖的扁桃体肿大)。牙齿损坏或牙龈炎可导致肺脓肿或肺炎。上腔静脉阻塞可导致面部充血或发绀。阻塞性睡眠呼吸暂停患者可能表现为肥胖,伴下颌后缩,咽腔狭小,脖子粗短。

胸部触诊应首先从触诊颈部的辅助呼吸肌(即斜角肌和胸锁乳突肌)开始。辅助呼吸肌肥大和收缩表明呼吸用力程度增加。气管触诊应显示气管位于颈部中线。若有偏离则提示肺萎陷或肿块。若有颈部肿块应予记录。

医生应将双手置于患者后胸的下半部,拇指相抵,手指分开。双手保持原位状态令患者深吸气数次。患者吸气时医生的拇指应稍微分开,双手应对称移动。出现不对称运动的原因包括疼痛、胸壁异常、肺实变和张力性气胸。

语音震颤是一种细微的振动。当患者说话时,用掌缘抵住患者的胸壁可以最好地感知这种振动。肺实变区域会出现语音震颤增强;胸腔积液时会出现语音震颤减弱。接下来,应对患者胸部进行叩诊,并确定双侧膈肌的位置。应从肺尖开始向下叩诊,并比较两侧的叩击音,包括胸壁前部、后部和侧面。胸腔积液、实变、肿块或膈肌抬高会导致叩击音变浊;气胸或肺气肿会导致叩诊过清音。

肺部听诊可用于评估呼吸质量并检查正常时于肺部听不到的额外声音。正常呼吸音有两种,肺泡呼吸音和支气管呼吸音。支气管呼吸音可在中央气道中闻及,比肺泡呼吸音更响亮、更粗糙;后者可在肺外周和肺底部闻及。支气管肺泡呼吸音是两者的结合,可在中等大小气道闻及。支气管呼吸音具有较长的吸气成分,而肺泡呼吸音具有较长的呼气成分,并且更为柔和。肺外周出现支气管呼吸音或支气管肺泡呼吸音是异常的,提示可能存在潜在的肺实变。在肺实变的情况下,会产生耳语音,也就是人声传输增强;还可以闻及羊鸣音,此时字母 e 的音在实变区域会听起来像字母 a,有时听起来像山羊的咩咩叫声。

Abnormal or extrapulmonary sounds are crackles, wheezes, and rubs. Crackles can be coarse rattles or fine, velcro-like sounds. Airway mucus or the opening of large- and medium-sized airways often causes coarse crackles. In bronchiectasis, alteration of crackles occurs with coughing. Fine inspiratory crackles, caused by the opening of collapsed alveoli, are most common at the bases and are often heard in pulmonary edema or interstitial fibrosis.

Wheeze is a higher-pitched sound suggestive of large airway obstruction when heard locally. Wheeze in the setting of asthma or congestive heart failure is lower in pitch and heard diffusely over all lung fields. Localized wheezing can be heard in conditions such as pulmonary embolism, bronchial obstruction by a tumor, and foreign-body aspiration.

A pleural rub is a sound generated by inflamed pleural surfaces rubbing together, often compared to the sound of pieces of leather rubbing against each other. Rubs, which are often transient and dependent upon the amount of fluid in the pleural space, can develop post large-volume thoracentesis, along with pleuritic chest pain.

A crunching sound timed with the cardiac cycle, called *Hamman crunch* or *Hamman sign,* is heard in patients with a pneumomediastinum. The complete absence of breath sounds on one side should cause one to consider pneumothorax, hydrothorax, or hemothorax; obstruction of a main stem bronchus; or surgical or congenital absence of the lung.

EVALUATION

A differential diagnosis should be established based on a comprehensive history and a thorough physical examination. The preliminary differential diagnosis determines the battery of tests requested, recognizing that these investigations may reveal disorders not considered in the initial assessment. The objective of this extended evaluation is twofold: to affirm a diagnosis or disregard other disorders and to assess the severity of the lung derangement.

Patients with a suggested lung disorder should undergo pulmonary function testing (see Chapter 15). Spirometry evaluates airflow and helps differentiate between the obstructive pattern characteristic of COPD, asthma, and related disorders and the restrictive pattern observed in fibrotic lung disease. Spirometry also illustrates the severity of the physiologic alteration.

Lung volume measurements are effective in assessing hyperinflation or confirming a restrictive process. Calculating the diffusing capacity of the lung for carbon monoxide (D_{LCO}) elucidates alterations in gas-exchanging capability. The recording of oxygen saturation via pulse oximetry can be utilized to further assess gas exchange.

Information regarding oxygenation and acid-base status is obtained from arterial blood gas determination. A 6-minute walk test, which evaluates oxygenation during exertion, can demonstrate that patients require supplemental oxygen. Other, more specialized tests (e.g., bronchoprovocation, cardiopulmonary stress testing, polysomnography) may be necessary, depending on the context.

Imaging studies of the chest are beneficial in evaluating pulmonary structure. The chest radiograph displays the lung parenchyma and pleura, the cardiac silhouette, mediastinal structures, and body habitus. Examining old chest radiographic images is essential to assess for disease progression.

Computed tomography (CT) provides a more comprehensive assessment of the pulmonary and mediastinal structures and is essential in the evaluation of interstitial lung disease, lung masses, and other disorders. Together with ventilation-perfusion scanning and pulmonary angiography, CT is one of several resources used to evaluate the lung vasculature. Positron emission tomography is used to assess metabolic activity of lung masses and can indicate a diagnosis of malignancy.

Standard blood tests such as the blood counts and blood chemistry point to specific disorders or may provide information about the severity of a lung disorder (e.g., polycythemia in chronic hypoxemia, leukocytosis in lung infection). Some specialized tests should be reserved for specific diagnoses such as connective tissue disorders (e.g., rheumatoid factor, antinuclear antibodies) or hypersensitivity pneumonitis (hypersensitivity profile).

Together with the history and physical examination, these investigations are useful for narrowing a diagnosis to establish a specific management plan that can often be devised in a single visit. However, patients frequently require several follow-up visits in which the physician assesses disease progression, patient compliance, and response to treatment.

If noninvasive tests do not yield a diagnosis of the problem, more invasive tests may be necessary. Fiberoptic or rigid bronchoscopy allows direct visualization of the airways and acquisition of valuable clinical samples for examination. Transthoracic percutaneous needle aspiration or navigational bronchoscopy is useful in evaluating peripheral lung lesions. Ultimately, surgery may be required to obtain tissue through open or video-assisted thoracoscopically guided lung biopsy.

For a deeper discussion on this topic, please see Chapter 78, "Imaging in Pulmonary Disease," and Chapter 93, "Interventional and Surgical Approaches to Lung Disease," in *Goldman-Cecil Medicine,* 26th Edition.

PROSPECTUS FOR THE FUTURE

The predictive values of various facets of the history and physical examination need to be clarified. The role of quantitative CT analysis in the diagnosis and assessment of disability from lung diseases should be refined. The role of interventional pulmonary procedures must be ascertained for the diagnosis and treatment of lung diseases.

SUGGESTED READINGS

Davis JL, Murray JF: History and physical examination. In Mason RJ, Murray JF, Broaddus VC, et al, editors: Murray and Nadel's textbook of respiratory medicine, ed 6, Philadelphia, 2016, Elsevier.

Hollingsworth H: What's new in pulmonary and critical care medicine. https://www.uptodate.com/contents/whats-new-in-pulmonary-and-critical-care-medicine. Accessed August 5, 2019.

Ryder REJ, Mir MA, Freeman EA: An aid to the MRCP PACES, vol 1, ed 4, Chichester, 2012, Wiley-Blackwell Publishing.

Weiner DL: Causes of acute respiratory distress in children. Available at: https://www.uptodate.com/contents/causes-of-acute-respiratory-distress-in-children. Accessed August 5, 2019.

异常或肺外声音包括湿啰音、哮鸣音和摩擦音。湿啰音可以是粗糙的喀喇声，也可以是细小的捻发音。气道黏液或大中型气道的打开经常会引起粗湿啰音。在支气管扩张症患者，湿啰音会随着咳嗽发生变化。细小的吸气相湿啰音是由塌陷的肺泡打开引起的，最常见于肺底部，常在肺水肿或肺间质纤维化中闻及。

哮鸣音是一种音调较高的声音，在局部闻及时提示大气道阻塞。哮喘或充血性心力衰竭时产生的哮鸣音音调较低，可在整个肺部弥漫闻及。在肺栓塞、肿瘤阻塞支气管和异物吸入等情况下，则可闻及局部哮鸣音。

胸膜摩擦音是有炎症的胸膜表面相互摩擦产生的声音，与皮革相互摩擦的声音类似。胸膜摩擦音的存在往往是短暂的，取决于胸膜腔内的液体量，可在胸腔穿刺抽出大量胸水后出现，同时伴有胸膜性胸痛。

纵隔气肿患者可闻及一种与心动周期同步的嘎吱声，被称为哈曼（Hamman）摩擦音或哈曼征。如果一侧完全听不到呼吸音，则应考虑气胸、胸腔积液、血胸、支气管主干阻塞、手术导致的或先天性肺缺失。

检查评估

鉴别诊断应建立在全面的病史采集和彻底的体格检查基础之上。初步的鉴别诊断决定了下一步需要进行的一系列检查，并且医生应意识到这些检查可能会发现初步评估中未考虑到的问题。进一步评估的目的有两个：确定诊断或排除其他疾病，以及评估肺病的严重程度。

拟诊肺病的患者应接受肺功能检查（见第 15 章）。肺量计法可评估通气情况，有助于区分 COPD、哮喘和相关疾病导致的阻塞性通气功能障碍与纤维化肺病所致的限制性通气功能障碍。肺量计法还可明确呼吸生理改变的严重程度。

肺容积测定可有效评估肺过度充气情况或明确限制性肺病。计算肺的一氧化碳弥散量（D_{LCO}）可明确气体交换能力的变化。通过脉搏血氧仪记录氧饱和度可用于进一步评估气体交换能力。

通过动脉血气测定可获得有关氧合和酸碱状态的信息。6 分钟步行试验可评估运动时的氧合情况，可明确患者是否需要辅助吸氧。根据患者具体情况，还可能需要进行其他更专业的检查（如支气管激发试验、心肺运动功能测试、多导睡眠监测）。

胸部影像学检查有助于评估肺部结构。胸部 X 线片可显示肺实质和胸膜、心脏轮廓、纵隔结构和身体体型。检查患者既往 X 线片情况对于评估病情进展至关重要。

计算机断层成像（CT）可以更全面地评估肺部和纵隔结构，在评估间质性肺疾病、肺肿物和其他疾病方面起到关键作用。CT 与肺通气灌注扫描以及肺血管造影都是用于评估肺血管的手段之一。正电子发射断层成像（PET）用于评估肺肿物的代谢活性，并对诊断恶性肿瘤有提示意义。

常规血液检查（如血常规和血生化）可提示特定疾病或提供有关肺病严重程度的信息（例如，慢性缺氧导致的红细胞增多、肺部感染导致的白细胞增多）。一些专门的检查应限于特定疾病的诊断，例如结缔组织病（如类风湿因子、抗核抗体）或过敏性肺炎（过敏相关检测）。

这些检查与病史采集及体格检查相结合，有助于缩小诊断范围，制订特异的诊治计划，且常常只需要患者一次就诊就可以确定。然而，由于医生需要评估病情进展、患者依从性和治疗反应，往往需要患者多次随访。

如果非侵入性检查无法诊断出问题，则可能需要进行更具侵入性的检查。纤维支气管镜或硬质支气管镜可以直接观察气道并获取有价值的临床标本来进行检查。经胸壁针吸活检或导航支气管镜检查有助于评估肺外周病变。作为最后的手段，还可以通过开胸或胸腔镜下的肺活检获取肺组织标本。

有关此专题的深入讨论，请参阅 *Goldman-Cecil Medicine* 第 26 版第 78 章 "肺病影像学" 和第 93 章 "肺病的介入和外科手术方法"。 ❖

未来展望

我们需要明确病史采集和体格检查各方面的预测价值，应提高 CT 定量分析在肺病诊断和功能受损评估中的作用，必须进一步明确介入性肺部手术在肺病诊断和治疗中的作用。

推荐阅读

Davis JL, Murray JF: History and physical examination. In Mason RJ, Murray JF, Broaddus VC, et al, editors: Murray and Nadel's textbook of respiratory medicine, ed 6, Philadelphia, 2016, Elsevier.

Hollingsworth H: What's new in pulmonary and critical care medicine. https://www.uptodate.com/contents/whats-new-in-pulmonary-and-critical-care-medicine. Accessed August 5, 2019.

Ryder REJ, Mir MA, Freeman EA: An aid to the MRCP PACES, vol 1, ed 4, Chichester, 2012, Wiley-Blackwell Publishing.

Weiner DL: Causes of acute respiratory distress in children. Available at: https://www.uptodate.com/contents/causes-of-acute-respiratory-distress-in-children. Accessed August 5, 2019.

4

Evaluating Lung Structure and Function

Patrick Koo, F. Dennis McCool, Jigme Michael Sethi

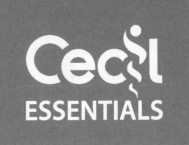

INTRODUCTION

The satisfactory functioning of all organ systems depends on their capacity to consume oxygen and eliminate carbon dioxide. The primary function of the lung is to deliver oxygen to the pulmonary capillary blood and to excrete carbon dioxide. To accomplish this, the lung must generate a flux of air into and out of the alveoli (ventilation) while absorbing oxygen into the pulmonary blood and eliminating carbon dioxide from alveolar air (gas exchange). This is accomplished in a manner that attempts to optimize gas exchange (ventilation-perfusion matching). This remarkably efficient process allows the human to maintain optimal oxygenation and acid-base balance over a range of activities, from resting breathing to moderately strenuous activity. This chapter provides an overview of the anatomy and physiology that enable the respiratory system to perform its life-sustaining functions as well as a discussion of tests available to evaluate lung structure and function.

ANATOMY

Airway

Inspired air travels through the nose and nasopharynx, where it is warmed to body temperature, humidified, and filtered of airborne particles greater than 10 μm in diameter. Air then enters a complex system of dichotomously branching airways that form a tree occupying the thorax. The first 15 divisions, beginning with the trachea, the mainstem bronchi, segmental and subsegmental bronchi down to the terminal bronchioles, are simply a set of conducting tubes that do not participate in gas exchange. Together, they constitute the *conducting zone* of the lung, also known as the *anatomic dead space* (about 1 mL per pound of ideal body weight, or approximately 150 mL) (Fig. 4.1). Cartilaginous rings help to maintain the patency of these large airways. In the mainstem bronchi, the rings are circumferential, whereas in the trachea, the cartilaginous rings are U-shaped, with the posterior membrane of the trachea sharing a wall with the esophagus. The branching pattern of these first 15 divisions of the airways follows the principles of fractal geometry: The reduction of airway diameter and length between each generation is similar, by a factor of 0.79, serving to densely compact the airways into the available space of the thorax (Fig. 4.2 A and B). This geometry reduces bronchial path length from the trachea to the periphery and minimizes both dead space volume and resistance to convective airflow.

The remaining eight generations of airways comprise the respiratory bronchioles and alveolar ducts lined with alveolar sacs. This area of the lung is referred to as the *respiratory zone*, and the terminal respiratory unit is called the acinus. Gas exchange commences in the

Airway subdivision	Order No.	Cross-sectional area (cm^2)	Resistance (cm H$_2$O • L^{-1} • sec)
Larynx	0		0.5
Trachea	0	2.5	0.5
Bronchi	1	2.0	
	2		
		5.0	0.2
	16	1.8×10^2	
Respiratory bronchioles	17		
	19	9.4×10^2	
Alveolar ducts	22	5.8×10^3	
Alveoli	23	5.6×10^7	

Fig. 4.1 The subdivisions of the airways and their nomenclature. (Modified from Weibel ER: Morphometry of the human lung, Berlin, 1963, Springer.)

肺的结构与功能评估

陈茹萱　陈闽江　译　王孟昭　徐燕　审校　黄慧　王辰　通审

引言

各器官的正常运转都依赖于它们消耗氧气和清除二氧化碳的能力。肺的主要功能是将氧气输送到肺毛细血管内的血液中并排出二氧化碳。为此，肺必须产生气流进出肺泡（通气），同时将氧气吸收到肺血液中并经肺泡排出二氧化碳（气体交换），通过通气-血流灌注匹配优化气体交换效率。通过这一高效的生理过程，使人体在从平静呼吸到中等强度运动的不同活动状态下都能够维持理想的氧合和酸碱平衡。本章将对呼吸系统解剖及其如何实现维持生命的生理功能进行概述，并介绍可用于评估肺结构和功能的检查方法。

解剖

气道

吸入的空气通过鼻和鼻咽，被加热至体温水平，进行湿化，并过滤掉直径大于 10 μm 的可吸入颗粒物，随后流经胸腔内一个逐级分叉的复杂支气管系统，即支气管树。前 15 级分支起自气管，包括主支气管、段和亚段支气管，直至终末细支气管，只作为传导气体的通道，不参与气体交换。它们共同构成肺的传导区，也被称为解剖无效腔［每磅（约 0.45 kg）理想体重约 1 ml，共约 150 ml］（图 4.1）。软骨环的支撑有助于维持大气道的开放。主支气管内的软骨环是环形结构，而气管内的软骨环为 U 形结构，后壁膜部与食管相邻。前 15 级气道的分支结构遵循分形几何学原理：每级气道的直径和长度以相同的比例减少，缩减系数均为 0.79，以便在胸腔有限的空间内密集地容纳更多的气道（图 4.2A 和 B）。这种几何形状减少了从气管到外围的支气管路径长度，最大限度地减少了无效腔体积和对传导气流的阻力。

后 8 级气道包括呼吸性细支气管和排列着肺泡囊的肺泡管，该区域被称为肺呼吸区；终末呼吸单位被称为肺腺泡。气体交换从呼吸区起始部位即开始出现，

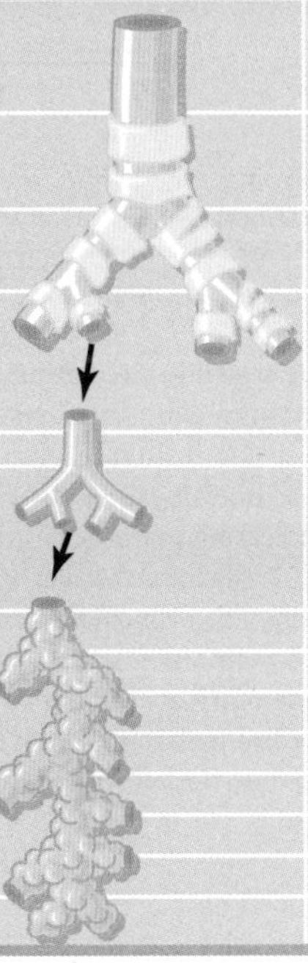

气道分级	级数	横截面积（cm²）	阻力 (cm H₂O·L⁻¹·s⁻¹)
喉	0		0.5
气管	0	2.5	0.5
支气管	1	2.0	
	2		
细支气管		5.0	0.2
	16	1.8×10^2	
呼吸性细支气管	17		
	19	9.4×10^2	
肺泡管	22	5.8×10^3	
肺泡	23	5.6×10^7	

图 4.1　气道分级及命名（改编自 Weibel ER：Morphometry of the human lung，Berlin，1963，Springer.）

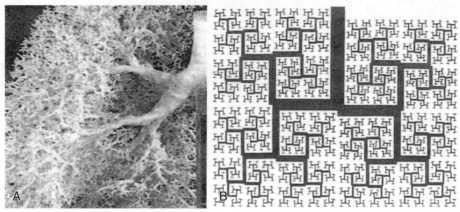

Fig. 4.2 (A) Cast of the right lung demonstrates branching of airways. (B) The branching airways can be modeled by use of the principles of fractal geometry, which allow for efficient filling of the thoracic space.

respiratory zone but primarily occurs in the alveoli. Inspired air moves down the conducting zone primarily by bulk convective flow, whereas the movement of oxygen in the respiratory zone is by diffusion.

In total, there are an average of 23 subdivisions of the airway from the trachea to the alveolar ducts. Although it might be suspected that resistance to convective flow would be highest in the small airways because of their small diameter, the opposite is the case. The enormous number of small airways together provide a huge net cross-sectional area for airflow. For example, the cross-sectional area of the trachea is 2.5 cm^2, compared with a total cross-sectional area of 300 cm^2 for all of the alveolar ducts combined. As a result, 80% of the resistance to airflow occurs in the first seven generations of bronchi, and the remaining "small" airways (diameters <2 mm) contribute only 20% of the resistance to airflow (Fig. 4.3). As the lung expands during inspiration, the net cross-sectional area of the alveolar ducts doubles, further reducing resistance to airflow.

Alveoli

The alveoli are the grapelike clusters of air sacs that interface with the pulmonary capillaries. There are about 300 million individual alveolar sacs, or 10,000 in each of the 30,000 acini. The alveoli are thin-walled structures with a total surface area of about 130 m^2. This is roughly half the size of a doubles tennis court. The surface of the alveoli is lined by two types of cells. The flat type I pneumocytes constitute 95% of the cells. Type II pneumocytes, which account for about 5% of the alveolar lining cells, secrete surfactant, a complex lipoprotein whose role in lowering surface tension in the alveolar space is critical to reducing the forces needed to expand the lung. Surfactant is also important in preventing alveolar collapse at low lung volumes and thereby promoting normal gas exchange. The capillaries run in the exceedingly thin septa that separate the alveoli and are therefore exposed to the air from surrounding alveoli. The epithelial lining of the alveoli, the endothelial lining of the capillaries, and the intervening fused basement membrane form the alveolar-capillary interface. Normally, this interface is less than 1 μm thick and does not significantly interfere with gas exchange.

Blood Vessels

The pulmonary artery arises from the right ventricle and branches until it terminates in a meshwork of capillaries that surround the alveoli. This creates a large surface area that facilitates gas exchange. Blood returns to the heart through pulmonary veins that course through the lungs, coalesce into four main pulmonary veins, and empty into the left atrium. The pulmonary circulation is a low-resistance circuit; pulmonary vascular resistance is about one tenth of the resistance in

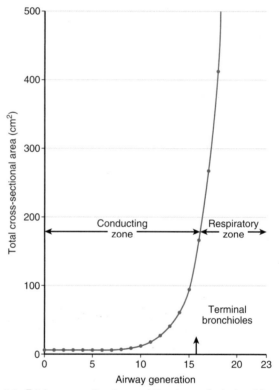

Fig. 4.3 Total cross-sectional area of the airways is depicted for several generations of airways. The total cross-sectional area increases dramatically in the respiratory zone. Consequently, the velocity of gas entering the respiratory zone decreases and resistance is low.

the systemic circulation. Pulmonary vessels can easily be recruited to accommodate increases in blood flow while maintaining low pressure and resistance. Accordingly, during exercise, any increase in cardiac output can be distributed through the lung without significantly increasing pulmonary arterial pressures.

A separate vascular system, the bronchial system, also supplies the lung. The bronchial arteries originate from the aorta and, in contrast to the pulmonary arteries, are under systemic pressure. These vessels provide nutrients to lung structures proximal to the alveoli. Two thirds of the bronchial circulation drains into the pulmonary veins and then empties into the left atrium. This blood, which has low oxygen content, mixes

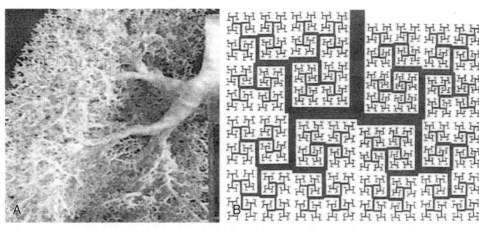

图 4.2 （A）右肺铸型标本展示了气道分支情况。（B）气道分支结构可以用分形几何学原理建模，该结构使得胸腔空间被充分利用

但气体交换的主要场所为肺泡。被吸入的气体主要以大量对流的方式流经传导区，而在呼吸区氧气以弥散的方式流动。

从气管到肺泡管，气道共有 23 级分支。由于小气道的直径较小，有人可能会猜测小气道产生的对流阻力最高，而事实正好相反。大量的小气道共同提供了巨大的净横截面积以供气流通过。例如，气管的横截面积是 2.5 cm²，而所有肺泡管加起来的总横截面积高达 300 cm²。因此，80% 的气流阻力来自于前 7 级的支气管，只有 20% 的气流阻力来自于剩下的"小"气道（直径 < 2 mm）（图 4.3）。随着吸气时肺的扩张，肺泡管的总横截面积加倍，气道阻力进一步减小。

肺泡

肺泡是与肺毛细血管相连的葡萄串样的气囊。肺内共有大约 3 亿个独立的肺泡囊，构成 3 万个肺腺泡，平均每个肺腺泡包含 1 万个肺泡囊。肺泡壁很薄，总表面积约有 130 m²，相当于半个双打网球场大小。肺泡表面由两种细胞覆盖，其中扁平的 I 型肺泡（上皮）细胞占 95%。II 型肺泡（上皮）细胞约占 5%，它们分泌表面活性物质，这种脂蛋白复合物对降低肺扩张时肺泡腔的表面张力起着重要作用。在肺容积缩小时，表面活性物质对于防止肺泡塌陷也发挥着重要作用，从而保证正常的气体交换。毛细血管在菲薄的肺泡间隔内走行，暴露于周围肺泡的气体中。肺泡上皮细胞、毛细血管内皮细胞及二者之间的基底膜共同构成肺泡-毛细血管界面。这一界面的厚度通常不超过 1 μm，不会对气体交换产生明显影响。

血管

肺动脉起源于右心室，不断分支而最终构成包绕肺泡的毛细血管网，其巨大的表面积有利于气体交换。肺静脉最终汇合成四支主肺静脉，将流经肺部的血液汇入左心房。肺循环是一个低阻力的回路，肺血管阻

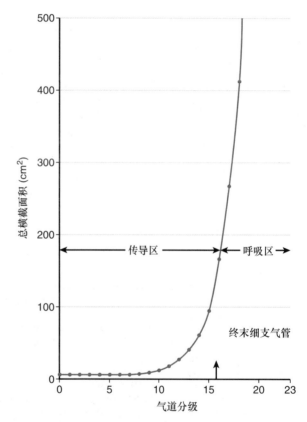

图 4.3 气道总横截面积在各级气道内的分布。相较于传导区，呼吸区的总横截面积明显增加。因此，气体进入呼吸区后，气体流速减慢，气流阻力降低

力大约只有体循环阻力的 1/10。肺血管的适应性较强，血流量增加时肺血管扩张，以保持低压和低阻力。因此，在运动时增加的心输出量可通过肺分布，而不会显著增加肺动脉压力。

还有一套单独的血管系统也为肺供血，即支气管动脉系统。与肺动脉不同，支气管动脉起源于主动脉，处于体循环压力下。这些血管为肺及其邻近结构提供营养。2/3 的支气管动脉循环回流到肺静脉内，然后汇入左心房。这一部分血液含氧量较低，与肺静脉引流的新鲜

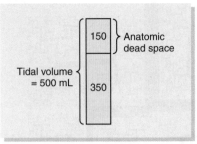

Fig. 4.4 Schematic diagram of the inspired volume of air that participates in gas exchange (VA, 350 mL) and the volume of anatomic dead space (VD, 150 mL), which together provide a tidal breath (VT) of 500 mL.

with the freshly oxygenated blood from the pulmonary veins to lower the oxygen content of the blood that enters the systemic circulation.

PHYSIOLOGY

Ventilation

Ventilation refers to the bulk transport of air from the atmosphere to the alveolus. The product of tidal volume (VT) and breathing frequency (f) represents the total volume of air delivered to the lung per minute (minute ventilation). However, not all air entering the lung is in contact with gas-exchanging units. The portion of VT that fills the respiratory zone and alveoli and is available for gas exchange constitutes the alveolar volume (VA), whereas the portion remaining in the conducting airways is the anatomic dead space volume (VD) (Fig. 4.4). The ratio of VD to VT is called the *dead space ratio* (VD/VT). Normally, one third of a breath is dead space (VD/VT = ⅓). The amount of fresh air reaching the alveoli is VT − VD. With large breaths, the dead space becomes a smaller fraction of the total tidal volume. Therefore, for a given VT, slow, deep breathing results in greater VA and improved gas exchange compared with rapid, shallow breathing.

The VD/VT ratio can be calculated by the Bohr method, as follows:

$$V_D/V_T = (P_{aco_2} - P_{Eco_2})/P_{aco_2}$$

where P_{aco_2} is the arterial partial pressure of carbon dioxide and P_{Eco_2} is the partial pressure of carbon dioxide in mixed expired gas (i.e., the mixture of CO_2-rich gas that enters the alveoli from the pulmonary capillaries and dead space gas, which is devoid of CO_2). P_{Eco_2} increases during expiration, reaching a plateau at end-expiration. At end-expiration, the P_{Eco_2} represents exhaled alveolar gas that has been in equilibrium with pulmonary capillary blood. In healthy individuals, the P_{Eco_2} at end-expiration is equivalent to the P_{aco_2}.

Ventilation of the dead space is wasted ventilation, because only VA participates in gas exchange. Therefore, as the metabolic rate and carbon dioxide production increase, VA must increase to maintain an arterial P_{co_2} of 40 mm Hg. The relationship among these variables is described by the alveolar carbon dioxide equation:

$$P_{aco_2} = CO_2 \text{ production}/\dot{V}_A$$

where P_{aco_2} is the partial pressure of carbon dioxide in the alveolus and VA is alveolar ventilation. From this equation, one appreciates that the partial pressure of carbon dioxide in the alveolus is inversely proportional to alveolar ventilation.

The relationship described by the alveolar oxygen equation is similar:

$$P_{ao_2} = O_2 \text{ consumption}/\dot{V}_A$$

However, this relationship is more complicated because P_{ao_2} also is proportional to the fraction of inspired oxygen, the water vapor pressure, and the partial pressure of carbon dioxide in the alveolus (discussed later). The implications of the alveolar carbon dioxide and oxygen relationships are that (1) maintenance of a constant alveolar gas composition depends on a constant ratio of ventilation to metabolic rate; (2) if ventilation is too high (hyperventilation), alveolar P_{co_2} will be low and alveolar P_{o_2} will be high; and (3) if ventilation is too low (hypoventilation), alveolar P_{co_2} will be high and alveolar P_{o_2} will be low.

Mechanics of Breathing

Respiratory mechanics is the study of forces needed to deliver air to the lung and how these forces govern the volume and flow of gases. Mechanically, the respiratory system consists of two structures: the lungs and the chest wall. The lungs are elastic (spring-like) structures that are situated within another elastic structure, the chest wall. At end-expiration, with absent respiratory muscle activity, the inward recoil of the lung is exactly balanced by the outward recoil of the chest wall, representing the equilibrium position of the lung–chest wall unit. Normally, the recoil of the lung is always inward (favoring lung deflation), and the recoil of the chest wall is outward (favoring inflation); at high lung volumes, however, the chest wall also recoils inward (Fig. 4.5). The energy required to stretch the respiratory system beyond its equilibrium state (end-expiration during quiet breathing) is provided by the inspiratory muscles. With normal quiet breathing, gas flow out of the lung is usually accomplished by passive recoil of the respiratory system.

During a typical breath, inspiratory muscle contraction lowers the intrapleural pressure, which in turn lowers the intra-alveolar pressure. Once alveolar pressure becomes subatmospheric, air can flow from the mouth through the airways to the alveoli. At the end of inspiration, the inspiratory muscles are turned off, and the lungs and chest wall recoil passively back to their equilibrium states. This passive recoil of the respiratory system causes alveolar pressure to become positive throughout expiration until the resting position of the lung and chest wall are reestablished and alveolar pressure once again equals atmospheric pressure. During quiet breathing, pleural pressure is always subatmospheric, whereas alveolar pressure oscillates below and above zero (atmospheric) pressure (Fig. 4.6).

The major inspiratory muscle is the diaphragm. Others include the sternocleidomastoid muscles, the scalenus muscles, the parasternals, and the external intercostals. Diaphragm contraction results in expansion of the lower rib cage and compression of the intra-abdominal contents. The latter action results in expansion of the abdominal wall. The expiratory muscles consist of the internal intercostal muscles and the abdominal muscles. Expiratory flows can be enhanced by recruiting the expiratory muscles; this occurs during exercise or with cough.

To inflate the respiratory system, the inspiratory muscles must overcome two types of forces: the elastic forces imposed by the lung and the chest wall (elastic loads) and the resistive forces related to airflow (resistive loads). The elastic loads on the inspiratory muscles result from the respiratory system's tendency to resist stretch. The elastic forces are volume dependent; that is, the respiratory system becomes more difficult to stretch at volumes greater than the functional residual capacity (FRC) and more difficult to compress at volumes lower than the FRC. The elastic forces can be characterized by examining the relationship between lung volume and recoil pressure (Fig. 4.7). When either deflated or inflated, the lung and chest wall have characteristic recoil pressures. The slope of the relationship between lung volume and elastic recoil pressure of the chest wall or lung represents the

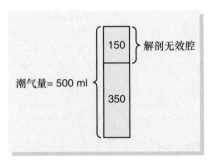

图 4.4　吸入空气体积示意图：参与气体交换的容积（V_A，350 ml）及解剖无效腔容积（V_D，150 ml）共同组成了潮气量（V_T，500 ml）

氧合血液混合后，降低了进入体循环内血液的氧含量。

生理学

通气

通气是指空气从大气到肺泡的输送过程。潮气量（tidal volume，V_T）和呼吸频率（f）的乘积体现了每分钟向肺里输送气体的总量（每分通气量）。然而，并非所有进入肺里的气体都参与气体交换。V_T 中进入呼吸区和肺泡的这部分气体可以进行气体交换，构成肺泡容积（alveolar volume，V_A），而停留在传导气道内的气体构成解剖无效腔容积（dead space volume，V_D）（图 4.4）。V_D 和 V_T 之比称为无效腔比（V_D/V_T），通常每次呼吸有 1/3 的气体构成无效腔（$V_D/V_T = 1/3$）。进入肺泡的新鲜气体体积为 $V_T - V_D$。深大呼吸时，无效腔占总潮气量的比例减小。因此，对于固定的 V_T 而言，与浅快呼吸相比，深而慢的呼吸可以获得更大的 V_A，从而改善气体交换。

V_D/V_T 比值可以用 Bohr 公式来计算，公式如下：

$$V_D/V_T = (PaCO_2 - P_ECO_2)/PaCO_2$$

其中，$PaCO_2$ 是动脉二氧化碳分压，P_ECO_2 是呼出的混合气体中二氧化碳分压（即，与肺毛细血管进行气体交换后的肺泡气体是富含 CO_2 的气体，而没有进行气体交换的无效腔气体是乏 CO_2 气体，此两者的混合气体）。呼气时 P_ECO_2 升高，在呼气末达到平台水平。呼气末的 P_ECO_2 代表了和肺毛细血管进行气体交换后达到平衡后呼出的肺泡气体。在健康个体中，呼气末 P_ECO_2 和 $PaCO_2$ 相近。

由于只有 V_A 参与气体交换，无效腔通气是无效通气。因此，随着代谢率升高、二氧化碳产生增加，必须增加 V_A 以维持动脉 PCO_2 在 40 mmHg 左右。这些变量间的关系可以用肺泡二氧化碳公式来计算：

$$P_ACO_2 = CO_2 \text{ 产生量} /\dot{V}_A$$

其中，P_ACO_2 是肺泡二氧化碳分压，$\dot{V}_A$ 是肺泡通气量。从此公式可以得出，肺泡中的二氧化碳分压与肺泡通气量成反比。

类似的还有肺泡氧公式：

$$P_AO_2 = O_2 \text{ 消耗量} /\dot{V}_A$$

然而，肺泡氧分压相关的变量关系更为复杂，因为 P_AO_2 还受吸入氧浓度、水蒸气分压及肺泡二氧化碳分压影响（详见后文）。肺泡二氧化碳和氧气的关系如下：①稳定的肺泡气体组成取决于通气和代谢率的恒定比例；②如果通气量过高（过度通气），肺泡 PCO_2 降低，肺泡 PO_2 升高；③如果通气量过低（通气不足），肺泡 PCO_2 升高，而肺泡 PO_2 降低。

呼吸力学

呼吸力学的研究对象是将气体输送至肺部所需的力，以及这些力如何控制气体的体积和流量。呼吸系统可以从机械的角度分为两部分：肺和胸壁，二者均为弹性（弹簧样）结构，肺是位于胸廓内的弹性结构。在呼气末，呼吸肌为放松状态，肺产生的弹性回缩力和胸壁产生的弹性扩张力达到平衡，是肺-胸廓的平衡位。正常情况下，肺的弹力回缩方向总是向内（有助于肺塌陷），胸廓的回弹方向总是向外（有助于肺充气）；而在高肺容积状态时，胸廓的弹力回缩方向也是向内（图 4.5）。吸气肌提供额外的力，使得呼吸系统过度扩张、超出平衡位（即平静呼吸的呼气末）。正常平静呼吸时，气体向肺外流出的动力来自于呼吸系统被动的弹性回缩。

在一次标准的呼吸周期里，吸气肌收缩时胸膜腔压力减小，从而降低肺泡内压力。当肺泡压低于大气压，气体可以从口腔经过气道流入肺泡。在吸气结束时，吸气肌不再收缩，肺和胸廓被动弹性回缩、恢复到平衡位。呼吸系统的被动弹性回缩力使得肺泡压在呼气时为正压，直到肺和胸廓回到静息位，肺泡压再次与大气压相等。在平静呼吸时，胸膜腔内压一直是负压，而肺泡压则在大气压上下呈周期性波动（图 4.6）。

人体最主要的吸气肌是膈肌，其他还包括胸锁乳突肌、斜角肌、胸骨旁肋间肌和肋间外肌。膈肌收缩引起下胸廓扩张，同时向下挤压腹腔内容物，进而引起腹壁向外扩张。呼气肌由肋间内肌和腹部肌构成。运动中或咳嗽时呼气肌收缩可增加呼气流速。

呼吸系统充气时，吸气肌必须克服两种阻力：来自肺和胸廓的弹性回缩力（弹性负荷）及气流相关的阻力（阻力负荷）。吸气肌承载的弹性负荷来自于呼吸系统抵抗伸展的倾向。弹性负荷与容积相关，即呼吸系统在容积大于功能残气量（FRC）时更难以继续扩张，而在容积小于 FRC 时更难以继续缩小。弹性回缩力可用肺容积和弹性回缩压来描述（图 4.7）。不论是呼气或吸气，肺和胸廓都有其特定的弹性回缩压。将肺容积与胸廓或肺弹性回缩压的关系作一曲线，其

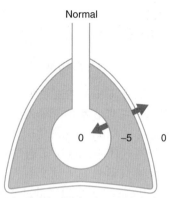

Fig. 4.5 Schematic diagram of the lung and chest wall at functional residual capacity (FRC). The *arrows* show that the expanding elastic force of the chest wall equals the collapsing elastic force of the lung. The intrapleural pressure is –5 at FRC because both forces are tugging on the pleural space in opposite directions.

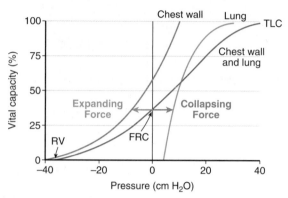

Fig. 4.7 Volume-pressure relationship of the respiratory system and its components, the lung and chest wall. Respiratory system recoil pressure at any volume is the sum of the lung and chest wall recoil pressures. Forces creating negative pressures expand the respiratory system, whereas forces creating positive pressures collapse the respiratory system. The slope of the volume-pressure curve represents the compliance of each structure. *FRC*, Functional residual capacity; *RV*, residual volume; *TLC*, total lung capacity.

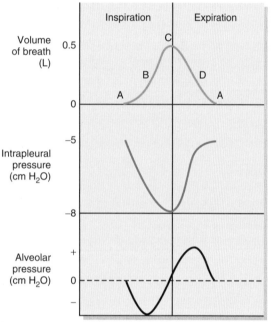

Fig. 4.6 Volume, intrapleural pressure, and alveolar pressure during a normal breathing cycle. The letters correspond to the various phases of the cycle: *A*, end-expiration; *B*, inspiration; *C*, end-inspiration; and *D*, expiration. Alveolar pressure is biphasic, with zero crossings at times of no flow (i.e., end-expiration and end-inspiration). Intrapleural pressure remains subatmospheric throughout.

compliance of each structure. The sum of the chest wall and lung recoil pressures represents the recoil pressure of the total respiratory system.

The elastic properties of the lung are related to two factors: the elastic behavior of collagen and elastin in the lung parenchyma and the surface tension in the alveolus at the air-liquid interface. Both factors contribute equally to lung elastic recoil. A surface-active substance called *surfactant* is produced by type II alveolar cells and lines the alveoli. This substance consists primarily of phospholipids. It lowers the surface tension of the air-liquid interface, making it easier to inflate the lung. The lungs are stiff (less compliant) and difficult to inflate in diseases that are characterized by a loss of surfactant (e.g., infant respiratory distress syndrome). Diseases such as pulmonary fibrosis, which

are characterized by excessive collagen in the lung, can make the lung stiff and difficult to inflate, whereas those such as emphysema, characterized by a loss of elastin and collagen, reduce lung recoil and increase lung compliance (Fig. 4.8). Normally, at FRC, it takes about 1 cm of water pressure (1 cm H_2O) to inflate the lungs 200 mL or to inflate the chest wall 200 mL. The lung and chest wall both need to be inflated to the same volume during inspiration, so 2 cm H_2O of pressure is required to inflate both to 200 mL. Therefore, normal respiratory system compliance is roughly 200/2 or 100 mL/cm H_2O and compliance of the lung or chest wall compliance is 200/1 or 200 mL/cm H_2O at volumes near FRC.

The second set of forces that the inspiratory muscles must overcome to inflate the lungs are flow-dependent forces; namely, tissue viscosity and airway flow resistance, the latter constituting the major component of the flow-dependent forces. Airway resistance during inspiration can be calculated by measuring inspiratory flow and the difference in pressure between the alveolus and the airway opening (ΔP_{A-ao}).

$$\text{Resistance} = \Delta P_{A-ao} / \dot{V}$$

The airflow velocity, the type of airflow (laminar or turbulent), and the physical attributes of the airway (radius and length) are the key determinants of airway resistance. Of the physical properties, the radius of the airways is the major factor. Resistance increases to the fourth power as the diameter decreases under conditions of laminar flow (streamline flow profile) and to the fifth power under conditions of turbulent flow (chaotic flow profile). Because airway diameter increases as lung volume increases, airway resistance decreases as lung volume increases (Fig. 4.9). Airway diameter also contributes to regional differences in airway resistance. Although the peripheral airways are narrower than the central airways, their total cross-sectional area is much greater than that of the central airways, as described earlier. Consequently, resistance to airflow of the peripheral airways is low relative to the central airways (see Fig. 4.3).

The type of airflow is another key determinant of airway resistance. Resistance is directly proportional to flow rate when flow is laminar. Resistance is much greater with turbulent flow because it is proportional to the square of the flow rate. The velocity of airflow determines,

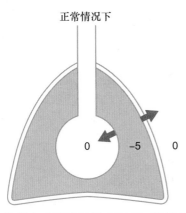

图 4.5　肺和胸廓在功能残气量（FRC）状态下的作用示意图。箭头方向提示胸廓向外扩张的弹力和肺向内塌陷的弹力相平衡。因为两个牵拉力作用于胸膜腔的方向相反，FRC 时胸膜腔内压为 −5 cmH₂O。（译者注：原文无单位，结合图 4.6 进行补充）

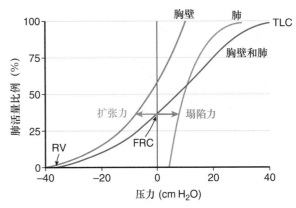

图 4.7　呼吸系统及其组分（肺和胸壁）的容积-压力曲线。任一容积下呼吸系统弹性回缩压均等于肺和胸廓的弹性回缩压之和。此压力产生负压从而扩张呼吸系统，而产生正压时则引起呼吸系统塌陷。容积-压力曲线的斜率反映各个结构的顺应性。FRC，功能残气量；RV，残气量；TLC，肺总量

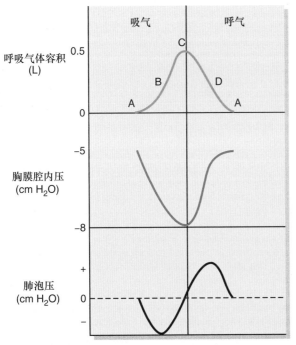

图 4.6　正常呼吸周期中的气体容积、胸膜腔内压和肺泡压的变化示意图。字母对应呼吸周期的不同阶段：A，呼气末；B，吸气；C，吸气末；D，呼气。肺泡压是双相变化的，在没有气流时（即呼气末和吸气末）为零。胸膜腔内压始终低于大气压

斜率反映的是相应结构的顺应性。胸廓和肺的弹性回缩压之和反映呼吸系统整体的弹性回缩压。

肺的弹力特性与两个因素有关：肺实质中胶原蛋白和弹性蛋白的弹力特性、肺泡气-液界面的表面张力。二者引起的肺弹性回缩力大致相当。Ⅱ型肺泡上皮细胞产生的表面活性物质分布于肺泡表面。表面活性物质主要由磷脂构成，能降低气-液界面的表面张力，使得肺更容易膨胀。一些由于表面活性物质缺失

引起的疾病（如新生儿呼吸窘迫综合征）会导致肺僵硬（顺应性下降）、难以膨胀。以肺内胶原蛋白过度增生为特征的肺病（如肺纤维化），同样会引起肺僵硬、难以膨胀；而肺气肿则是以弹性蛋白和胶原蛋白的破坏丢失为特点，导致肺弹性回缩力下降、肺顺应性增加（图 4.8）。在 FRC 状态下，肺或胸廓扩张 200 ml 通常各需要 1 cm 水柱（1 cmH₂O）压力。肺和胸廓在吸气时同时增加相等的容积，所以共需要 2 cmH₂O 的压力使其同时扩张 200 ml。因此，在临近 FRC 的容积时，正常呼吸系统的顺应性大约是 200/2 或 100 ml/cmH₂O，而肺或胸廓的顺应性是 200/1 或 200 ml/cmH₂O。

吸气时吸气肌必须克服的第二种阻力是气流相关的阻力，即组织的黏滞阻力和气道阻力，后者是气流相关阻力的主要构成部分。吸气时的气道阻力可以根据吸气流速和肺泡-气道开放压的差值（ΔP_{A-ao}）进行计算。

$$阻力 = \Delta P_{A-ao}/\dot{V}$$

气流速度、气流类型（层流或湍流）和气道的物理特性（半径和长度）是决定气道阻力的关键因素。在物理特性中，气道半径是主要决定因素。当气流为层流（平流）时，随着气道直径减小，阻力以四次方的级数增加；当气流为湍流（紊乱气流）时，阻力以五次方的级数增加。由于气道直径随着肺容积的增加而增加，气道阻力随着肺容积的增加而减小（图 4.9）。不同部位的气道阻力受气道直径影响存在一定差异。虽然外周气道比中央气道窄，但如前所述，它们的总横截面积远远大于中央气道的横截面积，因此外周气道的气流阻力比中央气道的更低（见图 4.3）。

气流类型是决定气道阻力的另一关键因素。当气流是层流时，阻力与气流速度成正比。而在湍流的情况下，阻力与气流速度的平方成正比，因此会明显增

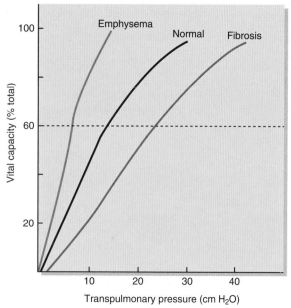

Fig. 4.8 Compliance curves for normal individuals and for patients with emphysema or pulmonary fibrosis. The transpulmonary pressure required to achieve a given lung volume is greatest for the patient with pulmonary fibrosis (notice the horizontal dashed line at 60% of the vital capacity). This increases the work of breathing.

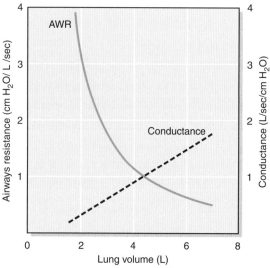

Fig. 4.9 As lung volume increases, the airways are dilated, and airways resistance (AWR) decreases. The reciprocal of resistance (conductance) increases as lung volume increases.

in part, whether the flow pattern is laminar or turbulent. Clinically, increased airway resistance can be seen in diseases associated with airway obstruction caused by an intrinsic mass, mucus within the airway, airway smooth muscle contraction, or extrinsic compression of the airways.

Lung elastic recoil also influences airway resistance and airflow. Decreased lung recoil increases resistance by promoting collapse of the small airways. Normal resistance when breathing at FRC at low flow rates is in the range of 1 to 2 cm H_2O/L per second.

Distribution of Ventilation

The distribution of inhaled volume throughout the lung is unequal. In general, more of the inhaled volume goes to the bases of the lung than to the apex when the individual is inhaling while in an upright body position. This pattern of volume distribution leads to greater ventilation of the bases than at the apices. This inhomogeneity of ventilation results largely from regional differences in lung compliance. The alveoli at the lung apex are relatively more inflated at FRC than the alveoli at the lung base. The difference in alveolar distention from apex to base is related to pleural pressure differences from apex to base. The weight of the lung causes pleural pressure to be more negative at the apex and less negative at the base. The normal difference in pleural pressure from apex to base in an adult is about 8 cm H_2O (Fig. 4.10). Because the apical alveoli are more stretched at FRC, they are operating on a stiffer, less compliant region of their volume-pressure curve than the alveoli at the bases, making them more difficult to inflate than the basilar alveoli. Therefore, at the beginning of inspiration, more volume is directed toward the base than to the apex of the lung.

Control of Ventilation

Maintenance of adequate oxygenation and acid-base balance is accomplished through the respiratory control system. This system consists of the neurologic respiratory control centers, the respiratory effectors (muscles that provide the power to inflate the lungs), and the respiratory sensors. The respiratory center that automatically controls inspiration and expiration is located in the medulla of the brain stem. The respiratory center in the brain stem has an intrinsic rhythm generator (pacemaker) that drives breathing. The output of this center is modulated by inputs from peripheral and central chemoreceptors, from mechanoreceptors in the lungs, and from higher centers in the brain, including conscious control from the cerebral cortex. The respiratory center in the medulla is primarily responsible for determining the level of ventilation.

Carbon dioxide is the primary factor controlling ventilation. Carbon dioxide in the arterial blood diffuses across the blood-brain barrier, thereby reducing the pH of the cerebral spinal fluid and stimulating the central chemoreceptors. A change in $Paco_2$ above or below normal will increase or decrease ventilation, respectively. During quiet, resting breathing, the level of $Paco_2$ is thought to be the major factor controlling breathing. Only when the Pao_2 (i.e., the partial pressure of oxygen dissolved in the blood that is not bound to hemoglobin) falls substantially does ventilation respond significantly. Typically, Pao_2 needs to fall to less than 50 mm Hg before ventilation dramatically increases (Fig. 4.11). Low oxygen levels in the blood are not sensed by the respiratory center in the brain but are sensed by receptors in the carotid body. These vascular receptors are located between the internal and external branches of the carotid artery. Changes in Pao_2 are sensed by the carotid sinus nerve. Neural traffic projects to the respiratory center through the glossopharyngeal nerve, which serves to modulate ventilation. The carotid body also senses changes in $Paco_2$ and pH. Nonvolatile acids (e.g., ketoacids) stimulate ventilation through their effects on the carotid body.

The outcome of this complex respiratory control system is that variables such as Pao_2, $Paco_2$, and pH are held within narrow limits under most circumstances. The respiratory control center also can adjust tidal volume and frequency of breathing to minimize the energetic cost of breathing and can adapt to special circumstances such as speaking, swimming, eating, and exercise. Breathing can be stimulated by artificial manipulation of the Pco_2, Po_2, and pH. For example, ventilation is increased by rebreathing of carbon dioxide, inhalation of a concentration of low oxygen, or infusion of acid into the bloodstream.

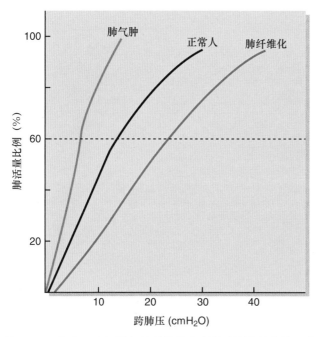

图 4.8　正常人、肺气肿和肺纤维化患者的肺顺应性曲线。在同样的肺容积下（图中水平虚线标示的肺容积是肺活量的60%），肺纤维化患者所需的跨肺压是最大的，相应的呼吸功增加

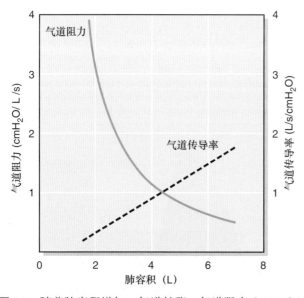

图 4.9　随着肺容积增加，气道扩张，气道阻力（AWR）减小，而气道阻力的倒数（气道传导率）随着肺容积的增加而增加

大。气流速度也部分决定了气流类型是层流或湍流。在临床上，引起气道阻塞的疾病都可以导致气道阻力增加，如气道内肿物、气道内黏液、气道平滑肌收缩或气道的外压性病变。

　　肺的弹性回缩也可以影响气道阻力和气流。在肺弹性回缩减弱时，通过促进小气道塌陷增加气道阻力。在 FRC 状态下以低气流速度呼吸时，正常气道阻力为每秒 1 ~ 2 cmH$_2$O/L。

通气的分布

　　被吸入的气体在肺内的分布并不均匀。在直立位状态，被吸入的气体通常更多地流入肺底部而不是肺尖。这样使得肺底部比肺尖通气更好。这种通气不均一性主要是由于肺顺应性存在区域差异。在 FRC 状态下，肺尖的肺泡比肺底部的肺泡处于更膨胀的状态。从肺尖到肺底肺泡膨胀程度的差异与从肺尖到肺底胸膜腔内压的差异有关。重力因素决定了肺尖的胸膜腔内压负压更大，而肺底部的负压较小。从肺尖到肺底部成人胸膜腔内压的正常压差大约是 8 cmH$_2$O（图 4.10）。由于 FRC 状态下，肺尖肺泡受到更明显的牵拉，所以它们处于容积-压力曲线上更僵硬、顺应性相对更差的区域，使得它们比肺底部肺泡更难膨胀。因此，在吸气开始时，更多的气体流向肺底部而不是肺尖。

通气的控制

　　充分的氧合和酸碱平衡的维持是通过呼吸控制系统来完成的。该系统由神经系统呼吸控制中枢、呼吸效应器（提供呼吸动力的肌肉）和呼吸传感器构成。自主控制吸气和呼气的呼吸中枢位于脑干髓质。脑干内的呼吸中枢有内源性的节律发生器驱动呼吸。呼吸中枢的输出受到多种调节，包括外周和中枢化学感受器的输入信号、肺内的机械感受器，以及大脑更高级的调节中枢如大脑皮质的意识控制等。脑干髓质内的呼吸中枢主要决定通气水平。

　　二氧化碳是控制通气的主要因素。动脉血中的二氧化碳以弥散的方式通过血脑屏障，降低脑脊液的 pH 值并刺激中枢化学感受器。PaCO$_2$ 的升高或降低会相应地增加或减少通气。在平静呼吸时，PaCO$_2$ 的水平是影响呼吸的主要因素。只有当 PaO$_2$（溶解在血液中而不与血红蛋白结合的氧分压）出现明显下降时，才会显著地增加通气。通常，只有当 PaO$_2$ 低于 50 mmHg 时才能引起通气量明显增加（图 4.11）。血液含氧量低的信号并非由大脑的呼吸中枢感知，而是通过颈动脉体的感受器感知。这些血管的感受器位于颈内动脉和颈外动脉的分叉处。PaO$_2$ 的改变通过颈动脉窦神经感知，通过舌咽神经传导至呼吸中枢而调节通气。颈动脉体还可以感知 PaCO$_2$ 和 pH 值的变化。非挥发性酸（如酮酸）也可以作用于颈动脉体而刺激通气。

　　复杂的呼吸控制系统确保了大多数情况下的 PaO$_2$、PaCO$_2$ 和 pH 值等变量都能保持在狭窄的范围内。呼吸控制中枢还能够调节潮气量、呼吸频率以将呼吸能耗降至最低，并适应各种特殊情况，如说话、游泳、进食和体育锻炼。人为地改变 PCO$_2$、PO$_2$ 和 pH 值也可以刺激呼吸。例如，通过二氧化碳的重复呼吸、吸入低浓度氧气或向血液中输入酸性物质均可增加通气。

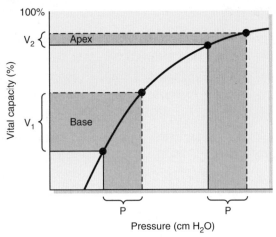

Fig. 4.10 Transpulmonary pressure and volume for lung units at the base and apex of the lung. Because pleural pressure is more negative at the apex of the lung, the alveoli in that region are stretched, placing them on a less compliant part of the volume-pressure curve. For a given change *(P)* in transpulmonary pressure during inspiration, the more compliant base inflates to a greater degree than the apex (V_1 and V_2, respectively).

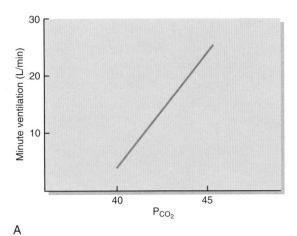

A

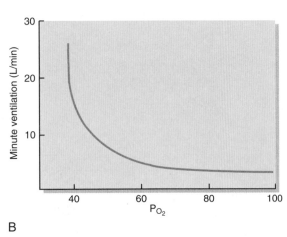

B

Fig. 4.11 (A) A rising partial pressure of carbon dioxide (P_{CO_2}) leads to a linear increase in minute ventilation. (B) The ventilatory response to hypoxemia is less sensitive and is clinically relevant only when the partial pressure of oxygen (P_{O_2}) has dropped significantly.

Perfusion

The pulmonary vascular bed differs from the systemic circulation in several respects. The pulmonary vascular bed receives the entire cardiac output of the right ventricle, whereas the cardiac output from the left ventricle is dispersed among several organ systems. Despite receiving the entire cardiac output, the pulmonary system is a low-resistance, low-pressure circuit. The normal mean systemic arterial pressure is about 100 mm Hg, whereas the normal mean pulmonary artery pressure is in the range of 15 mm Hg. The vascular bed can passively accommodate an increase in blood flow without raising arterial pressure by recruiting more vessels in the lung. During exercise, for example, there is little increase in pulmonary artery resistance despite a large increase in pulmonary blood flow. Hypoxic vasoconstriction, another feature unique to the pulmonary vascular system, regulates regional blood flow. This regulation aids in matching blood flow to ventilation by reducing flow to poorly ventilated regions of the lung.

Perfusion ($\dot{Q}$) refers to the blood flow through an organ (i.e., the lung). In the upright individual, there is greater perfusion of the lung bases than of the apices (Fig. 4.12). In a low-pressure system such as the pulmonary circulation, the effects of gravity on blood flow need to be taken into account. The arterial-venous pressure difference usually provides the "driving" pressure for blood flow in the systemic circulation, but this is true only for certain regions of the lung. Pulmonary blood flow also needs to be considered in the context of alveolar pressure. Venous and arterial pressures are importantly affected by gravity, whereas alveolar pressure remains constant throughout the lung, assuming the airways are open. Therefore, as one descends from the apex to the base of the lung, arterial and venous pressures increase because of gravity but alveolar pressure remains constant.

At the apex, alveolar pressure may be greater than arterial pressure. This region of the lung is referred to as *zone 1*, and, in theory, it receives no blood flow. The alveolar pressure may be greater than arterial pressure, for example, in special circumstances such as hypovolemic shock, which lowers the arterial pressure, or with very high levels of positive end-expiratory pressure (PEEP), which increases alveolar pressure.

As one descends from the apex toward the midzone of the lung, arterial and venous pressures increase, whereas alveolar pressure remains

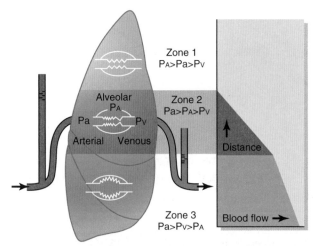

Fig. 4.12 Zonal model of blood flow in the lung. Because of the inter-relationship of arterial (Pa) and venous (Pv) vascular pressures and alveolar (PA) pressures, the lung base receives the most flow (see text for explanation). (From West JB, Dollery CT, Naimark A: Distribution of blood flow in isolated lung: relation to vascular and alveolar pressures, J Appl Physiol 19:713-724, 1964.)

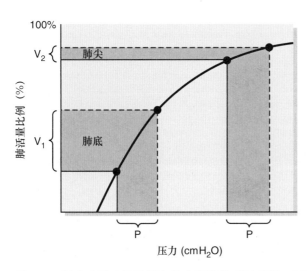

图 4.10　肺底和肺尖跨肺压与肺容积的关系示意图。因为胸膜腔内压在肺尖的负压更大，这一部位的肺泡受牵拉更明显，使得它们位于容积-压力曲线上顺应性较差的部分。吸气时，在同样的跨肺压变化（P）下，顺应性更好的肺底肺泡的扩张程度大于肺尖肺泡（分别对应 V_1 和 V_2）

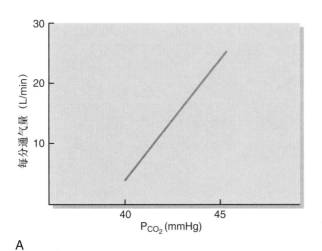

A

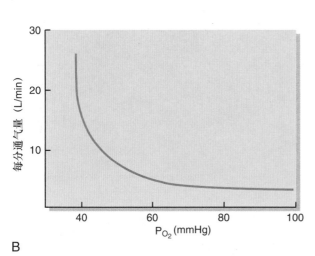

B

图 4.11　（**A**）二氧化碳分压（PCO_2）的升高可引起每分通气量的线性升高。（**B**）低氧引起的通气变化较小，只有当氧分压（PO_2）显著下降时才会引起通气明显增加

灌注

　　肺血管床和体循环在很多方面都存在差异。肺血管床接受右心室全部心输出量，而左心室的心输出量分布在数个器官系统中。尽管接受了右心全部的心输出量，肺循环系统仍然保持低阻、低压状态。正常的体循环平均动脉压约为 100 mmHg，而正常的肺动脉平均压在 15 mmHg 左右。血管床可以通过增加肺内血管的开放而被动性适应血流的增加，以维持肺动脉压稳定。例如在运动时，虽然肺血流量明显增加，但肺动脉阻力基本不变。缺氧性血管收缩是肺血管系统另一个独有的特点，可以对局部血流进行调节。通过减少肺内通气不良区域的血流，有助于血流和通气间的匹配。

　　灌注（$\dot{Q}$）是指通过器官（如肺）的血流量。直立位时肺底的灌注比肺尖更多（图 4.12）。在肺循环这种低压系统中，必须考虑重力对血流的影响。动-静脉的压力差为体循环血液的流动提供"驱动"的压力，但这仅适用于肺内的部分区域。肺血流还受到肺泡压的影响。假设气道开放，整个肺内的肺泡压保持恒定，静脉压和动脉压受重力影响很大。因此，从肺尖到肺底的动脉压和静脉压由于重力因素而增加，但是肺泡压力保持恒定。

　　在肺尖，肺泡压可能会高于动脉压，该区域被称作 1 区，理论上这一区域没有血流灌注。在某些特殊情况，如低血容量性休克时动脉压降低，或呼气末正压（PEEP）水平很高时肺泡压升高，可引起肺泡压高于动脉压。

　　当从肺尖移动到肺中部，肺动脉和静脉压力增加，而肺泡压力保持恒定。当移动到某一部位，动脉压会高于肺泡压（静脉压仍低于肺泡压），此处血流的驱动压

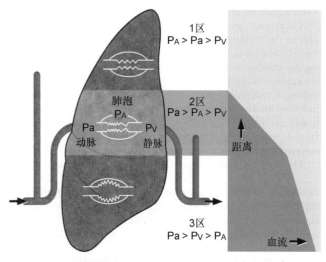

图 4.12　肺内血流的分区模型。由于动脉血管压力（Pa）、静脉血管压力（Pv）及肺泡压力（P_A）间的相互关系，肺底接受的血流量最大（详见正文）（引自 West JB, Dollery CT, Naimark A: Distribution of blood flow in isolated lung: relation to vascular and alveolar pressures, J Appl Physiol 19: 713-724, 1964. 因版权限制，中译文本图已作修改。）

constant. At some point, arterial pressure becomes greater than alveolar pressure. In this region, the driving pressure for blood flow is the arterial-alveolar pressure difference. This region is referred to as *zone 2* of the lung. Normally, zone 2 is very small because alveolar pressure is less than venous pressure in most of the lung. However, with high levels of PEEP, alveolar pressure becomes greater than venous pressure in more lung regions.

Further toward the base of the lung, the effects of gravity on arterial and venous pressures are more pronounced, venous pressure becomes greater than alveolar pressure, and the arterial-venous pressure difference provides the driving pressure for blood flow, as in the systemic circulation. This region is referred to as *zone 3* of the lung.

Normally, most of the lung is in zone 3, and most of the perfusion is to the lung base. This inequality in perfusion from apex to base is *qualitatively* similar to the inequality of ventilation from apex to base. However, blood flow increases from apex to base *more* than ventilation does, and this accounts for the small amount of ventilation-perfusion inequality that exists in the normal lung.

Gas Transfer

Oxygen and carbon dioxide are easily dissolved in plasma. Nitrogen is much less soluble and is not significantly exchanged across the alveolar-capillary interface. The driving force for the diffusion of a gas across a tissue barrier is the difference in partial pressure of the gas across the barrier. The partial pressure of oxygen in inspired room air entering the trachea is 150 mm Hg; this is derived from the equation, $P_{O_2} = (P_{atm} - P_{H_2O}) \times F_{IO_2}$, assuming that P_{atm} (atmospheric pressure) is 760 mm Hg, P_{H_2O} (the partial pressure of water vapor) is 47 mm Hg, and F_{IO_2} (the fraction of oxygen in inspired air) is 20.9%. In the alveolus, however, the partial pressure of oxygen is reduced to 100 mm Hg because the inspired V_T mixes with about 3 L of "oxygen-poor" air already in the lungs and is diluted by carbon dioxide moving into the alveolus from the pulmonary capillaries. The partial pressure of oxygen in the alveolus (P_{AO_2}) is set by the balance of these processes. Increasing minute ventilation increases the amount of oxygen added to the alveolus while lowering the P_{ACO_2}—the opposite result from hypoventilation. This reciprocal relationship between alveolar carbon dioxide and alveolar oxygen is described by the *alveolar gas equation*:

$$P_{AO_2} = [(P_{atm} - P_{H_2O}) \times F_{IO_2}] - (P_{ACO_2} / RER)$$

where RER is the respiratory exchange ratio, usually about 0.8.

The pressure gradient that drives diffusion of oxygen from the alveolus to the capillary is the difference between the alveolar P_{O_2} (100 mm Hg) and the arterial P_{O_2} (40 mm Hg) in the capillary blood entering the alveolus. By the time the blood leaves the alveolus, the P_{O_2} in the capillary blood has risen to 100 mm Hg. However, because small regions of ventilation-perfusion inequality and shunt exist in the normal lung, the P_{O_2} in the pulmonary veins from the lungs as a whole is usually about 90 mm Hg. Therefore, the difference between the alveolar and arterial partial pressures of oxygen, known as the *A-a gradient*, is typically about 10 mm Hg in health.

The pressure gradient that drives carbon dioxide from the mixed venous blood into the alveolus is the difference in partial pressure of carbon dioxide (45 mm Hg in mixed venous blood and 40 mm Hg in the alveolus). Despite the lower driving pressure for carbon dioxide compared with oxygen, the greater solubility of carbon dioxide allows complete equilibration between the alveolus and plasma during each respiratory cycle (Fig. 4.13).

Most of the oxygen contained in the blood is bound to hemoglobin; a small fraction is dissolved and measured as the P_{aO_2}. The amount of oxygen dissolved is about 3 mL/L in arterial blood, whereas the

amount of oxygen bound to hemoglobin is about 197 mL/L, assuming a normal hematocrit. Each molecule of hemoglobin is capable of carrying four molecules of oxygen. The shape of the oxyhemoglobin association curve reflects the cooperative binding of oxygen to hemoglobin (Fig. 4.14). In general, the hemoglobin saturation is between 80% and 100% with P_{aO_2} values greater than 60 mm Hg and drops dramatically when the P_{aO_2} is less than 60 mm Hg. Factors that decrease the affinity of hemoglobin for oxygen include a reduction in blood pH, an increase in temperature, an increase in P_{aCO_2}, and an increase in the concentration of 2,3-diphosphoglyceric acid (2,3-DPG) (Fig. 4.15). These factors facilitate unloading of oxygen into tissues, which is seen as a shift of the oxyhemoglobin dissociation curve to the right. The oxygen-carrying capacity of hemoglobin is also affected by competitive inhibitors

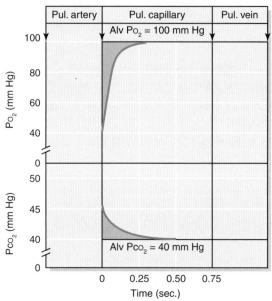

Fig. 4.13 Changes in the partial pressures of oxygen (P_{O_2}) and carbon dioxide (P_{CO_2}) as blood courses from the pulmonary artery through the capillaries and into the pulmonary veins. The diffusion gradient is greater for O_2 than for CO_2. However, equilibration of capillary and alveolar gas occurs for both molecules within the 0.75 second it takes for blood to traverse the capillaries. *Alv*, Alveolar; *Pul*, pulmonary.

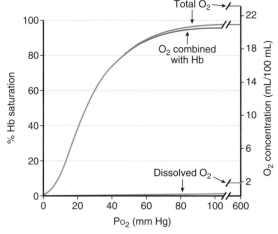

Fig. 4.14 The oxyhemoglobin dissociation curve. The bulk of the oxygen (O_2) is combined with hemoglobin (Hb). Little is dissolved in plasma. *P_{O_2}*, Partial pressure of oxygen.

为动脉-肺泡压力差。此区域被称为肺的 2 区。通常情况下，2 区非常小，因为肺内大多数肺泡内的压力低于静脉压。然而，在高 PEEP 水平的情况下，肺内大部分区域的肺泡压高于静脉压。

在肺底，重力对动脉压和静脉压的影响更为显著，静脉压开始高于肺泡压，与体循环相似，该区域血流的驱动压即是动-静脉压力差。此区域被称为肺的 3 区。

正常情况下，肺内大部分区域都处于 3 区，肺底部接受了大部分的血流灌注。这种从肺尖到肺底血流灌注的不均一性与从肺尖到肺底通气的不均一性类似。然而，从肺尖到肺底部血流量的增加比通气量增加得更多，因此正常肺也存在轻度的通气-血流灌注不匹配。

气体转运

氧气和二氧化碳易溶于血浆。氮气的溶解度很低，在肺泡-毛细血管界面处无显著气体交换。气体穿过组织屏障进行扩散的驱动力是屏障两侧气体的压差。吸入空气时，气管内的氧分压为 150 mmHg，可由公式 $PO_2 = (P_{atm} - P_{H_2O}) \times FiO_2$ 推算获得：假设 P_{atm}（大气压）为 760 mmHg，P_{H_2O}（水蒸气分压）为 47 mmHg，FiO_2（吸入空气中氧气的比例）为 20.9%。然而，被吸入的空气会与肺内约 3L 的"乏氧"气体混合，且二氧化碳从肺毛细血管弥散到肺泡内会导致氧气浓度被进一步稀释，肺泡中氧分压会降至 100 mmHg。这些过程达到平衡后的氧分压即是肺泡氧分压（P_AO_2）。增加每分通气量可以增加进入肺泡的氧气量同时降低 P_ACO_2，这与通气不足引起的改变相反。肺泡二氧化碳分压和肺泡氧分压之间的相互关系可以用肺泡气体方程来描述：

$$P_AO_2 = [(P_{atm} - P_{H_2O}) \times FiO_2] - (P_ACO_2/RER)$$

其中，RER 是指呼吸交换率（respiratory exchange ratio），通常为 0.8 左右。

驱动氧气从肺泡弥散到毛细血管内的压力梯度为肺泡氧分压（100 mmHg）和毛细血管内氧分压（40 mmHg）的差值。血液流经肺泡后，毛细血管内血液 PO_2 升至 100 mmHg。然而，由于正常肺中的小部分区域存在通气-灌注不匹配和分流，混合后的肺静脉内 PO_2 通常约为 90 mmHg。因此，A-a 梯度（即肺泡和体循环动脉的氧分压差）在健康人中约为 10 mmHg。

驱动二氧化碳从混合静脉血弥散到肺泡内的压力梯度为二者间的二氧化碳分压差（混合静脉血为 45 mmHg，肺泡内为 40 mmHg）。与氧气相比，二氧化碳弥散的驱动压力虽然较小，但由于其溶解度较大，二氧化碳仍然能够在每次呼吸周期内在肺泡和血浆之间达到完全平衡（图 4.13）。

血液中的氧气大部分与血红蛋白结合；只有一小部分溶于血浆，即被测量到的 PaO_2。在动脉血中氧气

的溶解量约为 3 ml/L，而在正常血细胞比容下，与血红蛋白结合的氧气量约为 197 ml/L。每个血红蛋白分子能携带四分子氧气。氧合血红蛋白解离曲线的形状反映氧与血红蛋白的协同结合情况（图 4.14）。通常，PaO_2 大于 60 mmHg 时，血红蛋白饱和度在 80%～100%，而当 PaO_2 小于 60 mmHg 时，血红蛋白饱和度则明显下降。可引起血红蛋白对氧亲和力降低的因素包括血液 pH 值降低、体温升高、$PaCO_2$ 增高及 2,3-二磷酸甘油酸（2,3-DPG）浓度增加（图 4.15）。这些因素有助于氧气解离到组织中，即氧合血红蛋白解离曲线右移。血红蛋白的携氧能力也受到一氧化碳等作用于结合位

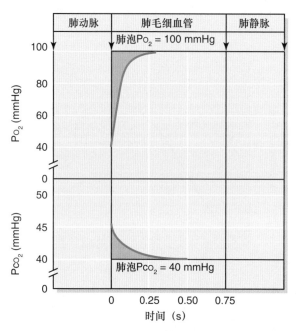

图 4.13　血液从肺动脉流经毛细血管到肺静脉过程中氧分压（PO_2）和二氧化碳分压（PCO_2）的变化。氧气的弥散梯度大于二氧化碳。然而，在血液通过肺毛细血管的 0.75 s 内，毛细血管与肺泡间可达到氧气和二氧化碳的交换平衡

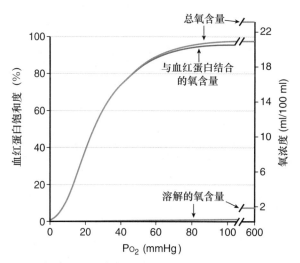

图 4.14　氧合血红蛋白解离曲线。大部分氧气与血红蛋白结合，只有极少部分溶于血浆。PO_2，氧分压

for binding sites, such as carbon monoxide. Carbon monoxide has an affinity for hemoglobin that is 240 times greater than that of oxygen and preferentially binds to the hemoglobin molecule. However, this does not affect the amount of oxygen dissolved in the blood. Someone with carbon monoxide poisoning may have a normal Pao_2 but a very low blood oxygen content because of the high amount of desaturated hemoglobin.

About 5% of carbon dioxide in the blood is dissolved in plasma, and about 10% is bound to hemoglobin. However, carbon dioxide does not exhibit cooperative binding; therefore, the shape of the carbon dioxide–hemoglobin dissociation curve is linear. Carbon dioxide binds to the protein component of the hemoglobin molecule and to the amino groups of the polypeptide chains of plasma proteins to form carbamino compounds. About 10% of carbon dioxide is transported in this fashion. Most of the carbon dioxide is transported as bicarbonate ion: As carbon dioxide diffuses from metabolically active tissue into the blood, it reacts with water to form carbonic acid. This reaction primarily occurs in the red blood cells because

it is catalyzed by the enzyme carbonic anhydrase, which resides in those cells. Carbonic acid then dissociates to bicarbonate and hydrogen ion. Although there is more carbon dioxide dissolved in blood than oxygen, it is still a small fraction of the total carbon dioxide transported by blood.

Abnormalities of Pulmonary Gas Exchange

The arterial Po_2 and Pco_2 are determined by the degree of equilibration between the alveolar gas and capillary blood, which depends on four major factors: ventilation, matching of ventilation with perfusion, shunt, and diffusion. *Hypoxemia* refers to a reduction in the oxygen content of the blood and is determined by measuring the Po_2 of arterial blood. In contrast, *hypoxia* refers to a decrease in oxygen content of an organ, for example, myocardial hypoxia. Aberrations in the four factors listed can result in hypoxemia. A fifth cause of hypoxemia is a low inspired Po_2, which may occur at altitude.

Hypoventilation is defined as ventilation that is inadequate to keep Pco_2 from increasing above normal. Hypoxemia may occur when increased carbon dioxide in the alveoli displaces alveolar oxygen. As alveolar ventilation falls and $Paco_2$ rises, Pao_2 will have to fall. Administration of supplemental oxygen (i.e., increasing the Fio_2) can reverse hypoventilation-induced hypoxemia. When one is breathing room air, the difference between alveolar oxygen and arterial oxygen (A-a gradient) is normally about 10 mm Hg. Typically, this difference increases when hypoxemia is present. However, if the hypoxemia is caused by hypoventilation, the A-a gradient will be within normal limits. Causes of hypoventilation are varied and range from diseases or drugs that depress the respiratory control center to disorders of the chest wall or respiratory muscles that impair respiratory pump function. Disorders associated with hypoventilation include inflammation, trauma, or hemorrhage in the brain stem; spinal cord pathology; anterior horn cell disease; peripheral neuropathies; myopathies; abnormalities of the chest wall such as kyphoscoliosis; and upper airway obstruction. Administration of a higher Fio_2 alleviates the hypoxemia but does little to improve the elevated $Paco_2$.

The most common cause of hypoxemia in disease states is ventilation-perfusion mismatch. In regions where the ratio of ventilation $\dot{V}$ to perfusion $\dot{Q}$ is low, the blood receives little oxygen from the poorly ventilated alveoli. By contrast, in regions where $\dot{V}/\dot{Q}$ is high, the blood is well oxygenated but receives little additional oxygen despite the higher ventilation because the shape of the oxyhemoglobin dissociation curve plateaus at levels of high Pao_2. As a result, lung units with high $\dot{V}/\dot{Q}$ cannot completely correct for the low oxygen content of blood flowing past units with low $\dot{V}/\dot{Q}$. Thus, the oxygen uptake of the whole lung is lowered, causing hypoxemia. In the ideal lung, ventilation and perfusion would be perfectly matched (i.e., $\dot{V}/\dot{Q} = 1$). However, the $\dot{V}/\dot{Q}$ normally ranges from 0.5 at the base to 3 at the apex, with an overall value of 0.8. If lung disease develops, ventilation-perfusion inequality may be amplified. If the $\dot{V}/\dot{Q}$ is less than 0.8, the A-a gradient is increased and hypoxia ensues. The $Paco_2$ is usually within the normal range but increases slightly at extremely low $\dot{V}/\dot{Q}$ ratios (Fig. 4.16). Typically, hypoxemia in diseases that affect the airways, such as chronic obstructive pulmonary disease (COPD), is caused by ventilation-perfusion mismatch. As with hypoxemia due to hypoventilation, administration of a higher Fio_2 improves hypoxemia by improving the Pao_2 in areas of *low $\dot{V}/\dot{Q}$*.

The third cause of hypoxemia is shunt. A right-to-left shunt occurs when a portion of blood travels from the right side to the left side of the heart without the opportunity to exchange oxygen and carbon dioxide in the lung. Right-to-left shunts can be classified as anatomic or physiologic. With an anatomic shunt, a portion of the blood bypasses the lung by traversing through an anatomic canal. In all healthy individuals, there

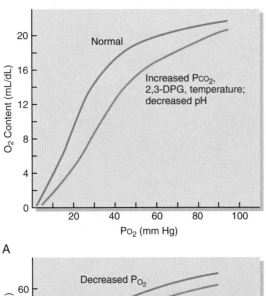

A

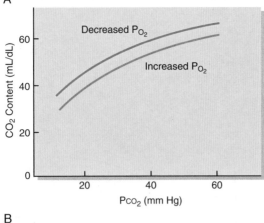

B

Fig. 4.15 (A) The various factors that decrease the oxygen affinity of hemoglobin are shown shifting the curve to the right. (B) The carbon dioxide dissociation curve is more linear than the oxyhemoglobin curve throughout the physiologic range. Increased partial pressure of oxygen in the arteries (Pao_2) shifts the curve to the right, decreasing the carbon dioxide content for any given arterial partial pressure of carbon dioxide ($Paco_2$) and thereby facilitating carbon dioxide off-loading in the lungs. The shift to the left at a lower Pao_2 facilitates carbon dioxide on-loading at the tissues. *2,3-DPG*, 2,3-Diphosphoglycerate.

点的竞争性抑制物的影响。一氧化碳与血红蛋白的亲和力比氧气高 240 倍，因此会优先与血红蛋白分子结合。然而，这并不影响溶于血液中的氧气量。一氧化碳中毒者可能 PaO_2 正常，但血氧含量非常低，因为大量血红蛋白呈未氧合状态。

血液中的二氧化碳大约有 5% 以直接溶解形式存在，另有大约 10% 以蛋白结合形式存在。由于二氧化碳没有协同结合的特点；因此，二氧化碳-血红蛋白解离曲线是线性的。以蛋白结合形式运输的二氧化碳，主要结合的是血红蛋白分子的蛋白质组分，以及血浆蛋白多肽链上的氨基（形成氨基甲酰化合物）。如前所述，约有 10% 的二氧化碳以这种形式运输。剩余的大部分二氧化碳则是以碳酸氢根形式运输的。二氧化碳分子从代谢活跃的组织扩散到血液中时，可以与水分子反应形成碳酸。这一反应主要由红细胞内的碳酸酐酶催化完成。反应生成的碳酸可进一步解离为碳酸氢根和氢离子。血液

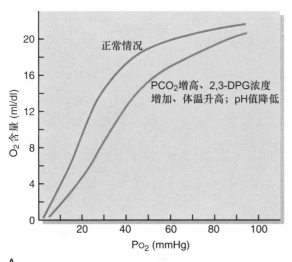

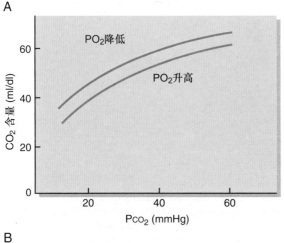

图 4.15　（**A**）多种降低血红蛋白对氧亲和力的因素引起曲线右移。（**B**）在生理状态范围内，二氧化碳解离曲线比氧合血红蛋白解离曲线更呈线性。动脉氧分压（PaO_2）升高使曲线右移，使得任一动脉二氧化碳分压（$PaCO_2$）下血液中的二氧化碳含量降低，从而促进二氧化碳在肺内解离而被排出。外周组织内 PaO_2 降低使曲线左移，有助于二氧化碳进入血液。2,3-DPG，2,3- 二磷酸甘油酸

中直接溶解的二氧化碳含量超过氧气，不过，该种形式在血液运输的全部二氧化碳中仅占一小部分。

肺气体交换异常

动脉氧分压和二氧化碳分压水平由肺泡内气体与毛细血管内血液间的平衡程度决定，主要受四种因素影响：通气、通气与灌注的匹配情况、分流和弥散。低氧血症（hypoxemia）是指血液中氧含量降低，可通过测量动脉血氧 PaO_2 判定。而缺氧（hypoxia）则是指器官内氧含量降低，如心肌缺氧。上述四种因素出现异常时可引起低氧血症。低氧血症的第五种原因是吸入气体的氧分压降低，可见于高海拔地区。

低通气是指通气量不足而导致 $PaCO_2$ 高于正常范围。当肺泡内二氧化碳含量增加，氧气含量随之减少，可引起低氧血症。随着肺泡通气降低、$PaCO_2$ 升高，P_AO_2 将会降低。补充氧气（即增加 FiO_2）可以纠正低通气引起的低氧血症。在吸入空气时，肺泡动脉氧分压差（A-a 梯度）通常为 10 mmHg 左右。当存在低氧血症时，这一差值往往增大。然而，如果是低通气引起的低氧血症，A-a 梯度将在正常范围内。低通气的病因多样，包括抑制呼吸中枢的疾病或药物、影响呼吸泵功能的胸壁或呼吸肌疾病等。可引起低通气的疾病包括脑干炎症、创伤或出血，脊髓病变，脊髓前角细胞病变，周围神经病，肌病，胸廓异常如脊柱侧后凸，及上气道梗阻。提供较高的 FiO_2 能改善低氧血症，但难以降低升高的 $PaCO_2$。

疾病状态下低氧血症最常见的原因是通气-灌注不匹配。在通气（$\dot{V}$）/ 灌注（$\dot{Q}$）比值低的区域，肺泡通气不良，血液难以氧合。与之相反，在 $\dot{V}/\dot{Q}$ 比值高的区域，血液氧合良好，但由于氧合血红蛋白解离曲线处于高 PaO_2 水平的平台部位，即使通气量更高，也难以进一步提高氧合。因此，肺内高 $\dot{V}/\dot{Q}$ 区域无法完全纠正低 $\dot{V}/\dot{Q}$ 区域引起的血氧含量降低。因此，整个肺脏的摄氧量下降，导致低氧血症。在理想情况下，肺内通气与灌注会完美匹配（即 $\dot{V}/\dot{Q}=1$）。但实际上，肺底的 $\dot{V}/\dot{Q}$ 通常为 0.5，而肺尖的 $\dot{V}/\dot{Q}$ 通常为 3，肺整体的 $\dot{V}/\dot{Q}$ 为 0.8。如果肺部出现病变，通气-灌注不匹配的影响会更明显。当 $\dot{V}/\dot{Q}$ 小于 0.8 时，A-a 梯度增加，从而导致人体缺氧。$\dot{V}/\dot{Q}$ 降低时，$PaCO_2$ 往往能维持在正常范围内，$\dot{V}/\dot{Q}$ 明显降低时才会引起 $PaCO_2$ 轻度升高（图 4.16）。通常，慢性阻塞性肺疾病（慢阻肺病，COPD）等影响气道的疾病中，低氧血症是由通气-灌注不匹配所致。与低通气引起的低氧血症类似，提供较高的 FiO_2 能提高低 $\dot{V}/\dot{Q}$ 区域的 P_AO_2，从而改善低氧血症。

低氧血症的第三个原因是分流。右向左分流是指一部分血液没有在肺内经过氧和二氧化碳的气体交换，而直接从右心流至左心。右向左分流可以分为解剖性分流和生理性分流。解剖性分流是指一部分血液通过解剖通道绕过肺流至左心。在健康人中，有一小部分血

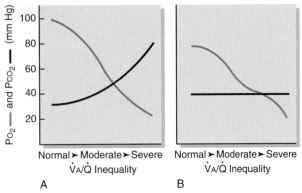

Fig. 4.16 (A) The effects of increasing inequality of alveolar ventilation and perfusion (decreasing $\dot{V}_A / \dot{Q}$) on the arterial partial pressures of oxygen (Po_2) and carbon dioxide (Pco_2) when cardiac output and minute ventilation are held constant. (B) The gas tensions change when minute ventilation is allowed to increase. Increased ventilation can maintain a normal arterial Pco_2 but can only partially correct the hypoxemia. (Modified from Dantzker DR: Gas exchange abnormalities. In Montenegro H, editor: Chronic obstructive pulmonary disease, New York, 1984, Churchill Livingstone, pp 141-160.)

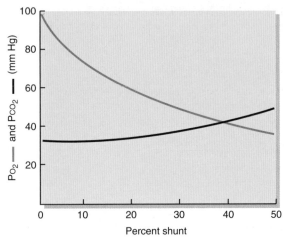

Fig. 4.17 The effects of increasing shunt on the arterial partial pressures of oxygen (Po_2) and carbon dioxide (Pco_2). The minute ventilation has been held constant in this example. Under usual circumstances, the hypoxemia would lead to increased minute ventilation and a fall in the Pco_2 as the shunt increased. (From Dantzker DR: Gas exchange abnormalities. In Montenegro H, editor: Chronic obstructive pulmonary disease, New York, 1984, Churchill Livingstone, pp 141-160.)

is a small fraction of blood in the bronchial circulation that passes to the pulmonary veins and empties into the left atrium, thereby reducing the Pao_2 of the systemic circulation. A smaller portion of the normal shunt is related to the coronary circulation draining through the thebesian veins into the left ventricle. Anatomic shunts found in disease states can be classified as intracardiac or intrapulmonary shunts. Intracardiac shunts occur when right atrial pressures are elevated and deoxygenated blood travels from the right atrium to the left atrium through an atrial septal defect or patent foramen ovale. Intrapulmonary anatomic shunts consist primarily of arteriovenous malformations or telangiectasias. With a physiologic right-to-left shunt, a portion of the pulmonary arterial blood passes through the normal vasculature but does not come into contact with alveolar air. This is an extreme example of ventilation-perfusion mismatch ($\dot{V}/\dot{Q} = 0$). Physiologic shunt can be caused by diffuse flooding of the alveoli with fluid, as seen in congestive heart failure or acute respiratory distress syndrome. Alveolar flooding with inflammatory exudates, as seen in lobar pneumonia, also causes a shunt. The fraction of blood shunted (Qs/Qt) can be calculated when the Fio_2 is 100% by the following equation:

$$Qs/Qt = (Cco_2 - Cao_2)/(Cco_2 - Cvo_2)$$

where Qs is the shunted blood flow, Qt is the total blood flow, Cco_2 is the end-pulmonary capillary oxygen content; Cao_2 is the arterial oxygen content; and Cvo_2 is the mixed venous oxygen content (amount of oxygen attached to hemoglobin in the blood returning from the body to right side of the heart).

If the shunt is severe enough, mechanical ventilation and PEEP are required to improve arterial oxygenation. At values less than 50% of the cardiac output, a shunt has very little effect on $Paco_2$ (Fig. 4.17). With shunting, the A-a gradient is elevated while the $Paco_2$ is within normal range or may be low. In contrast to hypoxemia due to hypoventilation or low $\dot{V}/\dot{Q}$, oxygen administration does not correct hypoxemia due to shunt because the shunted blood has no exposure to oxygen in the alveoli. However, the Pao_2 may increase somewhat because the higher Fio_2 improves oxygenation of blood traveling to low $\dot{V}/\dot{Q}$ areas that commonly coexist with shunt.

The fourth cause of hypoxemia is diffusion impairment. With normal cardiopulmonary function, the blood spends, on average, 0.75 second in the pulmonary capillaries. Typically, it takes only 0.25

second for the alveolar oxygen to diffuse across the thin alveolar capillary membrane and equilibrate with pulmonary arterial blood (see Fig. 4.13). However, if there is impairment to diffusion across this membrane, such as thickening of the alveolar capillary membrane by fluid, fibrous tissue, cellular debris, or inflammatory cells, it will take longer for the oxygen in the alveoli to equilibrate with pulmonary arterial blood. If the impediment to diffusion is such that it takes longer than 0.75 second for oxygen to diffuse, hypoxemia ensues, and the A-a gradient widens. Alternatively, if the time a red blood cell spends traversing the pulmonary capillary decreases to 0.25 second or less, hypoxemia may develop. Hypoxemia may be evident only during exercise in individuals with diffusion impairment because of the shortened red cell transit time. In these cases, the A-a gradient may be normal at rest but increases with exercise. With diffusion impairment, the $Paco_2$ usually is within the normal range. As with hypoxemia due to hypoventilation or ventilation-perfusion mismatch, administration of a higher Fio_2 improves hypoxemia due to impaired diffusion by raising the alveolar Po_2.

An additional cause of hypoxemia is low inspired oxygen. This may occur at high altitude: The Fio_2 is normal, but the Po_2 is low because the barometric pressure (P_{atm}) is low. Rarely, circumstances occur in which the Fio_2 is low (e.g., rebreathing air). Hypoxemia due to low inspired oxygen is associated with a normal A-a gradient and is usually accompanied by a low $Paco_2$. Supplemental oxygen corrects this form of hypoxemia. Finally, a low mixed venous Po_2 predisposes individuals to hypoxia (Fig. 4.18).

EVALUATION OF LUNG FUNCTION

Pulmonary function tests evaluate one or more major aspects of the respiratory system. Accurate measurements of lung volumes, airway function, and gas exchange require a pulmonary function laboratory. Pulmonary function tests are commonly used to aid in the diagnosis of disease and assess disease severity. In addition, they are helpful in monitoring the course of disease, assessing the risk for surgical procedures, and measuring the effects of varied environmental exposures (Table 4.1). The response to bronchodilators or other forms of treatment can also

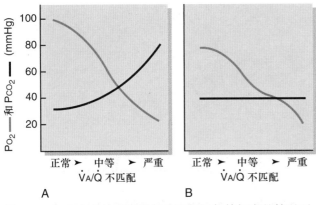

A　　　　　　　　　B

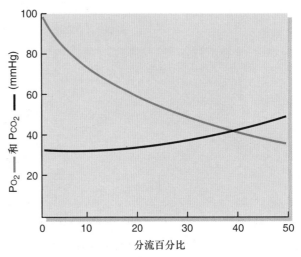

图 4.16 （**A**）在心输出量及每分通气量保持恒定的情况下，随着肺泡通气-灌注失调程度增加（$\dot{V}_A/\dot{Q}$ 降低），动脉氧分压（PO_2）及二氧化碳分压（PCO_2）相应变化。（**B**）当允许每分通气量增加时，气体张力有所改变。通气增加可维持动脉 PCO_2 正常，但仅能部分纠正低氧血症（改编自 Dantzker DR：Gas exchange abnormalities. In Montenegro H，editor：Chronic obstructive pulmonary disease，New York，1984，Churchill Livingstone，pp 141-160.）

图 4.17 分流比例增加对动脉氧分压（PO_2）及二氧化碳分压（PCO_2）的影响。此处假定每分通气量保持恒定。在通常情况下，随着分流量增加，低氧血症会引起每分通气量升高从而降低 PCO_2（引自 Dantzker DR：Gas exchange abnormalities. In Montenegro H，editor：Chronic obstructive pulmonary disease，New York，1984，Churchill Livingstone，pp 141-160.）

液通过支气管循环直接流入肺静脉而汇入左心房，降低了体循环的 PaO_2。一部分更小的正常分流来自于冠状动脉循环的引流，通过心最小静脉流入左心室。疾病状态下的解剖分流可分为心内分流或肺内分流。心内分流发生于右心房压升高时，未经氧合的血液通过房间隔缺损或卵圆孔未闭从右心房流入左心房。肺内分流主要包括动静脉畸形或毛细血管扩张。生理性右向左分流是指一部分肺动脉血液流经正常的脉管系统，但没有接触肺泡气体。这是通气-灌注不匹配（$\dot{V}/\dot{Q}=0$）的极端例子。生理性分流还可由肺泡内弥漫性液体填充所引起，可见于充血性心力衰竭或急性呼吸窘迫综合征。肺泡内填充炎性渗出物同样会导致分流，可见于大叶性肺炎。当 FiO_2 为 100% 时，可以通过以下公式计算肺内分流比例（Qs/Qt）：

$$Qs/Qt = (CcO_2 - CaO_2) / (CcO_2 - CvO_2)$$

其中，Qs 是分流血流量，Qt 是总血流量，CcO_2 是肺毛细血管末端氧含量，CaO_2 是动脉氧含量，而 CvO_2 是混合静脉血氧含量（从体内各脏器回流至右心的混合血液中血红蛋白所结合的氧含量）。

如果分流十分严重，则需要机械通气和 PEEP 来改善动脉氧合。在分流量小于心输出量 50% 的情况下，分流对 $PaCO_2$ 的影响很小（图 4.17）。在分流时，A-a 梯度升高，而 $PaCO_2$ 可维持在正常范围内甚至降低。与低通气或低 $\dot{V}/\dot{Q}$ 引起的低氧血症相反，吸氧并不能纠正分流引起的低氧血症，因为分流的血液在肺泡内并没有和氧气接触。然而，由于低 $\dot{V}/\dot{Q}$ 区域可以与分流并存，而提高 FiO_2 可以改善流经低 $\dot{V}/\dot{Q}$ 区域血液的氧合，因此 PaO_2 可能会有所增加。

低氧血症的第四个病因是弥散功能障碍。在心肺功能正常时，血液流经肺毛细血管的平均时间为 0.75 s。正常情况下，肺泡氧气弥散通过菲薄的肺泡毛细血管膜仅需 0.25 s 就能在血和肺泡间达到平衡（见图 4.13）。然而，如果通过此膜的弥散功能受损，如液体、纤维组织、细胞碎片或炎性细胞使肺泡毛细血管膜增厚，氧气在肺泡与肺动脉血间达到平衡则需要花费更长的时间。如果弥散障碍使得氧气弥散达到平衡的时间超过 0.75 s，就会导致低氧血症，并增大 A-a 梯度。或者，如果红细胞流经肺毛细血管的时间缩短到 0.25 s 以下，同样可能发生低氧血症。由于运动状态下血流速增快、红细胞通过时间缩短，存在弥散功能障碍的患者可能只会在运动后出现低氧血症。在这些患者中，A-a 梯度在静息状态下可能正常，但在运动时增加。弥散功能受损时，$PaCO_2$ 往往在正常范围内。与低通气或 $\dot{V}/\dot{Q}$ 失调引起的低氧血症一样，可以通过提高 FiO_2 来增加肺泡内 PO_2，改善弥散功能障碍引起的低氧血症。

低氧血症的另一个原因是吸入氧过少，可发生于高海拔地区：虽然 FiO_2 正常，但因为气压（P_{atm}）较低，所以 PO_2 较低。偶尔可见于低 FiO_2 的情况（如重复呼吸）。对于吸入氧过少引起的低氧血症，A-a 梯度正常，通常伴有 $PaCO_2$ 降低。补充氧气即可纠正这种类型的低氧血症。最后，混合静脉血 PO_2 降低可使人体容易发生缺氧（图 4.18）。

肺功能的评估

肺功能检查可以从一个或多个方面对呼吸系统进行评估。准确测量肺容积、气道功能和气体交换需要在肺功能实验室进行。肺功能检查常用于辅助诊断疾病和评估疾病严重程度。此外，还有助于监测病程发展、评估外科手术风险、评估各种环境暴露的影响（表 4.1）。还

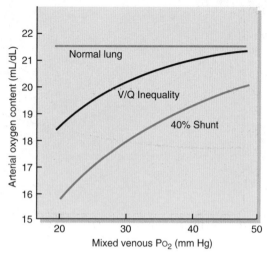

Fig. 4.18 The effects of increasing mixed venous partial pressure of oxygen (P_{O_2}) on the arterial oxygen content under three assumed conditions: a normal lung, severe ventilation-perfusion inequality ($\dot{V}/\dot{Q}$), and the presence of a 40% shunt. For each situation, the patient is breathing 50% oxygen and the mixed venous P_{O_2} is altered, keeping all other variables constant. (From Dantzker DR: Gas exchange in the adult respiratory distress syndrome, Clin Chest Med 3:57-67, 1982.)

TABLE 4.1   **Indications for Pulmonary Function Testing**
Evaluation of signs and symptoms:
Shortness of breath
Exertional dyspnea
Chronic cough
Screening of at-risk populations
Monitoring of pulmonary drug toxicity
Follow-up after abnormal study results:
Chest radiograph
Electrocardiogram
Arterial blood gases
Hemoglobin
Preoperative assessment:
Assess severity
Follow response to therapy
Determine further treatment goals
Assess disability

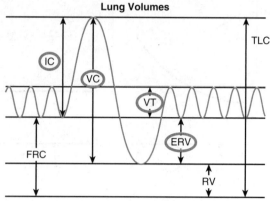

Fig. 4.19 Lung volumes and capacities. Although spirometry can measure vital capacity and its subdivisions *(red circles)*, calculation of residual volume (RV) requires measurement of functional residual capacity (FRC) by one of the following techniques: body plethysmography, helium dilution, or nitrogen washout. *ERV,* Expiratory reserve volume; *IC,* inspiratory capacity; *TLC,* total lung capacity; *VC,* vital capacity; *VT,* tidal volume.

be assessed with serial pulmonary function tests. Accurate interpretation of pulmonary function tests requires the appropriate reference standards. Variables that affect the predicted standards include age, height, gender, race, and hemoglobin concentration.

Spirometry, the simplest means of measuring lung function, can be performed in an office practice. A spirometer is an apparatus that measures inspiratory and expiratory volumes. Flow rates can be calculated from tracings of volume versus time. Typically, vital capacity (VC) is measured as the difference between a full inspiration to total lung capacity (TLC) and a full exhalation to residual volume (RV) (Fig. 4.19). Flow rates are measured after the patient is instructed to forcefully exhale from TLC to RV. Such a forced expiratory maneuver allows one to calculate the forced expiratory volume in 1 second (FEV_1) and the forced vital capacity (FVC) (Fig. 4.20). A value that is 80% to 120% of the predicted value is considered normal for FVC. Normally, people can exhale more than 75% to 80% of their FVC in the first second, and the majority of the FVC can be exhaled in 3 seconds. The ratio of FEV_1/FVC is normally greater than 0.80.

Spirometry can reveal abnormalities that are classified into two patterns: obstructive and restrictive. Obstructive impairments are defined by a low FEV_1/FVC ratio. Diseases that are characterized by an obstructive pattern include asthma, chronic bronchitis, emphysema, bronchiectasis, cystic fibrosis, and some central airway lesions. The reduction in FEV_1 (expressed as % predicted FEV_1) is used to determine the severity of airflow obstruction. Peak expiratory flow rate (PEFR) can be measured as the maximal expiratory flow rate obtained during spirometry or when using a handheld peak flowmeter. The lower the PEFR, the more significant the obstruction. A peak flowmeter can be used at home or in the emergency department to evaluate the presence of obstruction. Severe asthma decompensation, for example, is usually associated with PEFRs of less than 200 L/minute (normal, 500 to 600 L/minute). At home, a low PEFR can alert the patient to seek medical attention.

A restrictive pattern is characterized by loss of lung volume. With spirometry, both the FVC and the FEV_1 are reduced, so the FEV_1/FVC ratio remains normal. The restrictive pattern must be confirmed by measurements of lung volumes. Lung volumes are measured by body plethysmography or by dilution of an inert gas such as helium. Lung volumes that can be measured with these techniques include FRC, TLC, and RV (see Fig. 4.19). As described earlier, FRC is the lung volume at which the inward elastic recoil of the lung equals the outward elastic recoil of the chest wall. Changes in FRC reflect abnormalities in lung elastic recoil. Diseases associated with increased elastic recoil (e.g., pulmonary fibrosis) are associated with a reduction in FRC, whereas those with decreased recoil (e.g., emphysema) are associated with an increase in FRC. TLC is the amount of air remaining in the thorax after a maximal inspiration. It is determined by the balance of the forces generated by the respiratory muscles to expand the respiratory system and the elastic recoil of the respiratory system. Restrictive lung disease is defined as a TLC less than 80% predicted, whereas values of TLC greater than 120% predicted are consistent with hyperinflation. The lower the % predicted TLC, the more severe the restrictive impairment.

Restriction may be caused by disorders of the lung, chest wall, respiratory muscles, or pleural space. Lung diseases that cause pulmonary

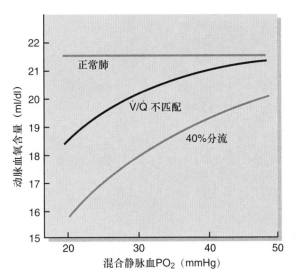

图 4.18　在正常肺、严重通气-灌注（V̇/Q̇）不匹配、肺内存在 40% 分流的三种假定的情况下，增加混合静脉血氧分压（PO_2）对动脉血氧含量的影响。在吸入氧浓度均为 50% 的情况下，改变混合静脉血 PO_2，保持其他指标相同（引自 Dantzker DR: Gas exchange in the adult respiratory distress syndrome, Clin Chest Med 3：57-67，1982.）

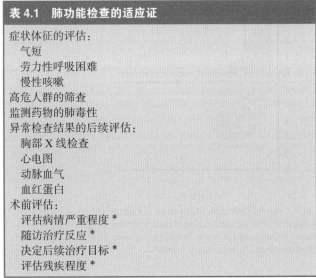

表 4.1　肺功能检查的适应证
症状体征的评估：
气短
劳力性呼吸困难
慢性咳嗽
高危人群的筛查
监测药物的肺毒性
异常检查结果的后续评估：
胸部 X 线检查
心电图
动脉血气
血红蛋白
术前评估：
评估病情严重程度 *
随访治疗反应 *
决定后续治疗目标 *
评估残疾程度 *

译者注：* 原文列于术前评估项下，译者认为应与术前评估处于同一级位置（不应缩进），因其应用场景不仅限于术前评估。

可以通过一系列肺功能检查来评估患者对支气管扩张剂或其他治疗的反应。肺功能检查结果的准确解读需要依据适当的参考值标准。影响预测值的变量包括年龄、身高、性别、种族和血红蛋白浓度。

　　肺量计法是评估肺功能最简单的方法，可以在诊室进行。肺量计是测量吸气和呼气容积的一种仪器。流量可以根据容积-时间曲线计算出来。通常，肺活量（VC）是充分吸气至肺总量（TLC）和充分呼气至残气量（RV）之间的差值（图 4.19）。在患者从 TLC 用力呼气至 RV 时测定流量。用力呼气时进行检测，可以计算出第 1 秒用力呼气容积（FEV_1）和用力肺活量

肺容积

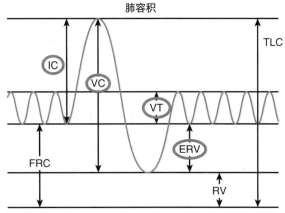

图 4.19　肺容积和容量。虽然肺量计法可以测量肺活量及其组分（如红圈所示），残气量（RV）的计算需要使用体积描记法、氦稀释法或氮冲洗法来测量功能残气量（FRC）而得出。ERV，补呼气容积；IC，深吸气量；TLC，肺总量；VC，肺活量；VT，潮气量

（FVC）（图 4.20）。FVC 占预计值百分比的正常范围是 80% ～ 120%。通常，人们可以在第 1 秒内呼出 FVC 的 75% ～ 80% 以上，在前 3 s 内可呼出绝大部分的 FVC。FEV_1/FVC 的比值通常大于 0.80。

　　肺量计法能够发现的异常分为两类：阻塞性和限制性。阻塞性通气功能受损的定义为 FEV_1/FVC 比值降低。以阻塞性通气功能受损为特征的疾病包括哮喘、慢性支气管炎、肺气肿、支气管扩张症、囊性纤维化和一些中央气道病变。FEV_1 的下降（用 FEV_1 占预计值百分比表示）可用来判断气流阻塞的严重程度。峰值呼气流速（PEFR）是呼气流速的最大值，可通过肺量计法或手持峰流速仪进行测量。PEFR 越低，说明阻塞越严重。在家中或急诊室可以使用峰流速仪判断是否存在气道阻塞。例如，严重哮喘发作时，PEFR 往往小于 200 L/min（正常范围为 500 ～ 600 L/min）。低 PEFR 可以提醒居家的患者寻求医疗救助。

　　限制性通气功能障碍的特点是肺容积减少。肺量计法测得的 FVC 和 FEV_1 均降低，所以 FEV_1/FVC 比值正常。限制性改变必须通过测量肺容积而进行确认。肺容积通过体积描记法或稀释惰性气体（如氦气）进行测定。可以测定的肺容积指标包括功能残气量（FRC）、TLC 和 RV（见图 4.19）。如前所述，FRC 是肺向内的弹性回缩力与胸廓向外的弹性牵拉力达到平衡时的肺容积。FRC 的改变反映肺弹性回缩异常。弹性回缩力增加的疾病（如肺纤维化）表现为 FRC 减小，而弹性回缩力下降的疾病（如肺气肿）则表现为 FRC 增加。TLC 是吸气到最大程度时胸腔内的气体量。它取决于呼吸肌扩张呼吸系统的牵拉力和呼吸系统本身的弹性回缩力之间的平衡。限制性肺疾病的定义是 TLC 小于预计值的 80%，而 TLC 大于预计值的 120% 则符合过度充气。TLC 占预计值百分比越低，提示限制性通气功能障碍越严重。

　　限制性通气功能障碍可以由肺、胸廓、呼吸肌或

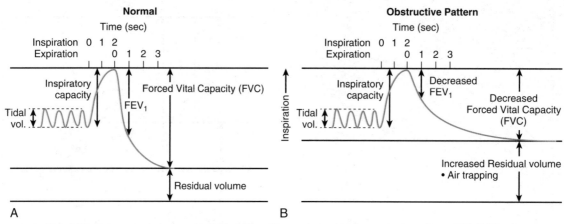

Fig. 4.20 Spirometry in a normal individual (A) and in a patient with obstructive lung disease (B). FEV_1 represents the forced expiratory volume in 1 second, and FVC represents the forced vital capacity. The FEV_1/FVC ratio is normally greater than 0.80. With obstruction, the FEV_1/FVC ratio is less than 0.70.

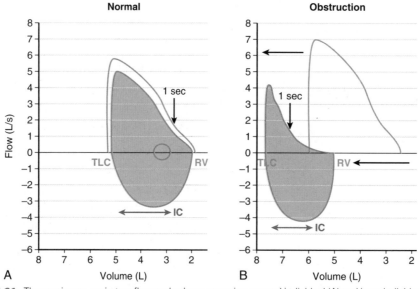

Fig. 4.21 The maximum expiratory flow and volume curve in a normal individual (A) and in an individual with obstructive lung disease (in this case, COPD) (B). Hyperinflation and air trapping *(arrows)* push the total lung capacity (TLC) and residual volume (RV) to the left (i.e., toward higher lung volumes). In addition, characteristic scalloping of the expiratory limb of the flow-volume curve develops. IC, Inspiratory capacity.

fibrosis cause a restrictive pattern because of the increased elastic recoil of the respiratory system. Diseases of the chest wall, such as kyphoscoliosis, obesity, or ankylosing spondylitis, can also cause restriction by reducing the elasticity of the chest wall. Weakness of the respiratory muscles causes restriction by reducing the force available to inflate the respiratory system. Myasthenia gravis, amyotrophic lateral sclerosis, diaphragm paralysis, and Guillain-Barré syndrome can be associated with weakness sufficient to cause restrictive lung disease. Finally, space-occupying lesions involving the pleural space, such as pleural effusions, pneumothorax, or pleural tumors, can cause restriction. Occasionally, RV and FRC may be elevated with no increase in TLC. This pattern is referred to as *air trapping* and can be seen with COPD or asthma.

The forced expiratory maneuver can be analyzed in terms of flow and volume by construction of a flow-volume loop (Fig. 4.21). Flow-volume loops are useful to identify obstructive and restrictive patterns. The characteristic appearance of obstructive impairment is concavity ("scooping") of the expiratory loop, whereas with restrictive impairments, the loops have a normal shape but are reduced in size. In addition, flow-volume loops are the primary means of identifying upper airway obstruction. Upper airway obstruction is characterized by a truncated (clipped) inspiratory or expiratory loop. A fixed obstruction produces clipping of both inspiratory and expiratory loops. Variable intrathoracic upper airway obstruction exhibits clipping of the expiratory loop, whereas variable extrathoracic obstruction exhibits clipping of the inspiratory loop (Fig. 4.22).

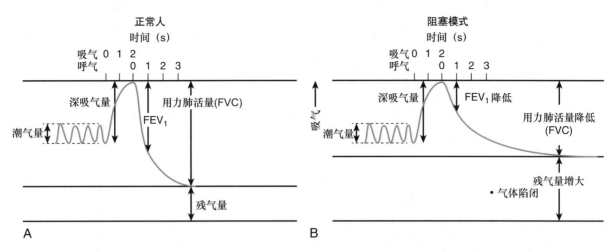

图 4.20　正常受试者（**A**）和阻塞性肺疾病患者（**B**）的肺量计测定结果示意图。FEV_1 是指第 1 秒用力呼气容积，FVC 是指用力肺活量。FEV_1/FVC 比值通常大于 0.80。存在阻塞性疾病时，FEV_1/FVC 比值小于 0.70

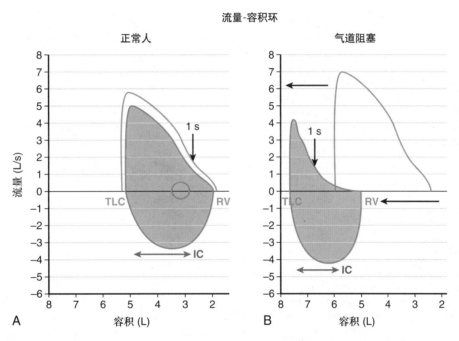

图 4.21　正常受试者（**A**）和阻塞性肺疾病（本例为慢阻肺病）患者（**B**）的最大呼气流量-容积曲线。过度充气和气体陷闭（箭头）使肺总量（TLC）和残气量（RV）左移（即肺容积增大）。此外，流量-容积环的呼气支上出现了特征性的凹陷。IC，深吸气量

胸膜腔病变引起。可以导致肺纤维化的肺病均可以导致限制性改变，因为呼吸系统的弹性回缩力增大。胸廓疾病如脊柱侧后凸、肥胖或强直性脊柱炎，也可以通过降低胸廓的弹性而引起限制性通气功能障碍。呼吸肌无力使得呼吸系统充气膨胀的力减弱而引起限制性通气功能障碍。重症肌无力、肌萎缩侧索硬化、膈肌麻痹及吉兰-巴雷综合征可导致呼吸肌无力，而引起限制性肺疾病。累及胸膜腔的占位性病变如胸腔积液、气胸、胸膜肿瘤等也可以导致限制性通气功能障碍。有时可能会出现 RV 和 FRC 升高而 TLC 正常的情况，这种情况被称为气体陷闭，可见于慢阻肺病或哮喘。

测量用力呼气的过程可以构建流量-容积环而分析流量和容积的变化情况（图 4.21）。流量-容积环可用于识别阻塞性及限制性改变。阻塞性通气功能障碍的特征表现是呼气环向内凹陷（"勺状"），而限制性通气功能障碍的曲线形态正常、但尺寸缩小。此外，流量-容积环是识别上气道梗阻的主要手段。上气道梗阻的特点是吸气环或呼气环的平台样表现（被削平）。固定型上气道阻塞表现为吸气和呼气环都呈平台样改变。可变胸内型上气道阻塞表现为呼气环出现平台样改变，而可变胸外型阻塞表现为吸气环平台样改变（图 4.22）。

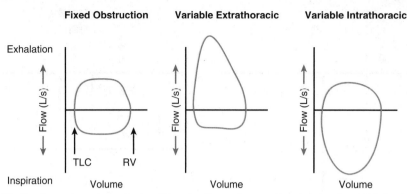

Fig. 4.22 The flow-volume loops display different patterns of upper airway obstruction. With fixed obstruction, both inspiratory and expiratory flows are reduced (clipped). With variable extrathoracic obstruction, only the inspiratory flows are clipped. With variable intrathoracic obstruction, only the expiratory flows are clipped. RV, Residual volume; TLC, total lung capacity.

Bronchoprovocation Testing

Bronchoprovocation testing is typically used to determine the presence or absence of hyperreactive airways disease. Some individuals with a clinical suspicion of asthma have normal expiratory flow rates and lung volumes. Bronchoprovocation testing in these individuals can be important to identify hyperreactive airways disease and support the diagnosis of asthma. Methacholine is a cholinergic agonist that causes bronchoconstriction. During the bronchoprovocation test, the subject inhales increasing concentrations of methacholine. Measurements of FEV_1, FVC, and specific airways conductance are obtained after the inhalation of each concentration until the maximal dose of methacholine has been administered. If the FEV_1 is reduced by 20% or more or the specific airways conductance is reduced by 40% or more, a diagnosis of hyperreactive airways disease is established. Patients with asthma demonstrate a fall in FEV_1 at considerably smaller doses than in normal individuals (Fig. 4.23).

Lung Diffusion Capacity

The diffusion of oxygen from the alveolus into the capillary can be assessed by measuring the diffusion capacity for carbon monoxide (D_{LCO}). To calculate the diffusion capacity for oxygen, one would need to know the alveolar volume and the partial pressures of oxygen in the alveolus and in the pulmonary capillary. Because it is not practical to measure the oxygen tension of pulmonary capillary blood, carbon monoxide is used rather than oxygen to assess diffusion capacity. Carbon monoxide diffuses across the alveolar capillary membranes much as oxygen does. However, carbon monoxide has the advantage of binding completely to hemoglobin. Therefore, the partial pressure of carbon monoxide in the pulmonary venous blood is negligible. The D_{LCO} is then measured as the rate of disappearance of carbon monoxide from the alveolus and is used as a surrogate for oxygen diffusion capacity.

The D_{LCO} measurement provides an overall assessment of gas exchange and depends on factors such as the surface area of the lung, the physical properties of the gas, perfusion of ventilated areas, hemoglobin concentration, and the thickness of the alveolar-capillary membrane. Therefore, an abnormal value may not only signify disruption of the alveolar-capillary membrane but may also be related to a reduction in surface area of the lung (pneumonectomy), poor perfusion (pulmonary embolus), or poor ventilation of alveolar units (COPD). A low D_{LCO} may be seen in interstitial lung diseases that alter the alveolar-capillary membrane or in diseases such as emphysema that destroy

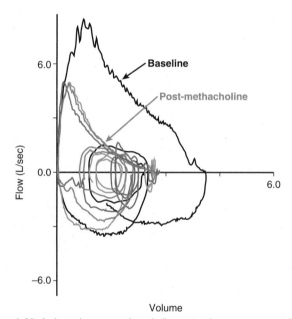

Fig. 4.23 In bronchoprovocation challenge, patients are exposed to increasing concentrations of an inhaled challenge (e.g., methacholine, histamine), followed by evaluation of the forced expiratory volume in 1 second (percentage of baseline value) or airways conductance. The FEV_1 falls by more than 20% (compared to baseline), and airways conductance by more than 40%, at lower concentrations of the challenge drug in individuals with asthma.

both alveolar septa and capillaries. Anemia lowers the D_{LCO}. Most laboratories provide a hemoglobin correction for diffusion capacity. An increased D_{LCO} may be associated with engorgement of the pulmonary circulation by red blood cells or polycythemia.

Arterial Blood Gases

The measurement of Pao_2 and $Paco_2$ provides information about the adequacy of oxygenation and ventilation. This requires arterial blood sampling through arterial puncture or indwelling cannula (Table 4.2). Oxygenation also can be measured through noninvasive devices such as the pulse oximeter, which measures hemoglobin oxygen saturation, and through transcutaneous devices that measure Pao_2 and $Paco_2$. These devices are particularly useful for measuring oxygenation during exertion or sleep.

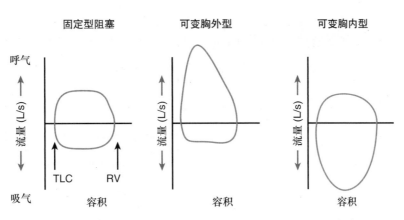

图 4.22　不同类型上气道阻塞的流量-容积环示意图。存在固定型阻塞时，吸气和呼气流量都降低（呈平台样改变）。可变胸外型阻塞时，只有吸气流量呈平台样改变。而可变胸内型阻塞时，只有呼气流量呈平台样改变。RV，残气量；TLC，肺总量

支气管激发试验

　　支气管激发试验通常用于确定是否存在高反应性气道疾病。一些临床怀疑哮喘的患者呼气流速和肺容积正常，在这一人群中进行支气管激发试验对于识别气道高反应性疾病、支持哮喘的诊断均十分重要。乙酰甲胆碱是胆碱能受体激动剂，可引起支气管收缩。在支气管激发试验中，受试者吸入浓度递增的乙酰甲胆碱，在每次吸入特定浓度的药物后测量 FEV_1、FVC 和气道传导率，直至吸入了最大剂量的乙酰甲胆碱。如果 FEV_1 减少 20% 以上，或气道传导率降低 40% 以上，则可以诊断气道高反应性疾病。与正常人相比，哮喘患者在吸入较低剂量的药物后即可出现 FEV_1 下降（图 4.23）。

肺弥散功能检查

　　氧气从肺泡进入毛细血管的弥散能力可以用肺—氧化碳弥散量（diffusion capacity for carbon monoxide of lung，D_{LCO}）（译者注：D_{LCO} 中的 L 应是 lung 的缩写，因此，英文全称应包括"of lung"，而原文中无）进行评估。为了计算氧弥散量，需要知道肺泡容积、肺泡氧分压和肺毛细血管氧分压。直接测量肺毛细血管血液中的氧气张力是不实际的，因此使用一氧化碳替代氧气来评估弥散量。一氧化碳弥散通过肺泡毛细血管膜的过程和氧气类似。但是，一氧化碳可以完全与血红蛋白结合，因此肺静脉血中的一氧化碳分压可以忽略不计。通过测量一氧化碳从肺泡内清除的速度来测量 D_{LCO}，作为氧弥散量的替代评估指标。

　　D_{LCO} 能够对气体交换情况进行整体评估，其影响因素包括肺的表面积、气体的物理特性、通气区域的灌注情况、血红蛋白浓度、肺泡-毛细血管膜厚度等。因此，数值异常时可能不仅提示存在肺泡-毛细血管膜受损，还可能与肺表面积减小（如肺切除术）、灌注减少（如肺栓塞）或肺泡单位通气不良（如慢阻肺病）等有关。D_{LCO} 降低可见于累及肺泡-毛细血管膜的间质性肺疾病、破坏肺泡间隔和毛细血管的肺气肿。贫血

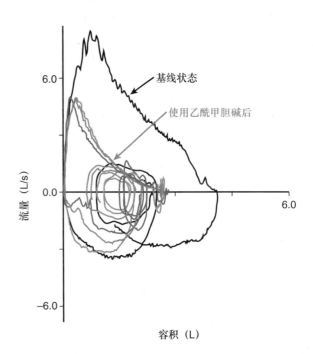

图 4.23　在支气管激发试验中，患者吸入浓度逐渐增加的激发药物（如乙酰甲胆碱、组胺），随后测量第 1 秒用力呼气容积（占基线值的百分比）或气道传导率。在哮喘患者中，吸入较低浓度的激发药物即可出现 FEV_1 下降超过 20%（与基线相比），气道传导率较基线下降超过 40%〔译者注：横坐标 Volume 的单位应为（L），原文未标注单位〕

同样可使 D_{LCO} 降低。大部分实验室可以根据血红蛋白校正弥散量的数值。D_{LCO} 升高可能和肺循环淤血或红细胞增多症有关。

动脉血气分析

　　测量 PaO_2 和 $PaCO_2$ 可用于评估氧合及通气的充分性，需要通过动脉穿刺或动脉置管进行动脉血液采样进行检测（表 4.2）。氧合情况还可以通过无创装置测量，如测量血红蛋白氧饱和度的脉搏血氧饱和度仪，以及经皮测量 PaO_2 和 $PaCO_2$ 的装置。这些装置尤其适用于运动或睡眠中测量氧合情况。

TABLE 4.2   Normal Values for Arterial Blood Gases
Partial pressure of oxygen (Pao_2): 104 – (0.27 × age)
Partial pressure of carbon dioxide ($Paco_2$): 36-44
pH: 7.35-7.45
Alveolar-arterial O_2 difference = 2.5 + (0.21 × age)

6-Minute Walk Distance

Often, alterations in oxygenation are not detected at rest but are unveiled during exertion. The 6-minute walk test is a standardized test in which the patient walks for 6 minutes while the oxygen hemoglobin saturation is measured. A decrease in saturation is abnormal and suggests impaired gas exchange capabilities, and a reduction in distance walked is a means of detecting deterioration of overall function due to lung disease. However, the 6-minute walk distance (6MWD) is primarily validated for following exercise capacity over time and in response to interventions. There is a "learning effect" that increases distance walked after the first attempt, and the minimal clinically important distance for this test is established as 30 meters. The 6MWD correlates well with peak oxygen consumption (VO_2 max) measured with maximal exercise testing.

In summary, pulmonary function tests, in conjunction with the history and physical examination, can be used to diagnose pulmonary disorders and assess severity and response to therapy.

EVALUATION OF LUNG DISEASE

Analysis of Exhaled Breath

Endogenously produced monoxides (nitric oxide and carbon monoxide) and volatile organic compounds (VOCs), collectively called the "volatolome," can be detected in the exhaled breath and may serve as biomarkers of pulmonary inflammation or cancer. Exhaled nitric oxide is elevated in asthma, and the US Food and Drug Administration has approved the test for exhaled nitric oxide for the diagnosis and evaluation of asthma exacerbations. The VOCs can be detected by gas chromatography or mass spectroscopy but more recently electronic "noses" have been developed that use changes in electrical resistance of polymers that bind VOCs to detect unique patterns of exhaled VOCs. These provide a "fingerprint" that may identify lung cancer, various pneumoconioses, obstructive sleep apnea, active pulmonary tuberculosis, and pulmonary hypertension. Cytokines and other similar compounds in the condensate phase of exhaled breath are being investigated for possible applications in inflammatory lung diseases (e.g., cystic fibrosis, bronchiectasis). Other nonpulmonary diseases such as malabsorption syndromes and *Helicobacter pylori* infection are also detected by analysis of exhaled breath.

Chest Radiography

Generally, the evaluation of a patient with lung disease begins with routine chest radiography and then proceeds to more specialized techniques such as computed tomography (CT) or magnetic resonance imaging (MRI). Ideally, the chest radiograph consists of two different films, a posteroanterior (PA) radiograph and a lateral radiograph. Many pathologic processes can be identified on a PA chest radiograph, and the lateral view adds valuable information about areas that are not well seen on the PA projection. In particular, the retrocardiac region, the posterior bases of the lung, and the bony structure of the thorax (e.g., the vertebral column) are better visualized on the lateral radiograph. The PA chest radiograph is obtained with the patient standing with his or her back to the x-ray beam and the anterior chest wall placed against the film cassette. The chest radiograph should be obtained while the patient takes the deepest breath possible. If the patient is too weak to stand or too sick to travel to the radiology department, the chest radiograph is performed at bedside (portable chest radiograph). The cassette is placed behind the patient's back while the patient is semi-supine in bed, and the x-ray beam travels from anterior to posterior (AP film). The quality of a portable film is not that of a standard PA film, but it still provides valuable information.

The examination of a chest radiograph should be systematic so that subtle abnormalities are not missed. It should include evaluation of the lungs and pulmonary vasculature, the bony thorax, the heart and great vessels, the diaphragm and pleura, the mediastinum, the soft tissues, and the subdiaphragmatic areas. Abnormalities that are visible on a chest radiograph include pulmonary infiltrates, nodules, interstitial markings, vascular abnormalities, masses, pleural effusions and thickening, cavitary lesions, cardiac enlargement, abnormal airway structure, and vertebral or rib fractures. In addition to the PA and lateral chest radiographs, the lateral decubitus projection is often used to identify the presence or absence of pleural effusion. The decubitus view is particularly useful in determining whether blunting of the costal phrenic sulcus is caused by freely flowing pleural fluid or related to pleural thickening. Chest radiography, in concert with a good history and physical examination, allows the clinician to diagnose chest disease in many circumstances.

Fluoroscopy

Fluoroscopic examination of the chest is useful for evaluating motion of the diaphragm. This technique is particularly helpful in diagnosing unilateral diaphragm paralysis. A paralyzed hemidiaphragm moves paradoxically when the patient is instructed to inhale or to forcefully sniff. However, fluoroscopy is limited when evaluating for bilateral diaphragm paralysis. Apparently normal descent of the diaphragm during inspiration, caused by compensatory respiratory strategies employed by the patient with bilateral diaphragm paralysis, leads to false-negative results. False-positive results are caused by paradoxical hemidiaphragm motion, which can be seen in as many as 6% of normal subjects during the sniff maneuver.

Ultrasonography

Point-of-care ultrasonography (POCUS) has improved clinical care by providing more focused and visual examinations of vital organs to aid in prompt diagnosis and management of diseases. In ultrasonography, sound waves in the frequency range of 3 to 10 MHz are reflected off internal tissues to produce images of viscera such as the liver, kidney, and heart. The air-filled lung cannot be imaged directly, but over the last decade, an understanding of various *artifacts* generated by ultrasound beams traversing normal and abnormal lung have led to increased application of ultrasound for imaging of the lung, particularly in the intensive care unit. Protocols are available to help with detecting lung consolidation, pulmonary edema, and volume responsiveness. Additionally, ultrasonography can rapidly and reliably detect a pneumothorax, pleural effusion, consolidation, and pulmonary

表 4.2　动脉血气分析正常值
氧分压（PaO_2，mmHg）：104 －（0.27× 年龄） 二氧化碳分压（$PaCO_2$，mmHg）：36 ～ 44 pH 值：7.35 ～ 7.45 肺泡-动脉氧分压差（mmHg）：2.5 ＋（0.21× 年龄）

译者注：原文未注明分压的单位，应为 mmHg。

6 分钟步行距离

很多情况下，氧合的改变在静息状态下并不显著，但在活动后就能显现出来。6 分钟步行距离试验是在患者步行 6 分钟的同时测量血氧饱和度的一项标准测试。试验中出现血氧饱和度下降即为异常，提示气体交换能力受损，同时步行距离的减少提示肺病导致了整体功能恶化。6 分钟步行距离主要用于动态评价病程中及治疗干预后运动耐量的变化。在进行首次尝试后，"学习效应"会提高第二次试验的步行距离，因此两次试验的步行距离差值至少应超过 30 m 才被认定存在临床意义。6 分钟步行距离与最大运动试验中测得的峰值耗氧量（$VO_2\ max$）存在良好的相关性。

综上所述，肺功能检查结合病史和查体可用于诊断肺病、评估疾病的严重程度和对治疗的反应。

肺病的评估

呼出气分析

挥发物（volatolome）是呼出气中由人体产生的一氧化物（一氧化氮和一氧化碳）及挥发性有机化合物（VOC）的总称，这些成分可能作为肺部炎症或肿瘤性疾病的生物标志物。呼出气一氧化氮水平在哮喘患者中升高，该检查已经被美国食品药品监督管理局批准用于诊断和评估哮喘病情发作。挥发性有机化合物可以通过气相色谱法或质谱法进行检测。近年来研发了"电子鼻"传感技术，其内的聚合物结合挥发性有机化合物后电阻会发生相应变化，从而检测呼出气中挥发性有机化合物的成分，生成的"指纹图谱"可能用于识别肺癌、各种类型的尘肺、阻塞性睡眠呼吸暂停、活动性肺结核及肺动脉高压等疾病。还有研究尝试将呼出气体冷凝物中的细胞因子和其他类似化合物用于肺部炎症性疾病（如囊性纤维化、支气管扩张症）的评估。呼出气分析还可用于检测其他肺外疾病如吸收不良综合征、幽门螺杆菌感染等。

胸部 X 线检查

肺病患者的评估通常从常规的胸部 X 线检查开始，然后才选择更有针对性的专项检查，如计算机断层成像（CT）或磁共振成像（MRI）。理想情况下，胸部 X 线检查拍摄两个不同的体位，一张后前位（posteroanterior，PA）片和一张侧位片。后前位胸部 X 线片（胸片）可以显示很多病理改变，侧位片则对后前位投照时显示不佳的区域提供了额外有价值的信息。尤其是心脏后的椎前区域、肺的后基底部及胸腔的骨性结构（如脊柱）在侧位片上观察得更清楚。后前位的胸部平片是患者背对 X 线束、前胸贴在胶片盒上拍摄的，需在患者深吸气末摄片。如果患者过于虚弱而无法站立或因病无法前往放射科，也可以在床旁拍摄胸片。患者在床上取半仰卧位，将胶片盒放置在患者背后，X 线束从前向后背穿过身体（anterioposterior，AP 片）。床旁胸片的影像质量虽不如标准的后前位胸片，但也能提供有价值的信息。

胸片的阅片应系统化，以避免错过细微的异常。阅片时应评估肺和肺血管、胸部骨性结构、心脏和大血管、膈肌和胸膜、纵隔、软组织和膈下区域。在胸片上可观察到的异常包括肺部浸润影、结节、间质性改变、血管性异常、占位、胸腔积液和胸膜增厚、空洞性病变、心脏增大、气道结构异常及椎体或肋骨骨折。除了后前位和侧位胸片以外，常使用侧卧位胸片来判断是否存在胸腔积液。侧卧位胸片对于肋膈角变钝的判断十分有意义，可以鉴别其是由游离的胸腔积液还是胸膜增厚引起的。胸片联合完整的病史和体格检查，能够辅助临床医生在许多情况下诊断胸部疾病。

X 线透视检查

胸部 X 线透视检查对于评估膈肌运动情况十分有用。该技术对诊断单侧膈肌麻痹尤其有价值。当嘱患者吸气或用力用鼻吸气时，麻痹的患侧膈肌会出现矛盾运动。然而，在评估双侧膈肌麻痹时，X 线透视检查的作用有限。双侧膈肌麻痹的患者在吸气时会因为呼吸补偿机制使得膈肌表现为向腹部运动，导致假阴性结果。而在高达 6% 的正常人群中可以观察到 Sniff 动作（通过鼻子进行用力最快吸气）时单侧膈肌矛盾运动，出现假阳性结果。

超声检查

床旁即时超声（POCUS）能够对重要器官进行更有针对性的评估和图像呈现，有助于诊断和管理多种疾病，提高了临床照护水平。在超声中，频率在 3 ～ 10 MHz 的声波可以被人体内组织反射，使肝、肾、心脏等内脏显像。充满气体的肺脏无法直接成像，但在过去的十年中，随着对超声波穿过正常及异常肺组织所产生的各种伪像（artifact）的理解，肺部超声成像的应用越来越多，尤其是在重症监护病房。已经形成了将超声用于检测肺实变、肺水肿及容量反应性的实施方案。并且

edema with sensitivity and specificity similar to those of a chest radiograph (Fig. 4.24).

In addition to its diagnostic capabilities, ultrasound is routinely used in real time to direct invasive procedures, such as thoracentesis, pericardiocentesis, and placement of a pleural, central venous, or arterial catheter. Other applications of pulmonary ultrasound include assessment of volume status by imaging inferior vena cava collapsibility with respiration and assessment of right ventricular function. Two-dimensional B-mode ultrasound imaging of the diaphragm can be used to visualize diaphragm function during inspiration. Failure of the diaphragm to thicken by a minimum of 35% during inspiration when visualized from the infraaxillary view is indicative of diaphragm weakness.

Ultrasonography is noninvasive, rapidly and easily applied, relatively low-cost, readily portable to the bedside, and because it does not use radiation, safe for repeated use on a patient.

Computed Tomography

CT has many applications in pulmonary medicine and provides more detailed information about lung structure than chest radiography. With the use of this technique, cross sections of the entire thorax can be obtained, usually at 2- to 5-mm intervals. CT scanning allows visualization of airways up to the seventh generation and delineation of parenchymal anatomy, texture, and density. Image contrast can be adjusted to optimize visualization of the lung parenchyma, pleura, and

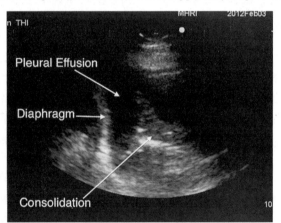

Fig. 4.24 Ultrasound image of the lung depicts the diaphragm, a pleural effusion, and an infiltrate.

mediastinal structures. The use of intravenous contrast material as part of the examination permits separation of vascular from nonvascular mediastinal structures. CT scans provide tremendous anatomic resolution when compared with chest radiography, but they expose the subject to about 70 times the radiation of a routine chest radiograph.

CT of the chest helps characterize pulmonary nodules and masses, distinguish between pleural thickening and pleural fluid, estimate the size of the heart and the presence of pericardial fluid, identify patterns of involvement of interstitial lung disease, detect cavities, and identify intracavitary processes such as mycetoma. It is also used to quantify the extent and distribution of emphysema, detect and measure mediastinal adenopathy for evaluating inflammatory diseases that involve mediastinal lymph nodes (e.g., sarcoidosis) and staging of lung cancer, and identify vascular invasion by neoplasm (Fig. 4.25). Newer generations of CT scanners are able to use multiple x-ray beams to create between 4 and 256 images simultaneously at a much faster rate (<10 seconds) than with the older models, which used only a single x-ray beam and detector. CT scans using much lower radiation doses are routinely advocated on a yearly basis for the early detection of lung cancer in older, high-risk smokers.

CT angiography allows for construction of three-dimensional images of the pulmonary vascular system. This imaging technique has emerged as the procedure of choice for identifying pulmonary embolism, supplanting pulmonary ventilation-perfusion scintigraphic lung scanning. The technique is used to identify pulmonary vascular abnormalities such as aortic dissection, pulmonary venous malformations, and aortic aneurysms. Additionally, three-dimensional construction of the airway and pulmonary parenchyma using CT images and specialized software has provided a means to electromagnetically guide a biopsy catheter through a bronchoscope (electromagnetic navigation bronchoscopy) to a distal pulmonary nodule or mass for biopsy. It could also be used to place a fiducial marker at the exact location of a lung cancer to accurately focus surgical or radiotherapy treatment.

Dynamic contrast-enhanced CT with single- or multi-detector scanner has been investigated as a modality to differentiate between a malignant and benign pulmonary nodule. First, baseline images are obtained using CT without contract enhancement. Subsequently, contrast is given over time while series of CT images are acquired. The difference time and contrast enhancement allow for evaluation of vascularity and blood flow patterns. Studies have confirmed high accuracy for differentiation.

High-resolution CT is a technique that generates thin (1-mm) anatomic slices to provide a high-contrast image of the pulmonary

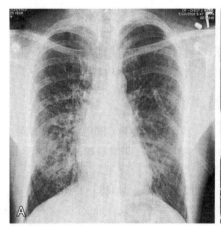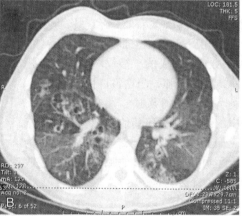

Fig. 4.25 Chest radiograph (A) and chest computed tomographic (CT) scan (B) of a patient with severe bronchiectasis. The abnormally dilated airways are better appreciated on the CT scan.

超声检查可以快速可靠地发现气胸、胸腔积液、实变及肺水肿，其灵敏性和特异性与胸片相近（图 4.24）。

除了其诊断价值，超声还被常规用于侵入性操作的实时引导，如胸腔穿刺、心包穿刺及胸腔置管、中心静脉或动脉导管置管。肺部超声的其他应用包括显示下腔静脉随呼吸塌陷率来评估容量状态、评估右心室功能。B 型二维超声成像能够可视化评估吸气时膈肌的收缩功能。从腋下角度观察吸气中膈肌收缩，若膈肌厚度增加不足 35% 提示膈肌无力。

超声成像无创、快速、易于操作、相对价廉，便于床旁检查；且因为超声检查没有辐射，可以安全地反复应用于同一患者。

计算机断层成像

计算机断层成像（CT）在呼吸病学中应用广泛，它提供了比胸部 X 线检查更详细的肺部结构信息。利用这种技术，可以获得整个胸部的横截面图像，层间距通常为 2 mm 到 5 mm。CT 扫描可以显示到第 7 级气道，展示肺实质的组织结构、纹理及密度。通过调整图像对比度可以更清晰地显示肺实质、胸膜及纵隔结

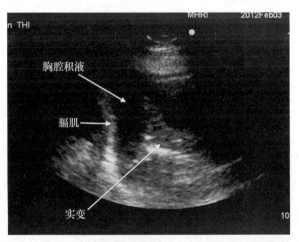

图 4.24　肺部超声图像显示了膈肌、胸腔积液和肺部浸润影

构。静脉注射造影剂后进行检查，能够区别纵隔内的血管与非血管结构。与胸部 X 线检查相比较，CT 扫描可以明显提高解剖分辨率，然而其辐射剂量约为常规胸部 X 线检查的 70 倍。

胸部 CT 有助于显示肺结节和肿块的特点，鉴别胸膜增厚和胸腔积液，估测心脏大小，判断有无心包积液，区分间质性肺疾病的受累模式，显示空洞及空洞内的病变（如真菌球）；还可用于量化评估肺气肿的程度和分布情况，显示并测量肿大的纵隔淋巴结用以评估累及纵隔淋巴结的炎症性疾病（如结节病）和进行肺癌分期，识别肿瘤是否侵犯血管（图 4.25）。新一代的 CT 扫描仪能够使用多个 X 线束，同时产生 4 ～ 256 个图像，比单一 X 线束及单一探测器的旧型 CT 扫描更快（< 10 s）。对于年龄较大的高危吸烟者，常规推荐年度低剂量 CT 检查，以早期发现肺癌。

CT 血管成像（CT 血管造影）可用于重建肺血管系统的三维成像。这种成像技术已经取代了肺通气-灌注闪烁显像扫描，成为诊断肺栓塞的首选检查手段。该技术还可用于显示有无胸部血管异常，如主动脉夹层、肺静脉畸形和主动脉瘤。此外，利用 CT 图像及专业软件对气道及肺实质进行三维重建，可经电磁引导活检导管通过支气管镜（电磁导航支气管镜）对远端肺结节或肿物进行活检。该技术还可以用于肺癌病灶的准确定位基准标记，以指导精确的外科切除或放射治疗。

单探测器或多探测器的动态增强 CT 扫描已被探索性应用于良恶性肺部结节的鉴别。首先采集平扫 CT 图像，之后注射造影剂，并在不同时间连续采集一系列的 CT 图像。病变强化程度随时间的变化可用于评估血管分布情况及血流模式。已有研究证实该方法鉴别良恶性肺结节具有高准确性。

高分辨率 CT 是一种可以生成薄层（1 mm）解剖切面图像的扫描技术，可以提供高对比度的肺实质显像。高分辨率 CT 采用特殊的重建算法，通过锐化软组

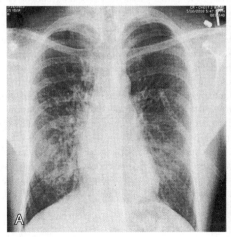
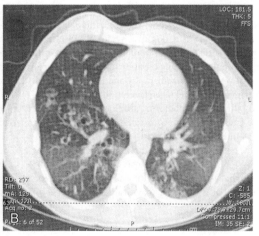

图 4.25　一位严重支气管扩张症患者的胸部 X 线检查（**A**）和胸部计算机断层成像（CT）检查（**B**）图像。异常扩张的支气管在 CT 扫描中显示得更清楚

parenchyma. With high-resolution CT, a special reconstruction algorithm sharpens the soft tissue interfaces to provide superior visualization of the pulmonary parenchyma. This technique is used primarily to identify interstitial lung disease and bronchiectasis. It is extremely useful for identifying interstitial lung disease that may not be apparent on a plain chest radiograph, and it has supplanted bronchography in the diagnosis of bronchiectasis.

Magnetic Resonance Imaging

MRI is a tomographic technique that uses radio waves modified by a strong magnetic field to produce an image resulting from the resonation of protons in tissue water. The chief advantage of MRI is that it does not entail the use of ionizing radiation. The ability of MRI to image pulmonary parenchyma is limited because of the low proton density in air-filled regions of the lung, which therefore cannot generate MRI images, artifacts arising from multiple air-tissue interfaces, and respiratory motion artifacts. However, vascular structures and pulmonary perfusion are well imaged by MRI, especially with the use of intravenous contrast agents such as gadolinium chelates. Therefore, MRI is very useful in the study of aortic dissection and may have a role in the evaluation of pulmonary emboli and chronic thromboembolic pulmonary hypertension. Three-directional velocity-encoded MRI allows three-dimensional, time-resolved cine reconstruction of blood flow patterns and pressures and is used in cardiac imaging. It may also have a role in the measurement of pulmonary blood flow. Infiltrative pulmonary diseases and pulmonary edema increase proton density in the lung, allowing better definition by MRI of honeycombing in pulmonary fibrosis and pulmonary edema in acute respiratory distress syndrome (ARDS). The use of inhaled hyperpolarized inert gases such as helium-3 or xenon-129 offers the ability to quantify peripheral airspace size, measure gas flow in lobar and segmental bronchi, and detect regional differences in ventilation. Ongoing studies are being completed to establish its utility. It has promising applications in the evaluation of emphysema and asthma and after lung transplantation, including assessment of bronchodilator responsiveness. In particular, MRI is very useful in delineating extension of malignant pleural mesothelioma to adjacent chest wall tissue or diaphragm, where it is much superior to CT imaging because of superior contrast resolution.

Pulmonary Angiography

Pulmonary angiography entails placement of a catheter in the pulmonary artery, followed by rapid injection of a contrast agent. In the past, this was "gold standard" for diagnosis of pulmonary thromboembolic disease. Pulmonary angiography still can be useful for detection of congenital abnormalities of the pulmonary vascular tree, but CT and MRI have largely supplanted it.

Pulmonary Ventilation-Perfusion Scanning

Ventilation-perfusion ($\dot{V}/\dot{Q}$) scintigraphy utilizes radiopharmaceuticals such as technetium-99m as a noninvasive means to evaluate regional blood flow and ventilation. Therefore, it has been used in the past as an alternative to pulmonary angiography to detect pulmonary embolism. With the advent of CT angiography and its improvements over the years, $\dot{V}/\dot{Q}$ imaging is no longer favored for the initial evaluation of suspected pulmonary embolism. Additionally, alteration of regional blood flow (pulmonary vasoconstriction and shunt) due to lung diseases such as pneumonia or interstitial lung disease limits its diagnostic accuracy. The PIOPED study in 1990 investigated the diagnostic accuracy of a $\dot{V}/\dot{Q}$ scan for the diagnosis of pulmonary embolism. The study found that a $\dot{V}/\dot{Q}$ scan is useful when the clinical pretest probability is high but that it has poor diagnostic accuracy. Despite

its limitations, $\dot{V}/\dot{Q}$ scan still has utility in certain clinical scenarios. These scenarios include patients who have abnormal renal function, patients who are allergic to CT contrast, and patients with suspected chronic thromboembolic pulmonary hypertension (higher sensitivity compared to CT angiography). Quantitative lung perfusion scanning is also very useful preoperatively to assess the predicted postoperative lung function remaining after planned lobectomy or pneumonectomy. Therefore, it is used by thoracic surgeons to evaluate a patient's suitability for undergoing lobectomy or pneumonectomy for curative resection of lung cancer.

Positron Emission Tomography

Positron emission tomography (PET) detects metabolically active pulmonary nodules greater than 0.8 cm in diameter. It is helpful in assessing whether a nodule is benign or malignant. However, it does not distinguish between inflammation and malignancy. Therefore, assessment of multiple pulmonary nodules by PET is limited because of false-positive findings due to active granulomatous disease, such as previous exposure to tuberculosis, sarcoidosis, or fungal infestation; or to active infection, such as bacterial or viral pneumonia, bronchiolitis, or aspiration.

Dual-modality integrated PET-CT combines morphologic and functional imaging. The combination of PET and CT is helpful for localizing solitary metastatic lymph nodes in the hila and extrapulmonary locations, allowing better staging of lung cancer. In addition, PET-CT is helpful in planning radiation therapy for patients who have lung cancer associated with atelectasis.

Bronchoscopy

Fiberoptic bronchoscopy is used for diagnostic or therapeutic indications. It is most commonly performed to directly visualize the nasopharynx, larynx, vocal cords, and proximal tracheobronchial tree for diagnostic purposes. The procedure is performed by sedating the patient and providing local anesthesia with inhaled and instilled lidocaine. The bronchial mucosa is assessed for endobronchial masses, mucosal integrity, extrinsic compression, dynamic compression, and hemorrhage. The bronchoscope is equipped with a channel for passing a variety of instruments including biopsy forceps for sampling endobronchial lesions or lung tissue (transbronchial biopsy), and fine 19- to 22-gauge needles for transbronchial aspiration biopsy from lymph nodes or lung masses. Saline also can be instilled through the channel for bronchial washings or bronchoalveolar lavage. Bronchial washings and bronchoalveolar lavage can be analyzed for cytology, culture, and special stains. A bronchial brush is used to scrape the bronchial mucosa and harvest cells for cytology. Bronchoscopes can also be adapted with a terminal ultrasound probe to provide ultrasound images of the airways and neighboring tissues. This technique, called endobronchial ultrasound (EBUS) uses high acoustic frequencies, in the range of 20 MHz, to provide high-resolution images of proximal tissue and provides accurate positional guidance for needle aspiration of mediastinal lymph nodes. It is now routinely used to detect lung cancer metastasis to mediastinal lymph nodes and for the diagnosis of granulomatous disorders of the lymph nodes. A different radial ultrasound probe inserted through the working channel of a bronchoscope can facilitate confirmation of the position of a transbronchial biopsy forceps near a lung mass during transbronchial biopsy of a lesion in the periphery of the lung parenchyma. A newer technique called transbronchial lung cryobiopsy (TBLC) uses a probe that traverses the working channel of a bronchoscope into the periphery of the lung near the chest wall. The probe is rapidly cooled to freeze the adjacent lung tissue, which adheres to the probe and is fractured off, resulting in biopsy specimens that are larger and less susceptible to the crush artifact noted on routine

织界面以优化肺实质显像。这种技术主要用于间质性肺疾病和支气管扩张症的识别，尤其是普通胸片难以显示的间质性肺疾病。该方法已取代了支气管碘油造影，成为诊断支气管扩张症的主要手段。

磁共振成像

磁共振成像（MRI）是利用组织水中的氢质子在强磁场中共振产生的信号波而生成图像的一种断层成像技术。MRI 的主要优点是没有电离辐射。由于充气的肺内氢质子密度低，无法产生 MRI 图像，空气-组织界面会产生大量伪像，且呼吸运动也会引起伪像，因而限制了 MRI 对肺实质的显像。然而，MRI 可清晰显示血管结构和肺灌注，尤其是在使用静脉造影剂如钆螯合物时。因此，MRI 在主动脉夹层的评估中非常有用，并且在肺栓塞和慢性血栓栓塞性肺动脉高压的评估中也能发挥相应作用。三维速度编码的 MRI 可以对血流模式和压力进行三维动态重建，因而可被用于心脏成像。该方法可能也可以用于肺血流的测量。浸润性肺疾病和肺水肿增加了肺内的氢质子密度，因此 MRI 可以更好地显示肺纤维化中的蜂窝影及急性呼吸窘迫综合征（ARDS）中的肺水肿。吸入超极化的惰性气体如氦-3 或氙-129 可以量化评估周边气腔大小，测量肺叶和肺段的气流量，评估不同部位的通气差异。该方法的临床实用性研究即将完成。吸入超极化惰性气体 MRI 成像在肺气肿、哮喘及肺移植术后的评估中具有广泛的应用前景，例如评估支气管扩张剂的反应性。此外，由于 MRI 的软组织对比分辨率明显高于 CT 成像，MRI 特别适用于勾画恶性胸膜间皮瘤对邻近胸壁组织或膈肌的侵袭范围。

肺血管造影

肺血管造影需要在肺动脉内放置导管，随后快速注射造影剂进行显影。在过去，这是诊断肺血栓栓塞性疾病的"金标准"。目前，肺血管造影仍然可用于发现肺血管树的先天性异常，但 CT 和 MRI 已在很大程度上将其取代。

肺通气-灌注扫描

通气-灌注（V̇/Q̇）闪烁显像是一种利用放射性药物如锝-99m 显像而评估区域性血流和通气情况的无创检查方法。因此，该方法曾在肺栓塞的诊断中被作为肺血管造影的替代手段。随着 CT 血管成像的出现及近年来的逐步优化，V̇/Q̇ 显像不再是疑诊肺栓塞时的首选评估手段。此外，肺炎或间质性肺疾病等肺病产生的区域性血流改变（肺血管收缩及分流）也限制了它的诊断准确性。1990 年发表的 PIOPED（Prospective Investigation of Pulmonary Embolism Diagnosis）研究探索了 V̇/Q̇ 扫描诊断肺栓塞的准确性。该研究发现，在肺栓塞的临床验前概率较高时，V̇/Q̇ 扫描价值较大，但其诊断准确性较差。尽管存在相应的局限性，V̇/Q̇ 扫描依然在特定临床情境中具有应用价值，如肾功能异常的患者、CT 造影剂过敏的患者及疑诊慢性血栓栓塞性肺动脉高压的患者（敏感性高于 CT 血管成像）。定量肺灌注扫描对于计划行肺叶切除或单侧全肺切除术的患者进行术前评估、估计术后肺功能保留情况也非常有用。因此，胸外科医生可使用该方法评估拟行肺癌根治性切除术的患者是否适合肺叶切除或单侧全肺切除术。

正电子发射断层成像

正电子发射断层成像（PET）可以检测直径大于 0.8 cm、有代谢活性的肺结节，有助于评估肺结节的良恶性。然而，PET 无法区分炎症和恶性肿瘤。由于活动性肉芽肿性疾病（如既往结核暴露、结节病或真菌感染）或活动性感染（如细菌性或病毒性肺炎、支气管炎或误吸）均可能出现假阳性结果，因此 PET 在肺部多发结节的评估中作用有限。

PET-CT 双模显像结合了形态和功能显像。PET 和 CT 的结合有助于肺门及肺外实性转移淋巴结的定位，以便对肺癌更精确地分期。此外，PET-CT 也能辅助对合并肺不张的肺癌患者制订放疗方案。

支气管镜检查

纤维支气管镜检查可用于诊断或治疗，最常用于直接观察鼻咽、喉、声带和近端气管支气管树以辅助诊断。操作过程中需要患者镇静，并使用吸入和局部滴注的利多卡因进行局部麻醉。检查中评估支气管黏膜是否存在支气管内肿物、黏膜完整性、有无外压性改变、动态压迫和出血。支气管镜配有通道可通过各种工具，包括用活检钳对支气管腔内病变或肺组织进行取样（经支气管活检），以及使用 19 至 22 号细针对淋巴结或肺肿物经支气管穿刺针吸活检。还可以通过该通道注射生理盐水，进行支气管冲洗或支气管肺泡灌洗，回收的液体可进行细胞学检查、培养和特殊染色分析。支气管毛刷可用于刮取支气管黏膜并采集细胞进行细胞学检查。支气管镜还可以配合末端超声探头，而对气道和邻近组织进行超声显像。这种技术被称为经支气管镜腔内超声（EBUS），它使用 20 MHz 范围内的高频声波，可提供邻近组织的高分辨率图像，为纵隔淋巴结的针吸穿刺提供精确的定位指导。该技术已被常规用于检测肺癌纵隔淋巴结转移情况，以及诊断淋巴结的肉芽肿性疾病。在对肺实质外周病变进行经支气管活检时，可以通过支气管镜的工作通道插入另一种径向超声探头，以辅助定位和确认活检钳到达肺肿物附近。一种被称为经支气管肺冷冻活检（TBLC）的新技术，探头通过支气管镜的工作通道进入邻近胸壁的肺外周区域，使用快速冷却的探头冷冻相邻的肺组织，这些肺组织黏附在探头上并被整体拔出，从而获得较大的活检标本，而且这些标

forceps biopsies. This technique, though often complicated by serious hemorrhage, is in use for the diagnosis of interstitial lung disease with the hope that it will obviate the need for surgical biopsy.

Common therapeutic indications for bronchoscopy include retrieval of foreign bodies, suctioning of secretions, reexpansion of atelectatic lung by removing obstruction, detection and localization of hemoptysis, and assistance with difficult endotracheal intubations. In special centers, bronchoscopy is used to perform yttrium aluminum garnet (YAG) laser therapy, argon plasma coagulation therapy, and cryotherapy for endobronchial lesions. It is also used to guide placement of catheters for brachytherapy in lung cancer or guide placement of stents. Lasers produce a beam of light that can induce tissue vaporization, coagulation, and necrosis. Argon plasma coagulation therapy uses heat from ionized argon gas to debulk the tumor while simultaneously coagulating to stop bleeding. Cryotherapy probes induce tissue necrosis through hypothermic cellular crystallization and microthrombosis. Cryotherapy and electrocautery have been used to treat and relieve airway obstruction caused by benign tracheal bronchial tumors, polyps, and granulation tissue. The goal of endobronchial brachytherapy is to relieve airway obstruction from central tumors. This is typically used as an adjunct to conventional external-beam irradiation. Tracheobronchial stenting can be performed to manage airway compression associated with malignant tumors, tracheoesophageal fistulas, or tracheobronchomalacia. Bronchoscopy is generally a safe procedure with major complications, including significant bleeding, pneumothorax, and respiratory failure, occurring in 0.1% to 1.7% of patients.

PROSPECTUS FOR THE FUTURE

Continued refinement and evolution of techniques and methods currently used to assess pulmonary structure and function will enhance the ability to diagnose and treat individuals with lung disease. Although pulmonary function testing has been performed for decades, advances in equipment design and better standardization of methods will improve accuracy and reproducibility. Further development of noninvasive techniques used to measure changes in lung volume from body surface displacements may allow for assessment of pulmonary function in settings outside the pulmonary function laboratory. Analysis of exhaled gas for biomarkers has tremendous potential for early diagnosis of many lung diseases, especially cancer.

Great strides in assessing lung structure will evolve from advances in CT, PET, and MRI technology. CT volume-rendering techniques will provide images of the central airways, enabling "virtual bronchoscopy." This technique will be useful to guide biopsy site selection in conventional bronchoscopy and to allow visualization of airways distal to an endobronchial obstruction. Volumetric measurements of pulmonary nodules using CT segmentation techniques will allow more accurate calculation of nodule volume and better assessment of tumor doubling times. This, in concert with PET-CT, may provide more accurate means of determining the malignant potential of a solitary pulmonary nodule. Also, dynamic contrast-enhanced CT may help with differentiating between malignant and benign pulmonary nodules that would further improve the lung cancer screening process.

MRI may evolve into the preferred method for evaluating pulmonary emboli, mediastinal disease, and regional ventilation-perfusion matching. Velocity-encoded MRI is a promising modality for assessment of pulmonary vascular blood flow and pressures and may prove to be more accurate than current noninvasive methods. Lymph node–specific magnetic resonance contrast agents and the development of PET molecular tracers targeting tumor proteins and receptors may better differentiate enlarged lymph nodes caused by hyperplasia from those due to neoplasia. Finally, new insights into the function of the respiratory control centers in the cortex and brain stem may be attained from the use of functional MRI studies of the brain.

SUGGESTED READINGS

McCool FD, Hoppin FG Jr: Respiratory mechanics. In Baum GL, editor: Textbook of pulmonary diseases, Philadelphia, 1998, Lippincott-Raven, pp 117-130.

McCool FD, Tzelepis GE: Current clinical aspects of diaphragm dysfunction, N Engl J Med 366:932-942, 2012.

Miller WT: Radiographic evaluation of the chest. In Fishman AP, editor: Fishman's pulmonary diseases and disorders, New York, 2008, McGraw-Hill, pp 455-510.

Pellegrino R, Viegi G, Brusasco V, et al: Interpretative strategies for lung function tests, Eur Respir J 26:948-968, 2005.

Wagner PD: Ventilation, pulmonary blood flow, and ventilation-perfusion relationships. In Fishman AP, editor: Fishman's pulmonary diseases and disorders, New York, 2008, McGraw-Hill, pp 173-189.

Weibel ER: It takes more than cells to make a good lung, Am J Respir Crit Care Med 187:342-346, 2013.

West JB: Respiratory physiology: the essentials, ed 5, Baltimore, 1995, Williams & Wilkins.

West JB, Wagner PD: Pulmonary gas exchange, Am J Respir Crit Care Med 157:S82-S87, 1988.

本并不易受到常规钳夹活检中存在的挤压伪影的影响。尽管这种技术常常因严重出血而复杂化，但它用于诊断间质性肺疾病以期能够避免外科活检的需要。

支气管镜下治疗的常见适应证包括异物取出、分泌物吸引、通过去除阻塞物使肺复张、发现和定位咯血，以及辅助困难气道的气管插管。在某些医疗中心，支气管镜还可用于钇铝石榴石（yttrium aluminum garnet，YAG）激光治疗、氩气等离子凝固治疗和支气管内病变的冷冻治疗。其还可用于引导放置肺癌近距离放疗的导管或支架置入。激光产生的光束可引起组织汽化、凝固和坏死。氩气等离子凝固治疗利用电离氩气产生的热量消融肿瘤，同时凝固止血。冷冻治疗探头通过低温细胞结晶和微血栓形成引起组织坏死。冷冻治疗和电灼术已被用于治疗和缓解由良性气管支气管肿瘤、息肉和肉芽组织引起的气道阻塞。支气管内近距离放疗的目标是缓解中央性肿瘤引起的气道阻塞，通常作为常规外照射放疗的辅助手段。气管支气管支架置入可用于治疗与恶性肿瘤相关的气道受压、气管食管瘘或气管支气管软化症。支气管镜检查通常是安全的，但会有一些严重并发症，包括大出血、气胸和呼吸衰竭，发生率为 0.1% ～ 1.7%。

未来展望

随着评估肺部结构和功能的技术和方法的持续优化和演变，肺病的诊断和治疗能力将继续增强。虽然肺功能检查的历史已经长达几十年，但设备的进步、检查方法的进一步标准化将提高结果的准确性和可重复性。随着测量肺容积的无创技术的进步，在肺功能实验室外也能够进行肺功能评估。呼出气生物标志物分析对于多种肺病（尤其是肺癌）的早期诊断具有巨大潜力。

在 CT、PET 和 MRI 技术的推动下，肺结构评估将取得巨大进步。CT 容积重建技术可以提供主气道的图像，从而实现"虚拟支气管镜检查"。这项技术将有助于指导传统支气管镜检查选择合适的活检部位，实现支气管内阻塞远端气道的可视化。在肺结节的体积测量方面，使用 CT 图像分割技术将有助于更精确地计算结节的体积、更好地评估肿瘤倍增时间。这一技术联合 PET-CT 将会有助于更精确地评估孤立性肺结节的恶性可能性。此外，动态增强 CT 可能有助于鉴别良恶性结节，这将进一步改善肺癌筛查的流程。

MRI 有可能会成为评估肺栓塞、纵隔疾病、区域性通气-灌注匹配程度的首选检查方法。速度编码 MRI 是一种评估肺血管血流和压力的方法，其应用前景良好，可能比目前的无创手段更准确。淋巴结特异的磁共振造影剂和以肿瘤蛋白和受体为靶点的 PET 分子示踪剂的发展，将有助于更好地区分由增生或肿瘤导致的淋巴结肿大。最后，大脑的功能 MRI 检查的应用可能有助于理解大脑皮质和脑干内的呼吸中枢的功能。

推荐阅读

McCool FD, Hoppin FG Jr: Respiratory mechanics. In Baum GL, editor: Textbook of pulmonary diseases, Philadelphia, 1998, Lippincott-Raven, pp 117-130.

McCool FD, Tzelepis GE: Current clinical aspects of diaphragm dysfunction, N Engl J Med 366:932-942, 2012.

Miller WT: Radiographic evaluation of the chest. In Fishman AP, editor: Fishman's pulmonary diseases and disorders, New York, 2008, McGraw-Hill, pp 455-510.

Pellegrino R, Viegi G, Brusasco V, et al: Interpretative strategies for lung function tests, Eur Respir J 26:948-968, 2005.

Wagner PD: Ventilation, pulmonary blood flow, and ventilation-perfusion relationships. In Fishman AP, editor: Fishman's pulmonary diseases and disorders, New York, 2008, McGraw-Hill, pp 173-189.

Weibel ER: It takes more than cells to make a good lung, Am J Respir Crit Care Med 187:342-346, 2013.

West JB: Respiratory physiology: the essentials, ed 5, Baltimore, 1995, Williams & Wilkins.

West JB, Wagner PD: Pulmonary gas exchange, Am J Respir Crit Care Med 157:S82-S87, 1988.

Obstructive Lung Diseases

Zoe G.S. Vazquez, Matthew D. Jankowich, Debasree Banerjee

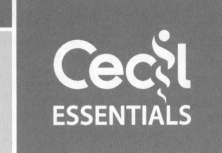

INTRODUCTION

The obstructive lung diseases are a group of pulmonary disorders that result in dyspnea characterized by an obstructive pattern of expiratory airflow limitation on spirometry. These disorders include chronic obstructive pulmonary disease (COPD), asthma, cystic fibrosis (CF), bronchiectasis, and bronchiolar disorders. In some cases, these disorders overlap clinically (Fig. 5.1), sharing several features aside from the presence of expiratory airflow limitation. These features may include symptoms of wheezing and sputum production, chronic airway-centered inflammation, presence of airway structural changes resulting in remodeling of the airways, and episodic periods of temporarily worsened clinical status, known as exacerbations. However, the causes, locations, and patterns of airway inflammatory changes and remodeling, as well as the treatments, prognoses, and natural histories, are often significantly different, making clinical distinction among these disorders important.

COPD is characterized by abnormal airway inflammation and lung structure in response to an inhaled irritant (typically cigarette smoke), resulting in irreversible or incompletely reversible airflow limitation that is typically progressive over time. *Asthma* is distinguished from COPD by characteristic smooth muscle hyperreactivity and reversible airflow limitation, by its variable clinical course, and by its frequent association with atopy. These disorders are epidemic in the general population worldwide and account for a significant proportion of the morbidity and mortality associated with the obstructive lung diseases. *Bronchiectasis* is a permanent abnormal dilation of the bronchi that results in chronic cough, purulent sputum production, and hemoptysis. Bronchiectasis is caused by diverse conditions including CF, a genetic disorder resulting from mutations in the *CFTR* gene. The *bronchiolar disorders*, also called *small airways disorders*, result from inflammation and/or fibrosis of the small airways of the lung that leads to dyspnea. They may be difficult to diagnose because loss or obstruction of a majority of the small airways must occur before the appearance of expiratory airflow limitation on spirometry.

The basis for expiratory airflow obstruction varies among these disorders. The flow of air through the bronchial tree is directly proportional to the driving pressure and inversely proportional to the resistance. In obstructive lung disease, alterations in one or both of these processes may be present. Loss of lung elastic tissue, frequently present in COPD, results in decreased lung elastic recoil on expiration and therefore decreased driving pressure for expiratory airflow. By contrast, airflow limitation in asthma is primarily caused by smooth muscle contraction resulting in bronchoconstriction that increases airway resistance. Increases in airway resistance are also present in COPD and are related to small airway inflammation and fibrosis as well as small airway collapse due to decreased "tethering" of the airways in the setting of loss of surrounding lung elastic tissue. Mucus obstruction of airway lumens contributes to increased airway resistance in all the obstructive lung diseases.

Obstruction to airflow causes characteristic changes in lung volumes. The residual volume (RV) and functional residual capacity (FRC) are increased, whereas the total lung capacity (TLC) remains normal or is increased. Vital capacity, and particularly inspiratory capacity, is eventually reduced by the increase in RV. Several factors may contribute to the increase in FRC and RV in obstructive lung disease. Decreased lung elastic recoil in COPD increases the FRC because of reduced opposition to the outward force exerted by the chest wall. Loss of airway tone and decreased tethering by the surrounding lung in COPD, as well as bronchoconstriction and mucus plugging in acute asthma, allow airways to collapse at higher lung volumes and trap excessive air. Finally, under demands for increased minute ventilation (e.g., during exercise), the increased resistance to airflow may not allow the lungs to empty completely in the time available for expiration; this leads to so-called dynamic hyperinflation of the lungs as the volume of trapped air progressively increases while the inspiratory capacity is progressively limited. This phenomenon contributes to symptoms of chest tightness and dyspnea during exercise and results in exercise limitation, especially in COPD.

Fig. 5.1 Classification of obstructive lung diseases. Although most patients with chronic obstructive pulmonary disease (COPD) have small airways disease, the bronchiolar disorders do not overlap with COPD. *CF*, Cystic fibrosis.

阻塞性肺疾病

曲木诗玮 译　代华平 审校　王辰 通审

引言

　　阻塞性肺疾病是一类导致呼吸困难的肺病，以呼气相气流阻塞为共同特征，包括慢性阻塞性肺疾病（慢阻肺病，COPD）、哮喘、囊性纤维化（CF）、支气管扩张症、细支气管疾病。上述疾病时有重叠（图5.1），除了呼气相气流阻塞，它们还具备以下共同点：喘息、咳痰，以气道为中心的慢性炎症、气道结构破坏及气道重塑，间断发作的临床状态恶化（又称为急性加重）。尽管如此，这些疾病在病因、病变部位、气道炎症与重塑特点、治疗、预后、自然转归这些方面又有显著不同，故而临床鉴别尤为重要。

　　慢阻肺病的主要特点为吸入性刺激物（如吸烟）所致气道炎症、肺结构异常，引起不可逆或不完全可逆的进行性加重的气流受限。支气管哮喘与慢阻肺病的不同之处在于平滑肌的高反应性与可逆性气流受限，病程中呈现多变性，且常与特应性有关。上述两

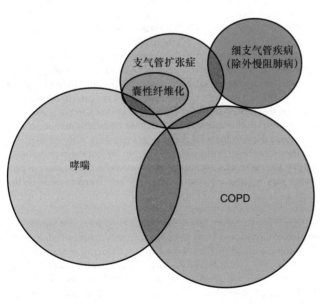

图5.1　阻塞性肺疾病分类。尽管多数慢性阻塞性肺疾病（COPD）患者常具有小气道病变（small airway disease），但慢阻肺病与细支气管疾病没有重叠

种疾病在世界范围总人群中十分流行，是阻塞性肺疾病相关患病率及死亡率的重要原因。支气管扩张症则是一种引起慢性咳嗽、咳痰、咯血症状的支气管永久性异常扩张。支气管扩张症是由多种疾病引起的，包括囊性纤维化，一种由CFTR基因突变引起的遗传性疾病。细支气管疾病，又称小气道疾病（small airway disorder），以小气道炎症和（或）纤维化，进而导致呼吸困难为特征。小气道疾病不易诊断，因为当患者测定肺通气功能出现呼气相气流受限时，绝大多数小气道已经丢失或发生阻塞。

　　在上述疾病中，呼气相气流阻塞的原因各不相同。支气管树内的气流与驱动压成正比，与气道阻力成反比。阻塞性肺疾病涉及上述1个或2个过程的改变。肺弹性组织的丧失（常见于慢阻肺病）导致呼气时肺弹性回缩力减小，从而降低呼气气流的驱动压力。相反，哮喘的气流受限主要源于平滑肌收缩导致的支气管痉挛，增加气道阻力。慢阻肺病中也存在气道阻力增加，相关因素包括小气道炎症、小气道纤维化、肺弹性组织丢失无法持续牵拉小气道从而导致小气道塌陷。在各种阻塞性肺疾病中，管腔内黏液阻塞均会导致气道阻力增加。

　　气流受阻会导致肺容积的特征性变化。残气量（RV）和功能残气量（FRC）增加，而肺总量（TLC）保持正常或增加。肺活量（VC），尤其是吸气量（IC），最终会随着残气量增加而降低。几种因素可能导致阻塞性肺疾病中FRC和RV的增加。慢阻肺病患者肺弹性回缩力降低，减轻了抵抗胸壁对肺所施加的外向牵拉力的程度，FRC增加。慢阻肺病患者气道张力丧失和周围肺组织牵拉作用减少，以及急性哮喘的支气管痉挛和黏液堵塞，均使得肺在较高容积下发生气道陷闭及气体潴留。最后，当每分通气量需求增加（如运动期间），气道阻力增加，肺难以在呼气时间内完全排空；上述因素引起了所谓的动态肺过度充气，即潴留的气体逐渐增加，吸气量逐渐减少。这一现象导致了活动后胸部紧缩感和呼吸困难症状，从而引发活动受限，以慢阻肺病尤甚。

TABLE 5.1   Features of Obstructive Lung Disease

Disorder	Clinical Features	Laboratory Findings
Chronic obstructive pulmonary disease	Chronic progressive dyspnea Cough, sputum production Periodic exacerbations	FEV_1/FVC <0.70 after bronchodilator use Often reduced D_{LCO}
Asthma	Episodic dyspnea, cough, and/or wheezing Nocturnal symptoms May have environmental trigger(s)	Variable airflow obstruction on spirometry Typically significant improvement in FEV_1 with bronchodilator use D_{LCO} normal or elevated Methacholine challenge shows airway hyperreactivity
Bronchiectasis	Chronic cough and purulent sputum production Hemoptysis	Chest radiograph: "tram track" shadows HRCT: dilated bronchi bigger than accompanying vessel, lack of tapering of bronchi, visible bronchi within 1-2 cm of lung border Sputum culture may grow *Haemophilus influenzae*, *Pseudomonas aeruginosa*, or atypical mycobacteria Laboratory evaluation may reveal specific etiology (e.g., decreased immunoglobulin levels in CVID)
Cystic fibrosis	Sinusitis, bronchiectasis, meconium ileus, malabsorption, infertility (in males, congenital absence of vas deferens)	Increased sweat chloride concentration, mutation in CFTR chloride channel, elevated fecal fat, abnormal nasal mucosal potential difference
Bronchiolar disorders	Progressive dyspnea Possible history of connective tissue disease, inflammatory bowel disease, lung transplantation, or hematopoietic stem cell transplantation	Fixed airflow obstruction on spirometry HRCT: mosaic attenuation pattern; centrilobular nodules; tree-in-bud opacities

CVID, Common variable immunodeficiency; *D_{LCO},* diffusing capacity for carbon monoxide; *FEV_1,* forced expiratory volume in 1 second; *FVC,* forced vital capacity; *HRCT,* high-resolution computed tomography.

There are two major consequences of the changes in lung volume in obstructive lung disease. First, breathing at higher lung volumes requires a higher change in pressure to achieve a smaller change in lung volume, and this requirement increases the work of breathing. Second, larger lung volumes place the inspiratory muscles at a mechanical disadvantage. The diaphragm is flattened, decreasing its ability to change intrathoracic volume, and all the inspiratory muscle fibers are shortened, decreasing the tension they are able to exert to effect changes in lung volume. The combination of a higher work of breathing and mechanical disadvantages of the respiratory muscles caused by lung hyperinflation can lead to respiratory muscle fatigue and failure in the setting of an abrupt worsening of airway obstruction, as during an acute exacerbation of COPD or asthma.

In addition to the clinical history and physical examination, spirometry is a key step in the diagnostic work-up for a patient with suspected obstructive lung disease. Although spirometry is readily available and inexpensive, it is often underutilized, and as a consequence, obstructive lung diseases are underdiagnosed. Assessment of the clinical and spirometric response to a bronchodilator is a simple and helpful step in distinguishing asthma from COPD. Measurement of the diffusing capacity of the lungs for carbon monoxide (D_{LCO}) can also be helpful in separating asthma, which is characterized by a normal or elevated diffusing capacity, from COPD in which the diffusing capacity is often reduced by loss of surface area for gas exchange. More sophisticated testing, such as high-resolution chest computed tomography (HRCT), may be needed to help diagnose less common causes of obstructive lung disease (e.g., bronchiectasis).

The clinical features and laboratory findings associated with the various obstructive lung disorders are summarized in Table 5.1.

CHRONIC OBSTRUCTIVE PULMONARY DISEASE

Definition and Epidemiology

The Global Initiative for Chronic Obstructive Lung Disease (GOLD) currently defines COPD as a common preventable and treatable disease characterized by persistent airflow limitation that is usually progressive and associated with an enhanced chronic inflammatory response in the airways and lungs to noxious particles and gases. The presence of airflow limitation is established by spirometry: If the ratio of the forced expired volume in 1 second (FEV_1) to the forced vital capacity (FVC) is less than 0.70 after administration of a bronchodilator, airway obstruction is indicated. Although in the past COPD was defined by the presence of either *emphysema* (a pathologic enlargement of the distal air spaces) or *chronic bronchitis* (a clinical syndrome characterized by the presence of cough and sputum production for at least 3 months in each of 2 consecutive years), the current definition is based on the presence of airflow limitation and not on the presence of these entities. Both emphysema and chronic bronchitis may occur with or without the simultaneous presence of expiratory airflow limitation, and therefore these entities overlap with but are not synonymous with COPD. The current definition of COPD highlights the presence of persistent, reproducible expiratory airflow limitation and emphasizes the progressive nature of COPD and the presence of abnormal inflammation in the lungs and airways.

COPD is a common disorder in populations across the world. The Burden of Obstructive Lung Disease study, in a sample of adults from 12 countries, found that 10.1% had at least moderate airway obstruction (FEV_1/FVC <0.70 and FEV_1 <80% predicted) after administration of a bronchodilator. Prevalence rates for COPD are correlated with increasing age, lower socioeconomic status, and smoking. Although COPD is more prevalent in men than in women, the prevalence of

表 5.1　阻塞性肺疾病的特点

疾病	临床特点	实验室检查特点
慢阻肺病	慢性进行性呼吸困难，咳嗽、咳痰，周期性加重	给予支气管扩张剂后 $FEV_1/FVC < 0.70$ D_{LCO} 通常降低
支气管哮喘	发作性呼吸困难、咳嗽和（或）喘息 夜间症状显著 可能有环境触发因素	肺通气功能检查提示可变气流阻塞 给予支气管扩张剂后 FEV_1 显著改善 D_{LCO} 正常或升高 乙酰甲胆碱激发试验提示气道高反应
支气管扩张症	慢性咳嗽、咳脓痰、咯血	胸部 X 线片："轨道征" HRCT：扩张的支气管直径大于伴随血管直径，支气管无逐渐变细，胸膜下 1～2 cm 范围内可见支气管 痰培养可生长流感嗜血杆菌、铜绿假单胞菌或非典型分枝杆菌 实验室检查可帮助查因（如 CVID 患者的免疫球蛋白水平下降）
囊性纤维化	鼻窦炎、支气管扩张症、胎粪性肠梗阻、吸收不良、不育症（男性先天性输精管缺失）	汗液氯化物浓度升高 CFTR 氯离子通道基因突变 粪便中脂肪增多 鼻黏膜电位差异常
细支气管疾病	进行性呼吸困难 可伴结缔组织病、炎症性肠病、肺移植病史或造血干细胞移植病史	肺通气功能检查提示固定气流受限 HRCT："马赛克"征；小叶中心结节；小树芽征

CFTR，囊性纤维化跨膜传导调节因子；CVID，普通变异型免疫缺陷；D_{LCO}，一氧化碳弥散功能；FEV_1，第 1 秒用力呼气容积；FVC，用力肺活量；HRCT，高分辨率计算机断层成像或高分辨率 CT。

　　阻塞性肺疾病的肺容积变化产生两种主要后果。首先，以较高的肺容积呼吸需要更高的压力变化才能实现较小的肺容积变化，而这种要求增加了呼吸功。其次，较高的肺容积使吸气肌处于机械劣势。膈肌低平，不利于其改变胸腔内容积，全体吸气肌纤维缩短，降低可施加的张力，不利于改变肺容积。肺过度充气引起的呼吸功增加和呼吸肌机械劣势相结合，在慢阻肺病急性加重、哮喘急性加重等气道阻塞突然恶化的情况下，可导致呼吸肌疲劳与呼吸衰竭。

　　除了病史和查体外，肺通气功能检查是疑似阻塞性肺疾病患者的诊断关键。尽管肺通气功能检查十分普及，并不昂贵，但常常没有被充分运用，导致阻塞性肺疾病诊断不足。区分哮喘和慢阻肺病可采用简单实用的临床评估、支气管舒张试验以及计算一氧化碳弥散量（D_{LCO}），哮喘患者弥散量正常或升高，而慢阻肺病患者弥散量往往因气体交换面积丢失而降低。有时需要用到高分辨率 CT（HRCT）等复杂检查，以诊断阻塞性肺疾病的相对少见病因（如支气管扩张症）。

　　表 5.1 总结了各种阻塞性肺疾病的临床特点和实验室检查。

慢性阻塞性肺疾病

定义和流行病学

　　慢性阻塞性肺疾病全球倡议（GOLD）目前将慢阻肺病定义为一种可防、可治的常见病，疾病特点是持续气流受限，常呈进行性加重，且与气道、肺对有毒颗粒、有毒气体的慢性炎症反应增强相关。通过肺通气功能检查明确是否存在气流受限：如果在支气管扩张剂给药后第 1 秒用力呼出气容积（FEV_1）与用力肺活量（FVC）之比小于 0.70，则提示气道阻塞。以前慢阻肺病的定义是存在肺气肿（远端气腔病理性增大）或慢性支气管炎（一种临床综合征，表现为连续 2 年中每年至少 3 个月出现咳嗽和咳痰），但当前定义已经不是基于上述两种疾病的存在，而是基于气流受限的存在。肺气肿和慢性支气管炎都可能同时伴或不伴呼气相气流受限，因此这两种疾病与慢阻肺病只是有所重叠，绝非同义词。目前慢阻肺病定义强调存在持续的、可重复验证的呼气相气流受限，进行性加重的自然病程，以及肺及气道的异常炎症。

　　慢阻肺病在世界各地人群中都属于常见病。阻塞性肺疾病负担研究（Burden of Obstructive Lung Disease study，又称 BOLD 研究）对来自 12 个国家的成年人进行抽样调查，发现 10.1% 的患者在给予支气管扩张剂后出现至少中等程度的气流阻塞 [$FEV_1/FVC < 0.70$ 且 $FEV_1 < 80\%$ 预计值（占预比 < 80%）]。慢阻肺病的患病率与年龄增长、低社会经济地位和吸烟相关。尽管慢阻肺病在男性中比在女性中更普遍，但女性的慢阻肺病发病率一直在增加，美国白人和黑人女性的慢阻肺病年死亡率一直在稳步上升。慢阻肺病在医保支

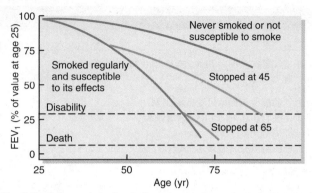

Fig. 5.2 Pattern of decline in forced expiratory volume in 1 second (FEV₁) with risks for morbidity and mortality from respiratory disease in a susceptible smoker compared with a normal patient and with a non-susceptible smoker. Although cessation of smoking does not replenish the lung function already lost in a susceptible smoker, it decreases the rate of further decline. (Data from Fletcher C, Peto R: The natural history of chronic airflow obstruction, BMJ 1:1645-1648, 1977.)

COPD in women has been increasing, and annual death rates for COPD have been steadily rising in both white and black women in the United States. COPD results in a significant economic burden in terms of health care expenditures and disability. In 2014, COPD accounted for 44.3 per 100,000 deaths in the United States. According to the World Health Organization, COPD is the fourth leading cause of death worldwide.

COPD is a complex disorder that results from a susceptibility to environmental factors brought about by a genetic predisposition. Cigarette smoking is the major environmental cause of COPD, although other factors may contribute, including outdoor air pollution, dust and fume exposure in the workplace, and indoor air pollution from use of biomass fuels for cooking and heat. Nonsmokers can and do develop COPD, highlighting the role of non–tobacco-related risk factors. A genetic predisposition is implied by the documentation of familial clusters of COPD. However, the only genetic disorder thus far definitively linked to COPD is α₁-antitrypsin deficiency resulting from mutations in *SERPINA1*, which accounts for approximately 1% to 2% of all COPD cases. Recent studies have highlighted other areas of the genome that are also associated with COPD susceptibility.

Several longitudinal studies have defined patterns of age-related decline in lung function and have documented the concept of age-related susceptibility to COPD. These studies showed that most adult nonsmoking men exhibit a decline in FEV₁ of 35 to 40 mL/year. This rate is increased to 45 to 60 mL/year in most cigarette smokers. However, the susceptible smoker may demonstrate losses of 70 to 120 mL/year (Fig. 5.2). This information allows the physician to project the rate of decrease of lung function in patients with COPD and to assess the effects of therapeutic interventions.

Pathology

Various structural changes have been observed in the airways and lungs of individuals with COPD. The current definition of COPD emphasizes the central role of chronic inflammation in the pathogenesis of COPD and in the development of pathologic lung and airway remodeling in the setting of COPD. Structural changes observed in COPD include emphysema and abnormalities of the small and large airways. There is increasing evidence that the small airways are the major site of airflow limitation and a central focus of pathology in COPD.

Emphysema in COPD

Emphysema is defined as a permanent enlargement of the air spaces distal to the terminal bronchioles. This is caused by destruction of the lung parenchyma in the absence of significant fibrosis. These changes result in an abnormal acinus with limited capabilities for gas exchange. Based on thin gross lung sections, emphysema can be classified as either centrilobular or panlobular. In centrilobular emphysema, the proximal part of the lobule (the respiratory bronchiole) is affected; this is the most common histologic feature observed in emphysema related to smoking. Panlobular emphysema is seen in α₁-antitrypsin deficiency.

α₁-Antitrypsin is a serine protease inhibitor that deactivates elastase molecules released by inflammatory cells that are capable of degrading connective tissue matrices. The observations that this enzyme was associated with emphysema and that emphysema could be reproduced in experimental models by the instillation of papain (a protease) into the lungs led to the hypothesis that emphysema is caused by an imbalance between protease and antiprotease systems in the lung. This theorized imbalance would favor proteolytic destruction of lung connective tissue, resulting in emphysema (the protease-antiprotease hypothesis). Research has focused on neutrophil elastase and its role in the destruction of lung elastin. Neutrophil elastase is the main target for inactivation by α₁-antitrypsin and has relatively unopposed effects. However, evidence for a primary role of this enzyme in cigarette smoke–induced emphysema is less clear, so the focus has broadened to include examination of the role of the matrix metalloproteinases (MMPs), produced by macrophages and other cells, in emphysema.

The inflammation induced by cigarette smoke is a trigger of the cycle of protease release and lung destruction resulting in emphysema. Macrophages are activated by cigarette smoke and recruit neutrophils and other inflammatory cells to the lung, leading to the release of elastase and MMPs. The destruction of elastin and other connective tissue elements in the lungs by these proteases leads over time to the loss of elastic recoil and destruction of alveolar structures characteristic of emphysema.

Cigarette smoke contains many oxidant molecules capable of inducing oxidative stress in the lung. Oxidative stress has diverse effects, including the oxidative inactivation of antiproteases in the lung and the acetylation of specific histones in the chromatin of lung cells and macrophages, allowing the expression of various pro-inflammatory genes. Histone deacetylase activity is reduced in COPD, and this in turn may result in an inability to control the pro-inflammatory response in this condition. Pro-inflammatory gene expression promotes cytokine production and release, contributing to further inflammatory cell recruitment and activation. Systemic inflammation, triggered by ongoing pulmonary inflammation, may lead to nonpulmonary abnormalities associated with emphysema, including cachexia and skeletal muscle alterations. Finally, increased apoptosis of pneumocytes and endothelial cells has been observed in lungs with emphysema and could contribute to the loss of alveoli.

Understanding of emphysema pathogenesis has improved with the recognition that inflammation, oxidative stress, protease-antiprotease balance, and apoptosis are linked in a complex interaction induced by cigarette smoke. This improved understanding has broadened the range of potential therapies that may be effective in ameliorating the destructive process. To date, however, therapies targeted at molecular pathways involved in emphysema pathogenesis have not been successful in altering disease progression, with the possible exception of α₁-antitrypsin replacement therapy in individuals with α₁-antitrypsin deficiency.

α₁-Antitrypsin, an acute phase reactant, is produced primarily in the liver, from which it travels to the lung. By its effect on elastases

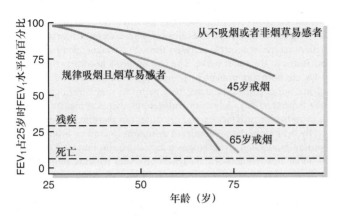

图 5.2　与正常患者和非烟草易感吸烟者相比，烟草易感吸烟者第 1 秒用力呼气容积（FEV_1）下降模式与呼吸疾病发病和死亡风险。虽然戒烟并不能提升烟草易感吸烟者已经丧失的肺功能，但可以延缓肺功能进一步下降的速度（引自 Fletcher C，Peto R：The natural history of chronic airflow obstruction，BMJ 1：1645-1648，1977.）

出和残疾方面造成了巨大经济负担。2014 年，美国每 100 000 例死亡中有 44.3 例死于慢阻肺病。根据世界卫生组织的数据，慢阻肺病是全球第四大死因。

慢阻肺病是一种复杂疾病，由遗传易感者受环境因素影响，进而致病。吸烟是慢阻肺病的主要环境原因，但其他因素也可造成影响，包括室外空气污染、工作场所扬尘及烟雾暴露、使用生物燃料做饭、取暖造成的室内空气污染。非吸烟者可以而且确实会患慢阻肺病，这突出体现了非吸烟相关危险因素的作用。家族聚集性慢阻肺病提示该病可能存在易感基因。然而，迄今为止唯一与慢阻肺病明确相关的遗传疾病是由 *SERPINA1* 突变引起的 α1- 抗胰蛋白酶缺乏，约占所有慢阻肺病病例的 1%～2%。最新研究强调了基因组的其他区域也与慢阻肺病易感性有关。

几项纵向研究已确定了年龄相关的肺功能下降模式，并记录了年龄相关慢阻肺病易感性的概念。这些研究表明，大多数成年非吸烟男性 FEV_1 每年下降 35～40 ml。大多数吸烟者 FEV_1 下降速度增加到每年 45～60 ml。然而，烟草易感吸烟者可能表现出每年 70～120 ml 的肺功能损失（图 5.2）。上述信息可助医生预测慢阻肺病患者肺功能下降速度，并评估治疗干预效果。

病理学

慢阻肺病患者的气道和肺部出现了各种结构改变。目前的慢阻肺病定义强调了慢性炎症在疾病发病机制、肺部病理进展及气道重塑中的核心作用。在慢阻肺病中观察到的结构变化包括肺气肿、小气道和大气道异常。越来越多的证据表明，小气道是气流受限的主要部位，也是慢阻肺病理学的核心特征。

慢阻肺病肺气肿

肺气肿的定义是终末细支气管远端气腔永久性扩大。这是由于肺实质破坏引起的，不伴明显纤维化。上述变化引起腺泡异常、气体交换能力受损。根据肺部大体病理薄层切片，肺气肿可分为小叶中心型肺气肿或全小叶型肺气肿。小叶中心型肺气肿是吸烟相关肺气肿最常见的组织学特征，受累部位为小叶近端部分（呼吸细支气管）。全小叶性肺气肿见于 α1- 抗胰蛋白酶缺乏。

α1- 抗胰蛋白酶是一种丝氨酸蛋白酶抑制剂，可灭活弹性蛋白酶分子，弹性蛋白酶来自于能够降解结缔组织基质的炎细胞。弹性蛋白酶与肺气肿有关，在实验模型中，将木瓜蛋白酶（一种蛋白酶）滴灌肺组织可构建肺气肿模型，由此得出假设，即肺部蛋白酶和抗蛋白酶系统之间的不平衡可引起肺气肿。这种不平衡引起了肺结缔组织的蛋白水解破坏，从而导致肺气肿（蛋白酶－抗蛋白酶假说）。有研究已经关注到中性粒细胞弹性蛋白酶及其如何破坏肺弹力纤维。中性粒细胞弹性蛋白酶是 α1- 抗胰蛋白酶灭活的主要靶标，相对而言不受抑制。但尚不清楚这种酶在香烟烟雾诱发的肺气肿中是否起到主导作用，因此研究进一步扩展，包括研究巨噬细胞和其他细胞产生的基质金属蛋白酶（MMP）在肺气肿中的作用。

香烟烟雾引起的炎症触发了蛋白酶释放-肺损伤-肺气肿这一循环。巨噬细胞被香烟烟雾激活，在肺部募集中性粒细胞和其他炎症细胞，导致弹性蛋白酶和 MMP 释放。随时间推移，这些蛋白酶破坏肺部弹性蛋白和其他结缔组织元件，导致弹性回缩力丧失和肺泡结构破坏，后者正是肺气肿的特征。

香烟烟雾含有许多氧化剂分子，能够在肺部诱导氧化应激。氧化应激作用众多，包括肺抗蛋白酶的氧化失活以及肺细胞、巨噬细胞染色质中特定组蛋白的乙酰化，从而允许机体表达各种促炎基因。慢阻肺病患者组蛋白去乙酰化酶活性降低，反过来可能导致疾病状态下促炎反应失控。促炎基因的表达增强了细胞因子的产生和释放，有助于炎细胞进一步募集和激活。持续的肺部炎症引发全身炎症，可能会导致与肺气肿相关的肺外病变，包括恶病质和骨骼肌异常。最后，肺气肿患者的肺泡细胞和内皮细胞凋亡增加，并可能引起肺泡丢失。

在香烟烟雾诱导下，炎症、氧化应激、蛋白酶-抗蛋白酶平衡和细胞凋亡等网络之间发生了复杂的相互作用，随着对这一问题的认识，人们对肺气肿发病机制的理解有所加深。随着理解加深，有潜力改善肺损伤过程的治疗方案也逐步增多。然而，迄今为止，针对肺气肿发病机制相关分子途径的治疗方案尚不能改变疾病进展，唯一例外的可能是针对 α1- 抗胰蛋白酶缺乏患者的 α1- 抗胰蛋白酶替代治疗。

α1- 抗胰蛋白酶是一种急性期反应物，主要在肝脏中产生，从肝脏进入肺部。α1- 抗胰蛋白酶通过影

in the lung, α_1-antitrypsin prevents the uncontrolled degradation of elastin in the lung parenchyma and protects against the development of emphysema. Individuals with the ZZ genotype of α_1-antitrypsin deficiency produce mutant forms of α_1-antitrypsin that have a tendency to inappropriately polymerize within the hepatocyte, leading to a deficiency in secreted α_1-antitrypsin and, in some cases, collateral damage to the liver caused by accumulation of intracellular misfolded, mutant α_1-antitrypsin. Patients who develop emphysema at a young age (<40 years) should be evaluated for this condition whether or not they smoke, as should patients with bronchiectasis and unexplained liver disease or cirrhosis. Testing shows reduced α_1-antitrypsin levels. Genotyping can reveal specific mutations (most commonly ZZ in severe deficiency). α_1-Antitrypsin supplementation has been used for patients with α_1-antitrypsin deficiency and appears to result in a decreased loss of lung density (surrogate for emphysema) by computed tomographic measurement.

Large and Small Airways Disease in COPD

Chronic bronchitis often coincides with emphysema in patients with COPD, but it may occur independently from either emphysema or COPD and is defined in clinical terms (described earlier). Cigarette smoking is the major cause, although exposure to pollutants such as dust and smoke may play a role. Pathologic findings are goblet cell hyperplasia, mucus hypersecretion and plugging, and airway inflammation and fibrosis (Fig. 5.3).

The disease mechanisms involved in the development of emphysema are also important in the pathogenesis of chronic bronchitis. However, in contrast to emphysema, chronic bronchitis is a disease of the large airways and not of the lung parenchyma. Therefore, the relationship of chronic bronchitis to airflow obstruction is less robust than for emphysema, and airflow limitation consistent with COPD in a patient with symptoms of chronic bronchitis may be more reflective of concomitant emphysema and small airways disease. Inflammation in chronic bronchitis leads to effects on the airway epithelium, including excess mucus production and impairment in mucociliary clearance.

Neurogenic stimuli are also important in the pathogenesis of airway obstruction in chronic bronchitis. The conducting airways are surrounded by smooth muscle, which contains adrenergic and

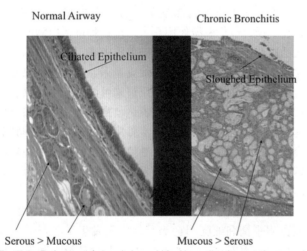

Fig. 5.3 Pathology of chronic bronchitis: Normally, airway submucosal serous glands outnumber mucous glands and the epithelium includes ciliated cells. In chronic bronchitis, mucous glands are more prevalent than serous glands and the epithelium is abnormal. (Courtesy Dr. Charles Kuhn.)

cholinergic receptors. Stimulation of β_2-adrenergic receptors by circulating catecholamines dilates airways, whereas stimulation of airway irritant receptors constricts airways through a cholinergic mechanism by means of the vagus nerve. The irritant bronchoconstrictive pathways are normally present to protect against inhalation of noxious agents, but in pathologic states these pathways may contribute to airway hyperreactivity. A host of endogenous chemical mediators such as proteases, growth factors, and cytokines can also affect airway tone.

By definition, the predominant symptom in chronic bronchitis is sputum production. Bronchospasm may also be prominent. Recurrent bacterial airway infections are typical. As with patients with COPD, the evaluation of patients with chronic bronchitis should include pulmonary function tests and a chest radiograph in addition to standard laboratory testing.

Damage to the small airways (those less than about 2 mm in diameter) is integral to the pathogenesis of COPD. The small airways are the major site of resistance to airflow in COPD. Respiratory bronchiolitis, in which there is an accumulation of pigmented macrophages in and around the bronchioles, may be an incidental finding in asymptomatic smokers without COPD. However, as COPD develops, other inflammatory cells are recruited to the small conducting airways, presumably in reaction to ongoing irritation from cigarette smoke or inhaled particles. With inflammation, the small airways in COPD can be affected by remodeling, leading to airway wall thickening and fibrosis, smooth muscle hypertrophy, and airway luminal narrowing, all of which contribute to airflow obstruction. Mucus plugs and inflammatory exudates can occlude the small airways, leading to increased resistance to airflow.

Recently, demonstration of profound decreases in small airway numbers and cross-sectional area in lungs of individuals with COPD has provided important evidence that loss of the small airways occurs with sufficient severity to result in detectable expiratory airflow limitation that characterizes COPD. Indeed, there is evidence that small airway loss may precede emphysema development in COPD.

Immune-mediated abnormalities are also seen at the level of the small airways in COPD. Lymphoid follicles may form around these airways in response to ongoing antigenic stimulation and bacterial infection, with a prominence of B cells and CD8+ T cells in more advanced COPD. These myriad changes at the small airway level contribute significantly to the physiologic abnormalities and altered local immune response in COPD.

Clinical Presentation

COPD related to chronic tobacco exposure is characterized by slowly progressive dyspnea that is first noticed during exertion but progresses over years until it is evident with minimal exertion (e.g., when dressing) or even at rest. Affected individuals complain of exercise intolerance and fatigue, and the disease eventually may lead to weight loss, depression, and anxiety as a result of increased work of breathing. Chronic cough can be present and is productive or dry, depending on the degree of mucus secretion (e.g., chronic bronchitis).

During the early stages of COPD, the physical examination may be normal. Normal examination results and the absence of symptoms often delay diagnosis. Inspection of the thorax and palpation may fail to reveal findings. As the disease progresses, the lungs may become hyperresonant to percussion, and auscultation may show diminished breath sounds with rhonchi or wheezes. The chest wall may begin to remodel, giving the patient the appearance of a "barrel chest." During the late stages of COPD, patients show evidence of increased work of breathing with use of accessory muscles, pursed-lip breathing, and weight loss. Skeletal muscle wasting may also become evident. Despite their respiratory insufficiency, some patients are able to sustain relatively

响肺内弹性蛋白酶，可防止肺实质中弹性蛋白不受控制的降解，从而延缓肺气肿进展。具有 α1- 抗胰蛋白酶缺乏 ZZ 基因型的个体会产生 α1- 抗胰蛋白酶突变，这些突变形式易在肝细胞内发生不恰当聚合，导致 α1- 抗胰蛋白酶无法分泌，甚至在某些情况下，由于细胞内错误折叠的 α1- 抗胰蛋白酶突变体不断积累，对肝脏造成附带损害。在年轻时（＜ 40 岁）发生肺气肿的患者，无论是否吸烟，都应对这方面病情进行评估，支气管扩张症合并不明原因的肝病或肝硬化的患者也应当进行评估。实验室检查显示患者 α1- 抗胰蛋白酶水平降低。基因检测可以揭示特定突变（在严重缺乏的患者中最常见的基因型是 ZZ）。α1- 抗胰蛋白酶补充剂已被用于 α1- 抗胰蛋白酶缺乏患者，并且可以改善患者 CT 的肺密度下降（肺气肿的等义词）。

慢阻肺病中的大气道和小气道疾病

慢性支气管炎是一个临床定义（如前所述），在慢阻肺病患者中常与肺气肿同时发生，但也可以独立于肺气肿或慢阻肺病发生。吸烟是主要原因，灰尘、烟雾等污染物暴露也可起作用。病理表现为杯状细胞增生、黏液高分泌、痰栓形成、气道炎症和纤维化（图 5.3）。

肺气肿进展的疾病机制在慢性支气管炎的发病机制中也很重要。与肺气肿的不同之处在于，慢性支气管炎是一种大气道疾病，而不是肺实质疾病。因此，慢性支气管炎与气流阻塞的关系不如肺气肿强，在有慢性支气管炎症状的患者中，符合慢阻肺病的气流受限其实更多反映伴随的肺气肿和小气道疾病。慢性支气管炎的炎症影响气道上皮，导致黏液过度分泌、黏膜纤毛清除能力受损。

神经源性刺激在慢性支气管炎的气道阻塞发病机制中发挥重要作用。传导气道被平滑肌包围，平滑肌

含有肾上腺素能和胆碱能受体。循环中的儿茶酚胺刺激 β2- 肾上腺素能受体，引起气道扩张，而气道刺激性受体一旦激活，可通过迷走神经胆碱能通路收缩气道。刺激性支气管收缩通路通常用于阻止有害物质吸入，但在病理状态下，这些通路可能导致气道高反应性。许多内源性化学介质，如蛋白酶、生长因子和细胞因子也会影响气道张力。

根据定义，慢性支气管炎的主要症状是痰液产生。支气管痉挛也可能是其突出表现。典型表现是反复发作的气道细菌感染。与慢阻肺病患者一样，慢性支气管炎患者的评估除了常规实验室检查外，还应包括肺功能及胸部 X 线片检查。

小气道（直径小于约 2 mm）的损伤是慢阻肺病发病机制的组成部分。小气道是慢阻肺病患者气流阻力的主要部位。一些没有慢阻肺病的无症状吸烟者可能会偶然发现呼吸性细支气管炎，色素巨噬细胞积聚在细支气管内部与周围。然而，随着慢阻肺病发展，其他炎细胞被募集到传导小气道，据推测可能是对香烟烟雾或可吸入颗粒物的持续刺激的反应。慢阻肺病患者的小气道可因炎症进而发生气道重塑，导致气道壁增厚和纤维化、平滑肌肥大、气道管腔狭窄等，这些均可导致气流阻塞。黏液栓和炎性渗出物会阻塞小气道，导致气流阻力增加。

最新证据表明，慢阻肺病患者肺部小气道的数量和横截面积大幅减少，证明小气道的丢失严重到足以导致呼气气流受限，这正是慢阻肺病的特征。有证据表明，在慢阻肺病中，小气道丢失可能先于肺气肿发生。

在慢阻肺病中，小气道也可以发生免疫调节异常。在持续的抗原刺激和细菌感染下，小气道周围形成淋巴滤泡，在较晚期的慢阻肺病中，这些淋巴滤泡以 B 细胞和 CD8[+] T 细胞为主。小气道的上述变化对于慢阻肺病的生理异常和局部免疫反应异常起到重要作用。

临床表现

慢性烟草暴露相关的慢阻肺病特征是缓慢的进行性呼吸困难，最先表现于患者劳力时，但随着数以年计的病情发展，患者在轻微劳力后（如穿衣时）甚至休息时即可明显表现出呼吸困难。患者主诉运动不耐受和疲劳，由于呼吸功增加，该疾病最终可能导致体重减轻、抑郁和焦虑；可出现慢性咳嗽，表现为咳痰或干咳，具体取决于黏液分泌程度（如慢性支气管炎）。

在慢阻肺病早期，体格检查可以正常。无症状且检查结果正常往往导致诊断延迟。胸部视诊和触诊可无特殊发现。随疾病进展，肺部叩诊呈过清音，听诊提示呼吸音下降，伴有鼾音或哮鸣音。患者胸壁发生重塑，呈现"桶状胸"外观。在慢阻肺病晚期，患者出现一系列呼吸功增加的表现，包括动用辅助呼吸肌、缩唇呼吸和体重下降。骨骼肌萎缩也愈发明显。尽管呼吸功能不全，但有一类患者能够维持血氧水平相对

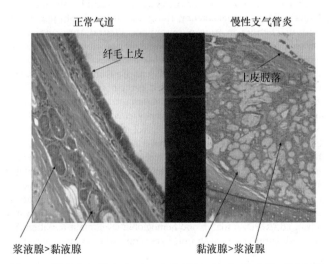

图 5.3 慢性支气管炎病理：正常情况下，气道黏膜下层内浆液腺多于黏液腺，气道上皮包含纤毛细胞。在慢性支气管炎中，黏液腺比浆液腺更常见，气道上皮异常（经 Dr. Charles Kuhn. 授权）

normal oxygen levels in blood until very late in the disease, leading to the classic clinical presentation of the "pink puffer." Other patients tend to retain carbon dioxide and diminish their work of breathing, resulting in chronic respiratory acidosis and, in extreme cases, polycythemia and cyanosis; this is the prototypical "blue bloater" phenotype. There is also an overlap of COPD with other respiratory disorders, such as obstructive sleep apnea, that may contribute to carbon dioxide retention.

Although COPD results in chronic, progressive dyspnea, periodic acute exacerbations are also characteristic. A rapid worsening of pulmonary function and an increased burden of respiratory symptoms such as dyspnea, cough, and sputum production characterize COPD exacerbations. Acute exacerbations are associated with various triggers, most importantly viral or bacterial respiratory infections, air pollution or other environmental factors, pulmonary embolism, and cardiac failure. Exacerbations are more common with increasing severity of COPD, with increasing age, and during the winter months. Exacerbations vary widely in severity. Severe exacerbations may lead to hospitalization, acute respiratory failure, and death. After an exacerbation, it may take weeks for the patient to return to a baseline level of function. Patients with frequent exacerbations of COPD experience an accelerated rate of decline in FEV_1. Patients who have experienced a COPD exacerbation are more likely to experience future exacerbations, suggesting that exacerbation is an important event in the natural history of COPD. On occasion, an exacerbation of COPD leading to acute respiratory failure is the first event leading to the diagnosis of COPD in an individual patient.

COPD is associated with a number of comorbid conditions, such as atherosclerotic heart disease, lung cancer, osteoporosis, and depression. These comorbidities may be related to smoking, to the chronic systemic inflammation present in patients with COPD, to the impaired quality of life resulting from COPD, or to treatments (e.g., corticosteroids) administered during the course of COPD. Monitoring for and appropriate management of these coexisting disorders is an important part of the ongoing assessment of patients with COPD.

As COPD progresses, the lung volumes increase (hyperinflation) and the diaphragms flatten, rendering inspiratory excursions inefficient. Tidal volume decreases and respiratory rate increases in an effort to decrease the work of breathing. In advanced disease, the cardiovascular system becomes affected as a result of the loss of vasculature in destroyed alveolar walls and vasoconstriction and vascular remodeling due to chronic hypoxia. With a limited area for blood flow, pulmonary vascular resistance is increased, leading to increased right ventricular afterload and development of pulmonary hypertension. This accelerates the development of right ventricular failure, which is referred to as cor pulmonale in the setting of lung disease. Right heart gallop, distended neck veins, hepatojugular reflux, and leg edema characterize cor pulmonale.

Diagnosis and Differential Diagnosis
Diagnosis
Pulmonary function tests, especially spirometry, are essential for the diagnosis of COPD. Classically, the diagnosis of COPD has been made using GOLD criteria, which defines COPD as an FEV_1/FVC ratio of less than 0.70 on post-bronchodilator spirometry. However, the American Thoracic Society (ATS)/European Respiratory Society (ERS) guidelines are coming into favor for diagnosing COPD. ATS/ERS defines COPD as FEV_1/FVC ratio less than the lower limit of normal based on the patient's sex and age. Although some degree of reversibility of the obstruction may be detected with bronchodilators, the obstructive defect is not entirely reversible in COPD. This characteristic and the consistent and progressive nature of the expiratory flow limitation

TABLE 5.2	GOLD Criteria
GOLD 1/mild COPD	$FEV_1 \geq 80\%$ predicted
GOLD 2/moderate COPD	$FEV_1 \geq 50\%$ but less than 80% predicted
GOLD 3/severe COPD	$FEV_1 \geq 30\%$ but less than 50% predicted
GOLD 4/very severe COPD	$FEV_1 < 30\%$ predicted

represent key features that help distinguish COPD from asthma, a major differential diagnostic consideration. The severity of disease and prognosis can be estimated by the FEV_1, as detailed in Table 5.2.

An FEV_1 of about 1 L (usually 50% predicted) suggests severe obstruction and, in the case of COPD, predicts a mean survival rate of 50% at 5 years. For a better predictor of mortality than FEV_1 alone, the BODE index can be used: *b*ody mass index, degree of *o*bstruction as measured by FEV_1, modified Medical Research Council *d*yspnea score, and *e*xercise capacity as denoted by 6-minute walk distance.

Lung volumes should be measured along with pulmonary function testing because the limitation to expired airflow and decreased elastic recoil lead to lung hyperinflation, as evidenced by increased RV, FRC, and, ultimately, TLC.

Destruction of alveoli decreases the surface area for gas exchange in emphysema. This loss of surface area, coupled with bronchial obstruction and altered distribution of ventilated air, results in ventilation-perfusion inequality or mismatch, a cause of hypoxemia. Hyperinflation leads to expansion of lung zone 1, the region of the lung in which alveolar pressure exceeds pulmonary arterial pressure. This process increases physiologic dead space because alveolar units ventilate areas that are not perfused. Hypercarbia can be avoided by increasing the minute ventilation, even with substantial ventilation-perfusion mismatching. However, eventually, the metabolic costs of increased ventilation become excessive, and respiratory muscles fatigue. Over time, chemoreceptors reset, allowing the level of partial pressure of carbon dioxide in arterial blood ($Paco_2$) to rise. Since $Paco_2$ is equal to alveolar partial pressure of carbon dioxide ($Paco_2$), the higher the $Paco_2$, the more CO_2 is exhaled with every breath, which increases the efficiency of ventilation. Significant individual variation is observed in relationship between the degree of mechanical impairment and in the magnitude of increase in $Paco_2$. Derangements in gas exchange can be detected by measuring arterial blood gases, by showing a decrease in D_{LCO}, or by evaluating hemoglobin oxygen desaturation during exertion. The degree of decrease in D_{LCO} correlates well with the radiologic extent of emphysema in COPD.

Chest radiography may fail to reveal abnormalities during the early stages of COPD, but in later stages, radiographic studies show hyperinflation, hyperlucency, flattening of the diaphragms, and bullous changes in lung parenchyma. Pleural abnormalities, lymphadenopathy, and mediastinal widening are not characteristic of emphysema and should point to other diagnoses, such as lung cancer. Computed tomography is more sensitive than plain radiography because it allows for a more detailed evaluation of the lung parenchyma and surrounding structures. Computed tomography is useful in assessing the distribution of emphysema in patients for whom operative interventions such as lung volume reduction surgery are being contemplated (see later discussion). High-resolution CT is highly sensitive for the detection of occult emphysema and can reveal the pattern of emphysematous changes. Electrocardiography might show evidence of right ventricular strain. Echocardiography can reveal evidence of right ventricular hypertrophy or dilation and can often provide an estimate of pulmonary arterial pressures in patients with advanced COPD. A high blood hemoglobin level might reveal erythrocytosis in the setting of chronic hypoxemia, whereas increased white

正常，直到疾病晚期，导致"红喘型"的经典临床表现。另一类患者则出现二氧化碳潴留、呼吸功减少的倾向，导致慢性呼吸性酸中毒，在极端情况下会继发红细胞增多症和发绀，即另一个经典表型"紫肿型"。慢阻肺病与其他呼吸疾病（如阻塞性睡眠呼吸暂停）也有重叠，导致二氧化碳潴留。

虽然慢阻肺病通常导致慢性进行性呼吸困难，但也经常出现反复发作急性加重，其特征为肺功能迅速恶化，伴有呼吸系统症状负担加重（如呼吸困难、咳嗽和咳痰）。急性加重的诱发因素很多，主要是呼吸道病毒或细菌感染、空气污染或其他环境因素、肺栓塞和心力衰竭。在慢阻肺病程度较重患者、高龄患者和冬季的情况下，急性加重会更频繁。急性加重的严重程度差异很大。重度急性加重可能导致住院、急性呼吸衰竭和死亡。急性加重后，患者可能需要数周时间才能恢复到基线肺功能水平。慢阻肺病频繁急性加重的患者 FEV_1 下降速度更快。经历过急性加重的患者更有可能在未来再次出现急性加重，这表明急性加重是慢阻肺病自然病程中的重要事件。有时以急性呼吸衰竭起病的急性加重可以是患者初诊慢阻肺病的首次事件。

慢阻肺病与许多合并症有关，如动脉粥样硬化性心脏病、肺癌、骨质疏松症和抑郁症。这些合并症可能与吸烟、慢性全身炎症状态、生活质量下降或慢阻肺病治疗药物（如糖皮质激素）有关。对共病的监测及正确管理是慢阻肺病患者动态评估的重要环节。

随着慢阻肺病进展，肺容积增加（过度充气）和膈肌低平，降低了吸气相膈肌位移效率。潮气量减少，呼吸频率增加，以减少呼吸功。疾病晚期肺泡壁毛细血管消失，长期缺氧引起肺血管收缩和血管重塑，使心血管系统受到影响。由于血流面积有限，肺血管阻力增加，导致右心室后负荷增加，发生肺动脉高压。这加速了右心室衰竭的进展，在合并肺病的情况下称为肺源性心脏病（肺心病）。肺心病典型体征包括右心奔马率、颈静脉扩张、肝颈静脉回流征和下肢水肿。

诊断和鉴别诊断
诊断

肺功能检查，尤其是肺通气功能，对于慢阻肺病诊断至关重要。传统上，慢阻肺病的诊断标准来自GOLD，该标准将慢阻肺病定义为应用支气管扩张剂后 FEV_1/FVC 比值小于 0.70。然而，越来越多人接受美国胸科学会（ATS）/欧洲呼吸学会（ERS）指南制定的诊断标准。ATS/ERS 将慢阻肺病定义为 FEV_1/FVC 比值低于性别年龄预测值的正常下限（LLN）。虽然给予支气管扩张剂后可以检测到一定程度的可逆性气流受限，但慢阻肺病患者的气流阻塞不完全可逆。慢阻肺病最需要鉴别诊断的就是哮喘，而区分慢阻肺病和哮喘的关键就在于气流阻塞不完全可逆以及呼出气流受限是否具有稳

表 5.2　GOLD 分级	
GOLD 1 级 / 轻度慢阻肺病	FEV_1 占预比 ≥ 80%
GOLD 2 级 / 中度慢阻肺病	FEV_1 占预比 ≥ 50% 但 < 80%
GOLD 3 级 / 重度慢阻肺病	FEV_1 占预比 ≥ 30% 但 < 50%
GOLD 4 级 / 极重度慢阻肺病	FEV_1 占预比 < 30%

定性和渐进性。慢阻肺病的严重程度和预后可以通过 FEV_1 来估计，详见表 5.2。

FEV_1 约为 1 L（通常占预比 50%）提示严重阻塞，在慢阻肺病中，可预测 5 年生存率为 50%。BODE指数在预测死亡率方面优于单独采用 FEV_1，BODE指数含义为：体重指数（B for body mass index）、由 FEV_1 体现的气流阻塞程度（O for obstruction）、mMRC（modified Medical Research Council）呼吸困难评分（D for dyspnea）以及由 6 分钟步行距离体现的运动耐量（E for exercise）。

肺功能检查应同时进行肺容积测定，因为呼出气流受限和弹性回缩力下降会引起肺过度充气，最初见于 RV 及 FRC 的增加，最终 TLC 也会增加。

在肺气肿中，肺泡破坏减少了气体交换面积。交换面积下降，加上支气管阻塞和气体分布改变，导致通气-灌注不均匀或不匹配，从而导致低氧血症。过度充气导致 1 区（Zone 1）扩张，1 区的肺泡压力超过肺动脉压。这一过程引起了生理无效腔增加，因为在无灌注区域，肺泡单位仍产生通气。即使存在严重的通气-灌注不匹配，增加每分通气量仍然可以防止高碳酸血症。但最终增加通气的代谢成本变得过高，呼吸肌疲劳。随着时间的流逝，化学感受器重新调定，使动脉二氧化碳分压（$PaCO_2$）升高。由于动脉二氧化碳分压等于肺泡二氧化碳分压（P_ACO_2），因此二氧化碳分压越高，每次呼吸呼出的 CO_2 就越多，从而提高通气效率。疾病程度与 $PaCO_2$ 增加幅度关系的个体差异较大。气体交换功能下降可体现在动脉血气异常、弥散功能下降或运动期间血氧饱和度下降。弥散功能（D_{LCO}）下降程度与慢阻肺病肺气肿的 CT 表现相关性良好。

在慢阻肺病早期，胸部 X 线可能无法发现异常，但在后期，影像学检查显示过度充气、透过度增加、膈肌低平和肺大疱。胸膜异常、淋巴结肿大和纵隔增宽并非肺气肿的特征，而是提示肺癌等其他疾病。CT比 X 线平片更敏感，因为它能更详细地评估肺实质和周围结构。CT 有助于评估拟行肺减容手术等外科干预（详见后文讨论）的住院患者的肺气肿分布情况。高分辨率 CT 对隐匿性肺气肿高度敏感，且能提示肺气肿类型。心电图可能提示右心室劳损。超声心动图可以显示右心室肥厚或扩大，并且能够估算晚期慢阻肺病患者的肺动脉压力。在慢性低氧血症的情况下，血红蛋白升高提示红细胞增多症，而白细胞增多可能提示感

blood cell counts might suggest infection. The arterial blood gas analysis may show hypoxemia, hypercarbia, or both, whereas acidemia due to acute hypercarbia may be present during an exacerbation.

Differential Diagnosis

The differential diagnosis of COPD includes the other major obstructive lung disorders: asthma, bronchiectasis, and the bronchiolar disorders. Asthma can occur at any age and sometimes overlaps with COPD, such as in patients with childhood asthma who smoke as adults. However, patients with COPD are typically older than 40 years of age and have a lengthy smoking history, whereas patients with asthma often have a history of atopy, have more variable symptoms that are often worse at night, and typically have marked improvements in lung function after bronchodilator administration. Patients with asthma may have normal pulmonary function during periods in which their asthma is well controlled, whereas those with COPD demonstrate ongoing airway obstruction even during periods of relative clinical stability.

It can be difficult to distinguish COPD with chronic bronchitis from bronchiectasis, and HRCT is necessary to assess for the abnormal bronchial dilation that is diagnostic of bronchiectasis.

Bronchiolar disorders can also be difficult to distinguish from COPD but should be considered in patients with risk factors, such as connective tissue disease or occupational exposures. Again, more sophisticated testing, such as HRCT with inspiratory and expiratory views to demonstrate peripheral areas of gas trapping and centrilobular nodules consistent with mucus impaction of the small airways, or even lung biopsy, may be needed to diagnose bronchiolitis.

Nonpulmonary causes of dyspnea on exertion, such as congestive heart failure or coronary artery disease, should also be considered in the differential diagnosis of COPD.

Treatment and Prevention

Because a cure for COPD does not exist, the best approach to this condition is prevention. Most cases of COPD in the United States are caused by cigarette smoking. Therefore, an appropriate major emphasis has been placed on the development of community education programs that focus on smoking prevention and promote smoking cessation. Legislative measures banning smoking in various public settings and levying increased taxes on cigarettes have been used to diminish the effects of environmental or second-hand exposure to tobacco smoke and to discourage smoking. Although smoking cessation interventions are effective in only a minority of patients, smoking cessation decreases mortality in patients with COPD who do succeed in quitting.

Most patients who are successful at smoking cessation have had at least one prior failed attempt, so physicians should encourage smoking cessation with at least brief interventions at every opportunity, even in patients who have tried but failed to quit in the past. Long-term physician and group support increase the success of cessation attempts, and pharmacologic smoking cessation aides, including nicotine replacement with gum or transdermal patches, bupropion, and varenicline, may provide additional benefit. Although there is considerable interest in the potential benefits and risk of E-cigarettes, further study is required to define its role.

Pharmacologic Therapies

After a diagnosis of COPD is established, therapy is guided primarily by symptoms of dyspnea and frequency of exacerbations. Dyspnea is assessed using subjective scoring systems. Patients are considered to be higher risk if they have a high dyspnea score or if they have had either one hospitalization for COPD or two exacerbations not requiring hospitalization in the past year. Overall treatment is directed at avoiding complications such as exacerbations, relieving airflow obstruction

through use of bronchodilators, and providing supplemental oxygen to patients with hypoxemia. Commonly used inhaled bronchodilators include sympathomimetic agents (β_2-adrenoreceptor agonists) and anticholinergic agents. Ipratropium bromide, a short-acting anticholinergic agent, is effective at decreasing dyspnea and improving FEV_1 in COPD. Albuterol is the most commonly used β_2-agonist; its bronchodilator effect is rapid in onset and relatively short lived. In practice, a combination of albuterol and ipratropium is frequently prescribed because these agents produce greater benefits when used in combination than when used individually.

Short-acting agents are typically prescribed for patients with mild disease or intermittent symptoms on an as-needed basis. Short-acting bronchodilators can be delivered by metered-dose inhaler (MDI) or by nebulizer. The MDI offers advantages of portability and ease of administration and convenience. When used correctly with a spacer, MDIs are as effective as nebulizers in delivering the drug. Nebulization has no advantage over the use of MDIs in the long-term management of obstructive lung disease except in patients who are unable to use an MDI properly.

Long-acting bronchodilators are effective for maintenance therapy in patients who have at least moderate COPD. Long-acting agents include the long-acting β_2-agonists (LABAs), which are available in once- or twice-daily formulations, and the long-acting anticholinergic/muscarinic antagonists (LAMAs), which are administered once daily. There have been several large studies evaluating the efficacy of long-acting bronchodilators and inhaled corticosteroids (ICS) in COPD, as detailed in Table 5.3. Initiation of either a LABA or a LAMA is reasonable for patients with COPD who require a long-acting bronchodilator. In more advanced disease, there is some evidence of additional benefits from the combination of a LABA and a LAMA. Tachycardia, hypokalemia, and tremor are potential adverse effects of LABAs, whereas dry mouth and urinary retention may occur with LAMA administration.

Current data suggest that the chronic use of inhaled corticosteroids improves symptoms and decreases the frequency of exacerbations.

TABLE 5.3 **Studies Evaluating the Efficacy of LABA, LAMA, and ICS**	
TORCH (2007): LABA/ICS vs ICS or LABA vs placebo	• n = 6112 • Length of study: 3 years • LABA/ICS associated with fewer COPD-related hospitalizations • No mortality benefit
INSPIRE (2007): LABA/ICS vs LAMA	• n = 1323 • Length of study: 2 years • No difference in exacerbation rates • More hospitalizations and deaths in LAMA group
UPLIFT (2008): LAMA vs placebo	• n = 5993 • Length of study: 4 years • No difference in decline of FEV_1
SPARK (2013): LAMA/LABA vs LAMA or LABA	• n = 2224 • Length of study: 64 weeks • LAMA/LABA was associated with fewer exacerbations than single agent
FLAME (2016): LABA/LAMA vs LABA/ICS	• n = 3362 • Length of study: 1 year • LABA/LAMA was associated with fewer COPD-related hospitalizations

染。动脉血气分析可表现为低氧血症、高碳酸血症或两者兼而有之，急性加重时可能出现呼吸性酸中毒。

鉴别诊断

慢阻肺病鉴别诊断包括其他常见阻塞性肺疾病：哮喘、支气管扩张症和小气道疾病。哮喘可发生于任何年龄，可与慢阻肺病重叠，例如童年哮喘且成年后吸烟的患者。慢阻肺病患者通常年龄超过 40 岁，吸烟史长，而哮喘患者常有特应性病史，症状多变，夜间显著，通常给予支气管扩张剂后肺功能得到明显改善。哮喘患者在良好控制期间肺功能可以正常，而慢阻肺病患者即使在临床相对稳定时期也表现出持续的气道阻塞。

支气管扩张症与伴有慢性支气管炎的慢阻肺病难以鉴别，HRCT 是评估支气管异常扩张所必需的检查，因而也是确诊支气管扩张症的关键。

细支气管疾病也很难与慢阻肺病相鉴别，但对于有危险因素（如结缔组织病或职业暴露）的患者，应考虑该疾病。同样，诊断细支气管炎可能需要更复杂的检查，例如吸呼双相 HRCT，用来显示外周区域的气体潴留，以及与小气道黏液嵌塞相匹配的小叶中心结节，有时甚至需要肺活检来诊断。

在慢阻肺病的鉴别诊断中，也应考虑劳力性呼吸困难的肺外原因，如心力衰竭或冠状动脉疾病。

治疗和预防

由于慢阻肺病无法治愈，因此重在预防。在美国，大多数慢阻肺病由吸烟引起。因此，重点制定了预防吸烟和促进戒烟的基层教育项目。为了减少环境暴露及二手烟暴露，政府立法禁止在任何公共场所吸烟，并对烟草增加征税。虽然戒烟干预措施仅对少数患者有效，但成功戒烟可成功降低慢阻肺病患者的死亡率。

大多数患者在成功戒烟之前至少会失败一次，因此即便是对于曾经尝试戒烟失败的患者，医生还是应当鼓励戒烟，利用一切机会进行哪怕很简短的干预。来自医生和戒烟团体的长期支持能够提高成功率，尼古丁咀嚼胶、尼古丁透皮贴剂、安非他酮和伐尼克兰等戒烟药能带来额外帮助。电子烟的潜在益处和风险均已引起相当高的关注，仍需要深入研究来明确其作用。

药物治疗

在确诊慢阻肺病后，治疗方案主要依据呼吸困难症状和急性加重频率而制订。呼吸困难使用主观评分系统进行评估。如果患者呼吸困难评分较高，或者在过去一年中因慢阻肺病住院治疗过一次、或有过两次不需要住院治疗的急性加重，则认为患者急性加重风险较高。总体而言，治疗目标是避免急性加重等并发

症，利用支气管扩张剂缓解气流阻塞，并对低氧血症患者进行氧疗。常用的吸入性支气管扩张剂包括拟交感神经药（β2-肾上腺素受体激动剂）和抗胆碱能药。异丙托溴铵是一种短效抗胆碱能药物，可有效缓解呼吸困难、改善慢阻肺病患者的 FEV_1。沙丁胺醇是最常用的 β2 受体激动剂，起效迅速，持续时间相对较短。这两个药物在联用时比单药使用获益更大，因此在临床工作中，沙丁胺醇和异丙托溴铵常常联合处方。

病情较轻或仅有间歇发作症状的患者多用短效制剂。短效支气管扩张剂可以通过定量吸入器（MDI）或雾化器给药。MDI 便携、易用、方便。如能配合储雾罐正确使用，MDI 与雾化器给药效果一样好。在阻塞性肺疾病的长期治疗中，除非患者无法正确使用 MDI，否则雾化与 MDI 相比没有优势。

对病情达到至少中度的慢阻肺病患者而言，长效支气管扩张剂是维持治疗的有效药物。长效药物包括长效 β2 受体激动剂（LABA），每日给药一次或两次，以及长效胆碱能/毒蕈碱拮抗剂（LAMA），每日给药一次。有几项大型研究评估了长效支气管扩张剂和吸入糖皮质激素（ICS）对慢阻肺病的疗效，详见表 5.3。对于需要长效支气管扩张剂的慢阻肺病患者，初始治疗采用 LABA 或 LAMA 都是合理的。当疾病进展，有证据表明 LABA 和 LAMA 的联合使用获益更多。LABA 可能出现的不良反应为心动过速、低钾血症和震颤，LAMA 则可能出现口干和尿潴留。

现有数据表明，长期使用 ICS 可改善症状并降低急性加重的频率。对于有急性加重病史的慢阻肺病患者，

表 5.3 评估 LABA、LAMA 和 ICS 疗效的研究

TORCH（2007） LABA/ICS 对比 ICS 或 LABA 对比安慰剂	• $n = 6112$ • 随访时间：3 年 • LABA/ICS 治疗与慢阻肺病相关住院率较低有关 • 在死亡率方面无优势
INSPIRE（2007） LABA/ICS 对比 LAMA	• $n = 1323$ • 随访时间：2 年 • 两组急性加重频率无差别 • LAMA 组的住院率、死亡率更高
UPLIFT（2008） LAMA 对比安慰剂	• $n = 5993$ • 随访时间：4 年 • 两组 FEV_1 下降无差异
SPARK（2013） LAMA/LABA 对比 LAMA 或 LABA	• $n = 2224$ • 随访时间：64 周 • 与单一药物相比，LAMA/LABA 治疗与急性加重频率较低有关
FLAME（2016） LABA/LAMA 对比 LABA/ICS	• $n = 3362$ • 研究时间：1 年 • LABA/LAMA 治疗与慢阻肺病相关住院率较低有关

Inhaled long-acting corticosteroids (e.g., beclomethasone, budesonide, fluticasone propionate) should be considered for individuals with COPD and a history of exacerbations but should not be used as monotherapy. Inhaled corticosteroids are less clearly effective in COPD than in asthma, and pneumonia occurs more frequently in patients with COPD treated with inhaled corticosteroids. Inhaled corticosteroids can be combined with LABAs; the combination salmeterol with fluticasone in patients with moderate to severe COPD was shown to improve health-related quality of life and to reduce exacerbations to a greater extent than either component alone.

Systemic use of corticosteroids is indicated during acute exacerbations, and intravenous corticosteroids are useful in the acute setting. Intravenous corticosteroids have also proved effective for the management of acute exacerbations of most obstructive lung diseases, including asthma (Fig. 5.4). Patients with acute exacerbations are usually transitioned from intravenous to oral steroids within 72 hours. While oral steroids were historically tapered over 14 days, more recent research suggests that a 5-day "burst" of steroids without a taper is noninferior to traditional tapering regimens. Other agents with anti-inflammatory capabilities, such as leukotriene inhibitors, are not indicated for treatment of COPD.

Theophylline, a methylxanthine, is a weak systemic sympathomimetic agent with a narrow therapeutic window. It is not a first-line drug in the treatment of COPD, although long-acting derivatives with improved safety profiles have been developed. Theophylline preparations have some anti-inflammatory activity and may provide additional bronchodilation in patients with COPD who do not respond adequately to inhaled β-agonists. When these preparations are used, blood concentrations should be maintained in the lower end of the therapeutic range (between 8 and 12 μg/mL). Toxicity is common at concentrations higher than 20 μg/mL. The metabolism of theophylline is decreased by many commonly used drugs (e.g., erythromycin), and toxic serum concentrations of theophylline can be reached quickly when these other drugs are administered unless the theophylline dose is adjusted appropriately. Toxic effects of theophylline may be observed in the gastrointestinal, cardiac, and neurologic systems. Severe theophylline toxicity can be fatal, and treatment with charcoal hemoperfusion may be required.

Phosphodiesterase type 4 (PDE4) inhibitors have been investigated for the treatment of COPD, and an oral PDE4 inhibitor was recently approved as add-on therapy for treatment of severe COPD with chronic bronchitis and a history of exacerbations. PDE4 inhibitors act to inhibit breakdown of cyclic adenosine monophosphate (cAMP), resulting in a weak bronchodilator effect (approximately 50 mL improvement in FEV_1); they should not be used as acute bronchodilators. However, roflumilast was demonstrated to reduce exacerbation rates in patients who had severe COPD with chronic bronchitis and a history of exacerbation in the prior year and were not using inhaled corticosteroids. Adverse effects include weight loss, nausea and loss of appetite, and an increase in psychiatric adverse reactions including suicidality.

Oxygen Therapy and Mechanical Ventilation

Continuous oxygen therapy has been shown to improve survival in patients with COPD and hypoxemia. Oxygen supplementation is recommended once the partial pressure of oxygen in arterial blood (Pao_2) drops below 55 mm Hg or the hemoglobin oxygen saturation decreases to 88%. Oxygen supplementation is indicated at higher levels of Pao_2 if end-organ damage, such as pulmonary hypertension, is present.

Oxygen therapy is frequently necessary for treatment of acute exacerbations of obstructive lung disease. In patients who hypoventilate chronically and therefore have an elevated $Paco_2$, elevating the inspired oxygen content may acutely worsen hypercarbia by inhibiting

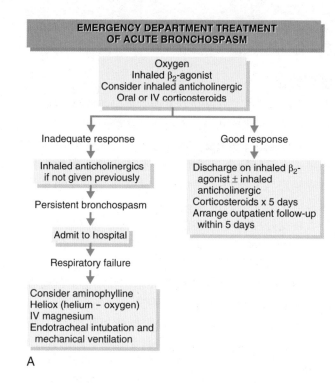

A

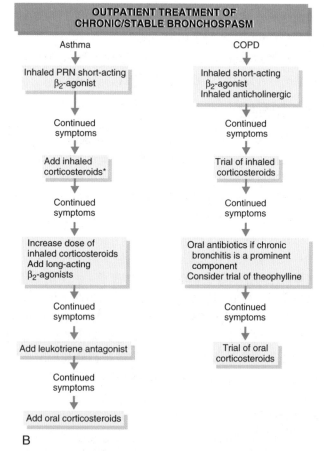

B

Fig. 5.4 Algorithms for the treatment of bronchospasm in patients in the emergency department (A) and in outpatients with stable disease (B). *IV,* Intravenous; *PRN,* as needed. *Leukotriene antagonists could be considered.

应考虑吸入 ICS（如倍氯米松、布地奈德、丙酸氟替卡松），但不应单药治疗。ICS 对慢阻肺病的疗效不如哮喘，ICS 治疗的慢阻肺病患者更常发生肺炎。ICS 可与 LABA 联合使用；沙美特罗与氟替卡松联合应用治疗中度至重度慢阻肺病患者，其结果显示与任一成分单独给药相比，可改善健康相关生活质量，并更好地减少急性加重。

急性加重发作时可以全身应用糖皮质激素，急诊处置静脉注射糖皮质激素十分有用。已证明静脉注射糖皮质激素可有效治疗大多数阻塞性肺病（包括哮喘）的急性加重（图 5.4）。急性加重患者通常在 72 h 内从静脉注射转为口服糖皮质激素。虽然向来习惯将口服糖皮质激素逐渐减量且疗程超过 2 周，但最新研究表明，连续 5 天短疗程、不减量的给药方案并不劣于传统减量方案。白三烯抑制剂等其他抗炎药物则不适用于治疗慢阻肺病。

茶碱是一种甲基黄嘌呤，是一种较弱的全身性拟交感神经药物，治疗窗较窄。尽管已经开发出较安全的长效衍生物，但它仍不是治疗慢阻肺病的一线药。茶碱制剂具有一定的抗炎活性，慢阻肺病患者如对吸入 β 受体激动剂反应不充分，则茶碱有助于进一步扩张支气管。在临床应用时，茶碱血液浓度应保持在治疗范围（8 ～ 12 μg/ml 之间）。浓度高于 20 μg/ml 时出现毒性。许多常用药物（如红霉素）会减慢茶碱的代谢，并且当给予这些其他药物时，如不及时调整剂量，茶碱可以迅速达到毒性血药浓度。茶碱的毒性作用可出现于胃肠道、心脏和神经系统。严重茶碱中毒可以致命，需用活性炭血液灌流进行治疗。

磷酸二酯酶 4 型（PDE4）抑制剂已被用于研究慢阻肺病治疗，最近一种口服 PDE4 抑制剂被批准作为附加疗法，用于治疗伴有慢性支气管炎和急性加重史的重度慢阻肺病。PDE4 抑制剂可抑制环磷酸腺苷（cAMP）的分解，导致较弱的支气管扩张作用（FEV_1 改善约 50 ml）；它们不能被当作速效支气管扩张剂使用。此外，罗氟司特被证明可以降低重度慢阻肺病患者的急性加重率，它适用于伴有慢性支气管炎、前一年有急性加重史、未使用 ICS 的重度慢阻肺病患者。不良反应包括体重减轻、恶心、食欲不振，以及包括自杀在内的精神不良反应。

氧疗和机械通气

连续氧疗已被证明可以提高慢阻肺病和低氧血症患者的生存率。当动脉血氧分压（PaO_2）降至 55 mmHg 以下或血氧饱和度降至 88% 时，建议吸氧。如果已存在终末器官损伤（如肺动脉高压），则需在 PaO_2 水平较高时启动吸氧。

氧疗通常用于治疗阻塞性肺疾病的急性加重。在长期低通气引起二氧化碳潴留的患者中，提高吸氧含量可能会引起高碳酸血症的急性加重，原因是提高吸氧含量

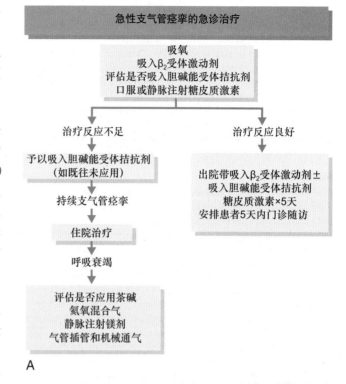

A

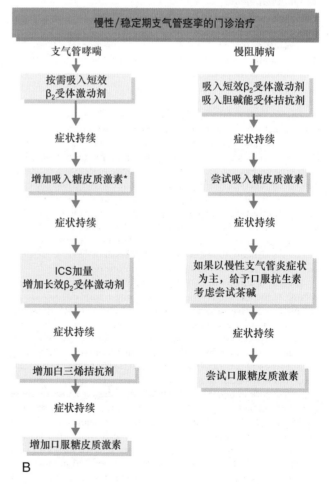

B

图 5.4　急诊（**A**）和门诊（**B**）支气管痉挛患者的治疗流程。
* 可以考虑应用白三烯拮抗剂

the hypoxic ventilatory drive and by promoting the dissociation of carbon dioxide from oxygenated hemoglobin (the Haldane effect). High-flow oxygen has been shown to be harmful in the setting of pre-hospital emergency treatment for COPD. Therefore, oxygen should be closely titrated to maintain normoxia and to avoid either hypoxemia or excessively elevated Pao_2. An oxygen saturation of 90% to 92% is a reasonable target in the absence of further data. During exacerbations of COPD leading to hypercarbic respiratory failure, noninvasive positive airway pressure ventilation has proved useful in reducing the work of breathing, alleviating diaphragm fatigue, and reducing the need for endotracheal intubation and mechanical ventilation.

Antibiotics

Exacerbations of airway obstruction may result most often from viral infections but also from bacterial infection. The most common bacterial pathogens in COPD are *Streptococcus pneumoniae*, *Haemophilus influenzae*, and *Moraxella catarrhalis*. Management of acute exacerbations with dyspnea and increased volume and purulence of mucus should include empiric administration of antibiotics, which have been shown to improve the success rate in exacerbation treatment. The role of chronic prophylactic antibiotic use in COPD is uncertain, and a trial of oral azithromycin resulted in a reduction in exacerbations but an increased risk of hearing loss. Immunization with influenza vaccines directed at specific epidemic strains reduces exacerbations of COPD. Pneumococcal vaccination is also recommended in patients with COPD.

Nonpharmacologic Therapies

Multiple airway clearance techniques aid in clearing of airway secretions, but their effectiveness in the management of emphysema and other obstructive lung diseases in adults is questionable. If needed, chest physiotherapy and postural drainage might be useful in patients with chronic bronchitis and increased sputum production. Few data support the use of specific mucolytics or expectorant agents for patients with COPD.

Patients with pulmonary disease of sufficient severity to compromise normal activities of daily living commonly demonstrate improved quality of life and less subjective dyspnea when enrolled in a comprehensive, high-quality pulmonary rehabilitation program. Pulmonary rehabilitation has not been shown to improve objective measures of pulmonary function, to affect the rate of decline in lung function, or to improve survival. However, it has been shown to improve the quality of life in motivated patients. An important part of pulmonary rehabilitation is nutritional assessment and careful attention to maintaining adequate nutrition. Malnutrition and cachexia are common in later stages of obstructive lung disease, and they result in decreased respiratory muscle strength and compromised immune function.

The role of surgery in COPD is generally limited. Bullectomy, lung volume reduction surgery (LVRS), and lung transplantation are all potentially effective surgical options for selected patients. Resection of nonfunctional areas of lung (e.g., bullectomy) may allow for compressed functional areas to expand and may improve symptoms, airflow, and oxygenation by improving ventilation-perfusion matching in a subgroup of patients. In addition, resection of bullae can decrease lung volumes, resulting in enhanced diaphragmatic function and decreased work of breathing. The best candidates for LVRS are those with predominantly upper lobe disease who have a low exercise tolerance despite rehabilitation and are without other major comorbidities. This subgroup may have reduced mortality after LVRS. In general, a high surgical mortality risk exists in patients referred for LVRS who have an FEV_1 or D_{LCO} of less than 20% predicted and in those who have more homogeneous distribution of emphysema. Patients with

high surgical risk may be candidates for endoscopic placement of endobronchial valves (EBV), which were FDA approved in 2018. EBVs are one-way valves that aim to deflate emphysematous regions of the lung by allowing air to flow out of but not into the affected alveoli.

Single or bilateral lung transplantation is an option for patients with end-stage airflow obstruction. The average survival after lung transplantation is 4 to 5 years. Rejection, viral infections, transplant-associated lymphoproliferative disease, and late occurrence of bronchiolitis obliterans remain significant problems, but the procedure can improve the quality of life in properly selected patients.

Palliative Care

Although the disease course can be unpredictable, discussion of end-of-life issues with the patient is an important component of longitudinal care as COPD progresses to an advanced stage. Preparation of advance directives regarding use of intensive care measures at the end of life may be desirable. Opioid narcotics can be highly effective for relieving dyspnea in patients with terminal complications of COPD.

Prognosis

COPD is a chronic and progressive disease with a variable and typically prolonged clinical course. As discussed previously, measurement of lung function (FEV_1 % predicted) has prognostic significance, and use of the multifactorial BODE index can improve prognostication compared with use of FEV_1 alone. Patients who have frequent exacerbations of COPD appear to have more rapid loss of lung function than those without exacerbations, suggesting that frequent exacerbations result in a worse clinical course.

At present, aside from smoking cessation and the addition of long-term oxygen therapy for patients with hypoxemia, interventions to improve survival in COPD are limited. No pharmacologic therapy for COPD has been definitively demonstrated to improve survival. In mild COPD, mortality is frequently related to comorbidities such as ischemic heart disease and lung cancer; in more advanced stages, a greater proportion of patients die from respiratory causes.

BRONCHIOLAR DISORDERS

Definition and Epidemiology

The bronchioles are defined as the small noncartilaginous airways (<2 mm in diameter). The bronchiolar disorders encompass a spectrum of diseases of widely varying causes primarily affecting these small airways. Bronchiolar disorders can be associated with cigarette smoking. For example, small airways disease contributes significantly to the syndrome of COPD. Respiratory bronchiolitis is also commonly found incidentally in smokers. However, bronchiolar disorders with etiologies other than cigarette smoking also exist. Bronchiolar disorders are associated with patchy inflammation and epithelial injury, fibrosis, mucoid impaction, or obliteration of the bronchioles. These changes result in airflow limitation due to increased airway resistance.

Acute bronchiolitis related to respiratory syncytial virus infection is epidemic among infants and young children, but primary bronchiolar disorders, including infectious or postinfectious bronchiolitis, are rare in the adult general population and tend to affect specific patient populations.

Pathology

The pathology of the bronchiolar disorders is complex. A variety of terms are used to describe or classify the various histopathologic patterns of small airways disease, including *cellular bronchiolitis* (inflammatory cell infiltration of the small airway wall resulting in small

可以抑制缺氧的通气驱动并促进二氧化碳与含氧血红蛋白的解离（霍尔丹效应）。在院前急诊处置中，有证据表明高流量氧疗对慢阻肺病患者有害。因此，应密切滴定氧气以维持常氧，避免氧分压过低或过高。在没有进一步数据的情况下，90% ～ 92% 的血氧饱和度是一个合理目标。在慢阻肺病急性加重导致高碳酸血症型呼吸衰竭的情况下，无创气道正压通气已被证明有助于减少呼吸功、减轻膈肌疲劳、减少气管插管和机械通气需求。

抗生素

气道阻塞加重的原因首先是病毒感染，也可以是细菌感染。慢阻肺病中最常见的细菌病原是肺炎链球菌、流感嗜血杆菌和卡他莫拉菌。如果慢阻肺病急性加重伴有呼吸困难、痰量增多、痰液变脓，则治疗应包括经验性抗生素，这一点已被证明可提高慢阻肺病急性加重的治疗成功率。长期预防性使用抗生素在慢阻肺病中的作用尚不确定，临床试验发现，口服阿奇霉素可减少急性加重，但会导致听力损伤。针对特定流行毒株的流感疫苗接种可减少慢阻肺病的急性加重。慢阻肺病患者接种肺炎球菌疫苗也是推荐的。

非药物治疗

各种气道清洁技术有助于清除气道分泌物，但在肺气肿及其他阻塞性肺疾病的成年患者中，气道清洁技术的有效性并不确切。对于慢性支气管炎和痰量增加的患者而言，如果需要痰液引流，胸部物理治疗和体位引流可能有用。化痰药或祛痰药的使用在慢阻肺病患者中鲜有数据支持。

如果患者的呼吸疾病已经严重到影响正常日常生活活动，则参加高质量的综合肺康复项目后往往会表现出生活质量的改善和主观呼吸困难的缓解。目前尚无证据支持肺康复能提高肺功能的客观指标、延缓肺功能下降的速度或提高生存率，但有证据表明康复可以改善积极活动的患者的生活质量。肺康复的重要组成部分之一是营养评估和重视维持营养充足。营养不良和恶病质在阻塞性肺疾病晚期很常见，它们会导致呼吸肌力量下降和免疫功能受损。

慢阻肺病的手术治疗作用有限。肺大疱切除术、肺减容手术（LVRS）和肺移植是面向特定患者可能有效的手术选择。切除肺非功能区（如大疱切除术）可使受压的功能区扩大，并可能通过改善部分患者的通气 - 灌注匹配，从而改善症状、气流与氧合。此外，大疱切除术可减少肺容积，从而增强膈肌功能并减少呼吸功。LVRS 最适合上叶受累为主、经肺康复治疗后运动耐量仍然较低，且没有其他严重合并症的患者。该亚组接受 LVRS 后死亡率可能降低。总体而言，LVRS 手术死亡风险较高的患者为 FEV_1 或 D_{LCO} 占预比低于 20% 以及均质型肺气肿患者。如果患者外科手术风险较高，可能适合行气管镜下支气管内瓣膜（EBV）置入术，EBV 已于 2018 年获得美国 FDA 批准。它是一种单向瓣膜，允许受累肺泡的气体流出、不允许气体流入，从而将肺气肿区域放气。

单肺移植或双肺移植是终末期气流阻塞患者的一种选择。肺移植后平均生存期为 4 ～ 5 年。排斥反应、病毒感染、移植相关淋巴增生性疾病、闭塞性细支气管炎仍然是重大难题，但该手术可以改善特定患者的生活质量。

缓和医疗

尽管病程未必可以预测，但随着慢阻肺病进展到晚期，与患者讨论临终问题是延续护理的重要环节，应采用预立医疗计划提前决定是否在生命终点采用重症监护手段。阿片类麻醉剂对于伴有终末期并发症的慢阻肺病患者非常有效。

预后

慢阻肺病是一种慢性进行性疾病，临床病程多变且迁延。如前所述，肺功能（FEV_1% 占预比）高度提示预后，与单独使用 FEV_1 相比，使用多因素的 BODE 指数可以提高预后判断准确性。慢阻肺病患者伴有频繁急性加重，会比不伴有急性加重的患者肺功能下降更快，频繁急性加重会导致更差的临床过程。

目前，除了戒烟和给低氧血症患者提供长期氧疗外，能提高慢阻肺病患者生存率的干预措施十分有限。慢阻肺病的药物治疗能否提高患者生存率尚未得到确切证明。在轻度慢阻肺病患者中，死亡率通常与缺血性心脏病及肺癌等共病有关；在疾病晚期，有更高比例的患者死于呼吸系统病因。

细支气管疾病

定义和流行病学

细支气管被定义为小的非软骨气道（直径 < 2 mm）。细支气管疾病包括一系列疾病，其病因各不相同，主要影响这些小气道。细支气管疾病可能与吸烟有关。例如，小气道疾病是慢阻肺病的重要特征。呼吸性细支气管炎也常见于吸烟者。然而也存在非吸烟病因的细支气管疾病。细支气管疾病与斑片状炎症、上皮损伤、纤维化、黏液嵌塞，或细支气管闭塞有关。上述变化导致气道阻力增高，引起气流受限。

与呼吸道合胞病毒感染相关的急性细支气管炎在婴幼儿中流行，但原发性细支气管疾病（包括感染性或感染后细支气管炎）在成年人中很少见，往往只影响特定患者群体。

病理学

细支气管疾病的病理学很复杂。描述或分类小气道疾病各种组织病理学特征的术语有很多，包括细胞性细支气管炎（小气道壁的炎症细胞浸润导致小气道

airway narrowing), *follicular bronchiolitis* (formation of abundant lymphoid follicles in close apposition to the small airways, resulting in airway compression), *obliterative* or *constrictive bronchiolitis* (fibrosis surrounding the small airways resulting in narrowing of the affected airways), and *bronchiolitis obliterans* (formation of endoluminal fibrous lesions, sometimes called *Masson bodies,* obstructing the small airway lumen). The histopathologic pattern of small airways disease may suggest a likely underlying etiology; for example, follicular bronchiolitis is often, although not exclusively, seen in the context of Sjögren's syndrome.

Clinical Presentation

In general, the bronchiolar disorders manifest nonspecifically with dyspnea, which may be severe or progressive, and in some cases accompanied by cough or sputum production. The physical examination may reveal inspiratory squeaks or wheezes but may be surprisingly normal. The possibility of a bronchiolar disorder should be considered in particular settings. For example, bronchiolitis may complicate the course of rheumatoid arthritis, Sjögren's syndrome, or inflammatory bowel disease.

Diffuse panbronchiolitis is a rare idiopathic disorder most common in Japan that is characterized by cough with purulent sputum, sinusitis, and dyspnea. Recurrent respiratory infections with bacterial organisms such as *Pseudomonas aeruginosa* complicate the course of diffuse panbronchiolitis.

Bronchiolitis obliterans can be a clinical syndrome (in addition to a histopathologic term) that is associated with chronic allograft rejection after lung transplantation, graft-versus-host disease after allogeneic hematopoietic stem cell transplantation, and occupational toxin exposures. For example, occupational clusters of bronchiolitis obliterans have been described after exposure to diacetyl, a flavoring chemical used in the manufacture of microwave popcorn. Constrictive bronchiolitis can be seen in war veterans who were exposed to burn pits in Iraq or Afghanistan.

Diagnosis and Differential Diagnosis

In general, the bronchiolar disorders cause an obstructive pattern of expiratory airflow limitation on pulmonary function testing without evidence of reversibility. The bronchiolitis obliterans syndrome is diagnosed clinically by a decline in FEV_1 of 20% from a stable baseline value on serial testing after lung transplantation. HRCT is valuable in the diagnosis and assessment of the bronchiolar disorders. Characteristic findings on HRCT include centrilobular nodules or tree-in-bud opacities, reflecting impacted inflammatory exudates or sloughed epithelial cells in the bronchioles. A "mosaic attenuation" pattern, with decreased attenuation in geographic regions of lung reflecting areas of air trapping distal to obstructed bronchioles, is often seen on inspiration. CT scanning during the expiratory phase can confirm that this finding is caused by air trapping rather than decreased perfusion from pulmonary vascular disease. Lung biopsy may be of limited value because of the scattered, patchy nature of the abnormalities present in the bronchiolar disorders. The differential diagnosis includes COPD, which also causes poorly reversible obstruction on spirometry.

Treatment

Treatment of the bronchiolar disorders is challenging. Acute bronchiolitis typically resolves without treatment; bronchodilators and steroids are not clearly beneficial, although they are often prescribed. The bronchiolitis obliterans syndrome responds poorly to increased immunosuppression and is a frequent cause of death after lung transplantation. Azithromycin has been reported to increase FEV_1 in the

bronchiolitis obliterans syndrome. Macrolide antibiotics have also been reported to positively affect the clinical course of diffuse panbronchiolitis, possibly reflecting immunomodulatory or antifibrotic effects of these medications. Lung transplantation may be necessary in progressive bronchiolitis obliterans, and retransplantation has sometimes been performed in patients affected by the bronchiolitis obliterans syndrome after transplant rejection.

Prognosis

These disorders may be self-limited, as in acute bronchiolitis caused by respiratory syncytial virus, or relentlessly progressive and fatal, as in the bronchiolitis obliterans syndrome occurring after lung transplantation.

BRONCHIECTASIS

Definition and Epidemiology

Bronchiectasis is defined as an abnormal dilation of the bronchi (the large airways containing cartilage within their walls) resulting from inflammation and permanent destructive changes of the bronchial walls. The incidence of bronchiectasis is unknown, but it may affect more than 100,000 individuals in the United States and is more frequent in older age groups. There is likely a higher incidence of bronchiectasis in developing countries where there are lower childhood vaccination rates and a higher prevalence of pulmonary tuberculosis.

Pathology

Bronchiectasis may be localized to a bronchial segment or lobe of the lung, or it may be diffuse. The involved bronchi are abnormally dilated and demonstrate chronic inflammation within the bronchial wall with neutrophilic inflammation and bacterial colonization and infection in the bronchial lumen. The inflammation in bronchiectasis is associated with structural changes in the walls of the bronchi, including destructive changes affecting the elastic fibers, smooth muscle, and cartilage. As with COPD, there is also involvement of the small airways. Small airway obstruction leads to increased resistance to airflow that results in airflow obstruction despite the dilation of the larger airways. The classic pathologic classifications of bronchiectasis are *tubular* (the most common form, in which there is smooth dilation of the bronchi), *varicose* (dilated bronchi with indentations reminiscent of varicose veins), and *cystic* (end-stage bronchiectasis with dilated bronchi ending in sac-like structures resembling clusters of grapes).

Bronchiectasis is hypothesized to result from an environmental insult leading to bronchial damage in a susceptible host. This in turn leads to impaired infection clearance, bacterial colonization and infection or reinfection, ongoing inflammation of the airways, and further bronchial damage, creating a classic vicious cycle. An inciting infection, sometimes occurring in childhood, is thought to initiate the development of bronchial damage leading to bronchiectasis in many cases (postinfectious bronchiectasis). This may be a viral infection (e.g., measles), a necrotizing pneumonia (e.g., *Staphylococcus aureus* pneumonia), tuberculosis, or infection with an atypical mycobacteria (e.g., *Mycobacterium avium-intracellulare*). Because infections such as *M. avium-intracellulare* also complicate the course of bronchiectasis, determination of whether a mycobacterial infection was an initiator or a consequence of bronchiectasis may be difficult.

Localized bronchiectasis may also result from anatomic obstruction by an endobronchial foreign body, tumor, or broncholith or from extrinsic compression by lymphadenopathy. Right middle lobe syndrome, for example, results from narrowing of the right middle lobe bronchial orifice, often by lymph node enlargement in the setting of tuberculosis, which leads to localized bronchiectasis distal to the site

狭窄）、滤泡性细支气管炎（形成大量淋巴样滤泡，紧贴小气道，导致气道压迫）、闭塞性或缩窄性细支气管炎（小气道周围的纤维化导致受累气道变窄）和闭塞性细支气管炎（形成腔内纤维病变，有时称为 Masson 小体，阻塞小气道管腔）。小气道病变的组织病理学可能提示其基础疾病；例如，滤泡性细支气管炎通常（尽管不限于）见于干燥综合征。

临床表现

一般来说，细支气管疾病临床表现为呼吸困难，并不特异，呼吸困难可能较严重或呈进行性加重，有时伴咳嗽或咳痰。体格检查可能会提示吸气性哮鸣音，但也可能出奇地正常。在特定情况下，应考虑细支气管疾病的可能性，如类风湿关节炎、干燥综合征或炎症性肠病可能并发细支气管疾病。

弥漫性泛细支气管炎是一种罕见的特发性疾病，在日本最常见，其特征是咳嗽、咳脓痰、鼻窦炎和呼吸困难，易反复并发呼吸道细菌感染（如铜绿假单胞菌）。

闭塞性细支气管炎（除了是一个组织病理学定义外）也是一种临床综合征，与肺移植后的慢性同种异体移植物排斥反应、同种异体造血干细胞移植后的移植物抗宿主病（GVHD）和职业毒素暴露有关。例如，有报道暴露于双乙酰（一种用于制造微波爆米花的调味化学品）的闭塞性细支气管炎职业聚集性病例。闭塞性细支气管炎亦可见于在伊拉克或阿富汗暴露于焚烧坑的退伍军人。

诊断和鉴别诊断

细支气管疾病在肺功能检查中通常表现出呼气相气流受限的阻塞性通气功能障碍，且不具备可逆性证据。闭塞性细支气管炎综合征（BOS）的临床诊断要求肺移植后连续检测的 FEV_1 较稳定基线值下降 20%。HRCT 在细支气管疾病的诊断和评估中很有价值。HRCT 特征性表现包括小叶中心结节或树芽征，反映了细支气管中炎性渗出物或脱落上皮细胞的嵌塞。吸气相 CT 常出现"马赛克"征，即呈现地图样密度下降，反映阻塞的细支气管远端存在气体陷闭区域。呼气相 CT 则可以证实形成病灶的原因为空气潴留，而不是由肺血管疾病引起的灌注下降。肺活检价值有限，因为细支气管疾病常呈散在、斑片状分布。鉴别诊断包括慢阻肺病，慢阻肺病的肺通气功能检查同样表现为阻塞性通气功能障碍，几乎不具备可逆性。

治疗

细支气管疾病的治疗很有难度。急性细支气管炎通常无需治疗即可恢复，处方上常用的支气管扩张剂和糖皮质激素其实并无明显获益。闭塞性细支气管炎综合征对免疫抑制剂反应不佳，且是肺移植后常见的死因。有研究报道阿奇霉素有助于闭塞性细支气管炎综合征患者 FEV_1 提高。另有研究报道大环内酯类抗生素对弥漫性泛细支气管炎的临床病程有改善作用，可能反映了上述药物的免疫调节或抗纤维化作用。进展的闭塞性细支气管炎患者可能需要肺移植。而肺移植术后患者发生排斥反应且出现闭塞性细支气管炎综合征时，有时会进行二次移植。

预后

这些疾病可能是自限性的，如呼吸道合胞病毒引起的急性细支气管炎，也可能是持续进展甚至致命的，如肺移植后发生的闭塞性细支气管炎综合征。

支气管扩张症

定义和流行病学

支气管扩张症被定义为支气管（气道壁含有软骨的大气道）的异常扩张，由支气管壁炎症及永久性破坏性变化引起。支气管扩张症的发生率尚不清楚，但在美国可能有超过 100 000 人发病，并且在老年群体中更常见。在儿童疫苗接种率较低、肺结核患病率较高的发展中国家，支气管扩张症的发病率可能更高。

病理学

支气管扩张症可能局限于支气管段或肺叶，也可能呈弥漫性分布。受累支气管异常扩张，支气管壁内出现慢性炎症，伴有中性粒细胞炎症、细菌定植以及支气管腔内感染。支气管扩张症的炎症与支气管壁的结构变化有关，包括弹性纤维、平滑肌和软骨的结构毁损。与慢阻肺病一样，小气道也受累。小气道阻塞导致气流阻力增加，尽管较大的气道呈现扩张，但总体仍会导致气流阻塞。支气管扩张症的经典病理分类是管状（最常见的形式，支气管平滑扩张）、串珠状（扩张的支气管存在凹陷，让人联想到静脉曲张）和囊状（终末期支气管扩张，支气管呈现葡萄串般的囊状结构）。

据推测，支气管扩张症起源于环境刺激诱发易感宿主的支气管损伤。这反过来又导致感染清除受损、细菌定植、感染或再感染、气道持续炎症以及支气管进一步损伤，形成典型的恶性循环。感染（有时发生在儿童期）会引发支气管损伤的发展，常常导致支气管扩张（感染后支气管扩张症），可能来源于病毒感染（如麻疹）、坏死性肺炎（如金黄色葡萄球菌肺炎）、结核病或非典型分枝杆菌感染（如鸟胞内分枝杆菌感染）。像鸟胞内分枝杆菌等病原引起的感染会使支气管扩张症的病程复杂化，很难确定分枝杆菌感染是支气管扩张的起因还是结果。

局限性支气管扩张也可能由解剖学阻塞引起，阻塞原因包括支气管内异物、肿瘤、支气管结石，或淋巴结肿大外压。例如，右中叶综合征是由右中叶支气管口狭窄引起的，通常是由于结核病情况下淋巴结肿大所致，这会导致该阻塞部位远端的局限性支气管扩

of obstruction. Anatomic obstruction results in chronic or recurrent bacterial infections and inflammation leading to bronchial distortion and destruction over time.

Diffuse bronchiectasis can result from various impairments in host defenses that create a vulnerability to persistent or recurrent lung infection leading to bronchial damage. For example, bronchiectasis may occur with congenital defects that impair mucus clearance in the airways such as CF (discussed later) or primary ciliary dyskinesia, a rare inherited abnormality of the ciliary microtubules (the classic triad of sinusitis, situs inversus, and infertility is diagnostic of Kartagener's syndrome, a form of primary ciliary dyskinesia). Immunodeficiency states, such as hypogammaglobulinemia in combined variable immunodeficiency, may also result in bronchiectasis. α_1-Antitrypsin deficiency is also associated with bronchiectasis. Bronchiectasis also complicates certain connective tissue disorders such as rheumatoid arthritis.

Finally, bronchiectasis overlaps with the more common obstructive lung disorders, COPD and asthma. Certain patients with COPD also have bronchiectasis, often in the lower lobes. Allergic bronchopulmonary aspergillosis is a condition that occurs in asthmatics with hypersensitivity to aspergillus fungi. It is associated with central bronchiectasis, high levels of immunoglobulin E (IgE), and precipitins for *Aspergillus* species.

Clinical Presentation

Patients with bronchiectasis exhibit chronic cough and copious, sometimes foul-smelling sputum. The sputum produced may be greater in volume and purulence than with COPD or asthma. Shortness of breath and fatigue may also be present. Blood-streaked sputum is common, and massive hemoptysis may occur during the course of bronchiectasis. Localized crackles and clubbing may be present. Periodic exacerbations due to infection with bacterial pathogens, including *H. influenzae* and *P. aeruginosa*, are common. Nontuberculous mycobacterial colonization or infection may also occur. Pulmonary function tests typically show mild to moderate obstruction. Evidence of bronchial hyperresponsiveness may occur.

Diagnosis and Differential Diagnosis

Chest radiographs may be normal or may show increased interstitial markings. The classic finding is parallel lines in peripheral lung fields, described as "tram tracks," which represent thickened bronchial walls that do not taper from proximal to distal sites. However, HRCT is more sensitive for the detection of dilated airways and is the diagnostic test of choice in the evaluation of suspected bronchiectasis. Bronchiectasis on HRCT is diagnosed by demonstration of lack of airway tapering, airways that are larger in diameter than their accompanying blood vessel, and the presence of visible bronchi at the lung periphery (outer 1 to 2 cm of the lung). Bronchoscopy may be indicated in localized bronchiectasis to assess for endobronchial abnormalities or foreign body. Sputum can be cultured to assess for fungal or mycobacterial organisms that may be causative or for identification of specific bacterial pathogens during exacerbations. Once the diagnosis of bronchiectasis is established, investigation to determine the underlying cause, such as assessment of immunoglobulin levels to rule out combined variable immunodeficiency, is indicated.

The differential diagnosis includes chronic bronchitis and COPD, asthma, and, in the setting of hemoptysis and clubbing, lung cancer.

Treatment

Treatment of the underlying cause of the bronchiectasis should be undertaken if possible. An anatomic obstruction, such as from a foreign body or benign tumor, should be relieved. Atypical mycobacterial infection should be treated with an appropriate multidrug regimen in symptomatic patients after confirmation of the diagnosis with multiple smears and cultures. Allergic bronchopulmonary aspergillosis is typically treated with corticosteroids; addition of azole antifungals may also be beneficial. Bacterial exacerbations of bronchiectasis should be treated with a broad-spectrum antibiotic that is effective against the likely pathogens, such as amoxicillin or, in patients known to be colonized or infected by *Pseudomonas*, a fluoroquinolone. Aerosolized antibiotics are of benefit to suppress bacterial growth in bronchiectasis associated with CF and may be beneficial in non-CF bronchiectasis if *Pseudomonas* infection is present or if frequent exacerbations occur. Chronic administration of macrolide antibiotics has been shown to reduce inflammation and exacerbations in bronchiectasis but may also promote development of macrolide-resistant bacteria. Immunoglobulin supplementation may aid in the host defense against bacterial infection in individuals with hypogammaglobulinemia.

Airway clearance and postural drainage are the mainstays of treatment in bronchiectasis (discussed in further detail under CF). Bronchodilators may provide symptomatic relief. Massive hemoptysis should be managed with airway protection and identification of the bleeding site; bronchial artery angiography with embolization of the causative bleeding vessels can be life-saving. The role of surgery is mainly in resection of obstructing lesions that are causing distal bronchiectasis, in removal of a badly damaged isolated segment of bronchiectatic lung, and, on occasion, as a salvage therapy in resection of a site with uncontrolled hemorrhage.

Prognosis

The prognosis of patients with bronchiectasis is generally thought to be favorable, although deterioration of lung function over time has been shown to occur. Quality of life may be affected adversely, for example by chronic production of copious sputum or frequent exacerbations. Massive hemoptysis is an emergency situation that requires intensive management and may be fatal.

CYSTIC FIBROSIS

Definition and Epidemiology

CF is an autosomal recessive genetic disorder that results from mutations in the *CFTR* gene. CF affects about 30,000 children and adults in the United States and 70,000 worldwide. This disorder affects many organs, including the lungs, pancreas, and reproductive organs, although most mortality related to CF is due to lung disease. It is the most common lethal genetic disorder in the Caucasian population, with a carrier frequency of about 1 in 29, affecting 1 in 3300 live births. About 1000 new cases of CF are diagnosed each year. Although 75% of patients with CF are diagnosed during their first two years of life, some patients are not diagnosed until adulthood. The prognosis has improved significantly with recent advances in therapy. Before 1940, infants with CF rarely lived to their first birthday, but today more than half of the CF population in the United States is older than 18 years of age. Currently, the median predicted life span for a person with CF is about 37 years.

Pathology

CF results from pathogenic mutations in both alleles of a single gene, *CTFR*, which encodes the CF transmembrane conductance regulator (CFTR), a cAMP-regulated chloride channel that is present on the apical surface of epithelial cells. The most common mutation is the ΔF508 mutation, a three-base-pair deletion that results in absence of the phenylalanine residue at the 508 position of the protein. However, more than 1900 mutations in CFTR have been identified to

张。解剖梗阻会导致慢性或复发性细菌感染和炎症，导致支气管变形和破坏。

弥漫性支气管扩张症可由宿主防御系统的各种损伤引起，这些损伤容易导致持续性或复发性肺部感染，从而导致支气管损伤。支气管扩张症可能继发于先天性缺陷，这些缺陷会损害气道中的黏液清除，例如囊性纤维化（详见后文）或原发性纤毛运动障碍，后者是一种罕见的纤毛微管遗传性异常（鼻窦炎、内脏转位、不孕症的经典三联征可诊断为 Kartagener 综合征，属于原发性纤毛运动障碍的一种）。免疫缺陷状态，例如普通变异型免疫缺陷病中的低丙种球蛋白血症，也可导致支气管扩张。α1- 抗胰蛋白酶缺乏也与支气管扩张症有关。支气管扩张症还会并发于某些结缔组织病，如类风湿关节炎。

最后，支气管扩张症可与更常见的阻塞性肺疾病、慢阻肺病和哮喘重叠。某些慢阻肺病患者也合并支气管扩张，常见于下肺叶。变应性支气管肺曲霉病（ABPA）发生于对曲霉菌过敏的哮喘患者中，表现为中央型支气管扩张、免疫球蛋白 E（IgE）水平升高和产生曲霉菌沉淀素。

临床表现

支气管扩张症患者表现为慢性咳嗽、大量咳痰，可伴恶臭气味。其产痰的量和脓性程度要比慢阻肺病或哮喘患者更多，可伴有气促和疲劳。痰中带血很常见，在支气管扩张发展过程中甚至可能发生大量咯血。可有局部湿啰音和杵状指。由于细菌病原体（包括流感嗜血杆菌和铜绿假单胞菌）感染导致的周期性加重很常见。也可能发生非结核性分枝杆菌定植或感染。肺功能检查通常显示轻中度阻塞，可能出现气道高反应的证据。

诊断和鉴别诊断

胸部 X 线片可能正常或显示间质纹理增加。典型表现是外周肺野中的平行线，称为"轨道征"（tram tracks），反映了支气管壁的增厚，以及支气管从近端到远端不能逐渐变细。然而，HRCT 对扩张的气道更敏感，是疑似支气管扩张症患者的首选诊断性检查。HRCT 下支气管扩张症的诊断依据是气道不能逐渐变细、气道直径大于伴随的血管，以及肺外周（胸膜下 1～2 cm 范围内）存在可见的支气管。支气管镜检查适应证包括局限性支气管扩张症，以评估支气管内异常或异物。痰培养可以评估致病的真菌或分枝杆菌，或在急性加重期间鉴定细菌病原体。一旦确诊支气管扩张症，就需要进一步查找基础病因，包括检查免疫球蛋白水平以除外联合变异型免疫缺陷病。

鉴别诊断包括慢性支气管炎、慢阻肺病、哮喘，对于有咯血和杵状指者还需要除外肺癌。

治疗

治疗要针对引起支气管扩张症的基础病因开展，应当解除异物或良性肿瘤等引起的解剖学梗阻。对于有症状的非典型分枝杆菌感染患者，在通过多次涂片和培养明确诊断后，应选用适当的多药联合方案。变应性支气管肺霉病常用糖皮质激素，加用唑类抗真菌药也可能获益。由细菌感染引起的支气管扩张症急性加重应当使用能有效覆盖可能病原的广谱抗生素，如阿莫西林，对于已知存在假单胞菌定植或感染的患者，应使用氟喹诺酮类药物。雾化抗生素有助于在囊性纤维化相关支气管扩张症中抑制细菌生长，如果存在假单胞菌感染或频繁的急性加重，则可能还有益于非囊性纤维化支气管扩张症。长期服用大环内酯类抗生素已被证明可以减轻支气管扩张症患者的炎症状态、减少急性加重，但也可能促进细菌对大环内酯类耐药。对于低丙种球蛋白血症患者，补充免疫球蛋白有利于宿主防御细菌感染。

气道清洁和体位引流是支气管扩张症的主要治疗手段（详见囊性纤维化一节）。支气管扩张剂可缓解症状。大咯血应进行气道保护和出血部位识别；通过支气管动脉造影对出血血管进行栓塞可以挽救生命。手术的作用主要包括切除引起远端支气管扩张的梗阻性病变、切除病损严重的支气管扩张的孤立肺段，以及作为挽救性治疗手段以切除无法控制出血的部位。

预后

支气管扩张症患者预后普遍较好，尽管随时间推移，肺功能恶化。长期大量咳痰或频繁急性加重可能导致生活质量受到不良影响。大咯血作为急症可致命，需要重症监护治疗。

囊性纤维化

定义和流行病学

囊性纤维化（CF）是一种常染色体隐性遗传病，由 CFTR 基因突变引起。在美国约有 30 000 名儿童和成人患 CF，在全世界约有 70 000 名儿童和成人患 CF。CF 影响许多脏器，包括肺、胰腺和生殖器官，不过大多数与囊性纤维化相关的死亡来自肺病。CF 是高加索人群中最常见的致命遗传病，携带频率约为 1/29，在活产新生儿中发病率为 1/3300。每年约确诊 1000 例新发 CF 病例。尽管 75% 的 CF 患者在出生后的前两年内能诊断，但有些人直到成年后才确诊。随着治疗手段的新进展，预后已显著改善。在 1940 年之前，患有 CF 的婴儿很少能活到 1 岁，但今天美国一半以上的 CF 患者年龄超过 18 岁。目前，CF 患者的预测寿命中位数约为 37 年。

病理学

CF 是由单基因 CTFR 的两个等位基因的致病突变引起的，CTFR 基因编码 CF 跨膜传导调节因子（CFTR），CFTR 是一种 cAMP 调节的氯离子通道，存在于上皮细胞的顶端表面。最常见的突变形式是 ΔF508 突变，这是一种三碱基对缺失，导致蛋白质 508 位缺乏苯丙氨酸残基。目前已发现 CFTR 中有 1900 多种突变。这些突

date. These mutations are categorized into five different classes based on their effects on CFTR. Class I and II mutations result in CFTR that is not present on the cell surface due to impaired translation or protein misfolding. Class III and IV mutations are associated with CFTR that is present on the cell surface but has abnormal function due to a gating defect or decreased conductivity. Class V mutations are associated with reduced expression of normally functioning CFTR.

Abnormal, reduced, or absent CFTR protein results in defective chloride transport and increased sodium reabsorption in airway and ductal epithelia; this leads to abnormally thick and viscous secretions in the respiratory, hepatobiliary, gastrointestinal, and reproductive tracts. The thick secretions do not easily clear from the airways, resulting in respiratory symptoms, and cause luminal obstruction and destruction of exocrine ducts in other organs, leading to exocrine organ fibrosis and dysfunction, including pancreatic damage.

Poor airway clearance predisposes CF patients to recurrent bacterial infection and eventual colonization with microorganisms such as *S. aureus* and *H. influenzae,* followed by *P. aeruginosa* in ensuing years. Persistent inflammation and infection cause bronchial wall destruction and bronchiectasis. Mucus plugging of small airways results in postobstructive cystic bronchiectasis and parenchymal destruction, progressive airflow obstruction, and eventually hypoxemia. The course of CF may additionally be complicated by the development of allergic bronchopulmonary aspergillosis or by nontuberculous mycobacterial infection. Colonization and infection with multidrug-resistant organisms such as the *Burkholderia cepacia* complex may occur in advanced CF, creating challenging management issues. The most common cause of death in CF is respiratory failure.

Clinical Presentation

Neonatal screening programs for CF exist nationwide in the United States to identify infants with possible CF who should undergo further testing (e.g., genotyping). Infants with CF may have meconium ileus or failure to thrive with steatorrhea. Salty-tasting skin may be noticed by caregivers. Patients with CF typically have chronic cough with thick sputum production, wheezing, and dyspnea. Pancreatic insufficiency and diabetes are common, and male patients may have azoospermia. Nasal polyps are often present, and clubbing is typical.

CF should be considered in the differential diagnosis of patients with unexplained chronic sinus disease, bronchiectasis, pancreatitis, malabsorption, or male infertility associated with absence of the vas deferens. Pulmonary function tests demonstrate hyperinflation and obstruction, with or without a bronchodilator response. Chest imaging studies show hyperinflation, bronchial wall thickening, and bronchiectasis.

Diagnosis and Differential Diagnosis

Measurement of the concentration of chloride in sweat (sweat test) is used to diagnose CF. The diagnosis is considered definitive if the clinical picture is consistent with CF and if the chloride concentration measured in a certified laboratory is greater than 60 mEq/L on at least two occasions. Genotyping can also confirm the diagnosis if known mutations are identified in both gene alleles and may be used if sweat testing is equivocal.

Treatment

The hallmark of CF treatment is aggressive airway hygiene. A typical airway clearance routine includes a series of therapies in the following order: First, patients use bronchodilators such as albuterol or ipratropium. Next, patients can use nebulized hypertonic (7%) saline to hydrate and loosen secretions, followed by aerosolized recombinant human deoxyribonuclease I (Dornase alfa) to decrease sputum viscosity. Then

patients should utilize a mechanical airway clearance technique. The specific technique is usually determined by patient preference. Available options include a vibratory vest, intrapulmonary percussive ventilation, or manual chest physiotherapy. The goal of the mechanical airway clearance techniques is to induce productive cough to clear mucous from the airways as much as possible. Lastly, patients can administer inhaled antibiotics (if applicable), such as tobramycin, colistin, or aztreonam, followed by inhaled steroids such as fluticasone propionate or budesonide.

Inhaled antibiotics are reserved for patients who are colonized with *Pseudomonas.* Inhaled tobramycin has been available as a nebulized solution since 1997 and as a dry powder inhaler since 2013. Inhaled tobramycin is typically prescribed as a 28-day course every other month. More recently, inhaled colistin and aztreonam have become available and can be used during tobramycin "off-months" or as alternatives to tobramycin if the patient is experiencing intolerable side effects or if their *Pseudomonal* resistance pattern warrants alternate therapy. Chronic anti-inflammatory therapy with azithromycin may be helpful in certain patients with CF.

Since 2012, there have been significant advancements in the treatment of CF due to the development of CFTR modulator drugs. As of 2019, there are three modulator therapies available, ivacaftor (Kalydeco®), lumacaftor/ivacaftor (Orkambi®), and tezacaftor/ivacaftor (Symdeko®). Ivacaftor is used in patients with class III genetic mutations. Ivacaftor binds CFTR causing the defective channel to remain open thus enabling chloride transport. In a large clinical trial, ivacaftor reduced sweat chloride by about 50%, increased FEV_1 by about 10%, and cut the incidence of pulmonary exacerbations in half. Ivacaftor can also be used in certain patients with class V mutations by increasing chloride transport through functioning CFTR to compensate for the reduced expression of these proteins.

Lumacaftor aids proper folding of CFTR and is used in combination with ivacaftor to treat patients who are homozygous for ΔF508 (class II mutation). Lumacaftor/ivacaftor was shown in clinical trials to improve FEV_1, increase BMI, and reduce pulmonary exacerbations. A common side effect of lumacaftor-ivacaftor is chest discomfort.

Tezacaftor can also be used in combination with ivacaftor in homozygous ΔF508 patients who cannot tolerate lumacaftor/ivacaftor due to side effects. In addition, tezacaftor/ivacaftor can also be used in patients with certain class II mutations other than ΔF508.

The first triple combination drug, Trikafta, was developed by adding elexacaftor to ivacaftor/tezacaftor. Trikafta was FDA approved in 2019 for patients with at least one ΔF508 mutation. It was shown to be superior to the other CF modulator therapies in improvement of lung function and quality of life as well as reduction in sweat chloride and frequency of exacerbations. As with other obstructive lung diseases, the ultimate therapy for patients with CF and end-stage lung disease is bilateral lung transplantation.

Prognosis

Although CF is still considered to be a fatal disease, significant advancements in therapy have led to considerable improvement in median survival time.

ASTHMA

Definition and Epidemiology

Asthma is described by the Global Initiative for Asthma as "a chronic inflammatory disorder of the airways in which many cells and cellular elements play a role. The chronic inflammation is associated with airway hyperresponsiveness that leads to recurrent episodes of wheezing, breathlessness, chest tightness, and coughing, particularly at night or in the early morning. These episodes are usually associated with

变根据它们对 CFTR 的影响分为五类。Ⅰ类和Ⅱ类突变导致 CFTR 由于翻译错误或蛋白质错误折叠而无法定位到细胞表面。Ⅲ类和Ⅳ类突变的 CFTR 可以存在于细胞表面，但由于门控缺陷引起电导率降低而发生功能异常。Ⅴ类突变与正常功能 CFTR 的表达量减少有关。

CFTR 蛋白异常、减少或缺失导致气道和导管上皮细胞中氯离子转运缺陷和钠重吸收增加；这会导致呼吸道、肝胆道、胃肠道和生殖道分泌物异常黏稠。黏稠的分泌物不易从气道中清除，引起呼吸系统症状、管腔阻塞和其他器官的外分泌管破坏，导致外分泌器官纤维化和功能障碍，包括胰腺损伤。

气道清洁不良使 CF 患者易反复发生细菌感染，并最终导致微生物定植，例如金黄色葡萄球菌、流感嗜血杆菌定植，随后数年又出现铜绿假单胞菌定植。持续炎症和感染会导致支气管壁破坏和支气管扩张。小气道黏液堵塞导致阻塞后囊性支气管扩张、肺实质破坏、气流阻塞进行性加重，最终导致低氧血症。囊性纤维化病程最终还可能因变应性支气管肺曲霉病或非结核分枝杆菌感染而复杂化。多重耐药微生物（如洋葱伯克霍尔德菌复合体）的定植和感染可能发生于晚期囊性纤维化患者，治疗难度高。囊性纤维化患者最常见的死因是呼吸衰竭。

临床表现

美国在全国范围内开展了囊性纤维化新生儿筛查计划，以识别应接受进一步检测（如基因分型）的可疑囊性纤维化婴儿。患有囊性纤维化的婴儿可能患有胎粪性肠梗阻或脂肪泻导致生长迟缓。照护者可能注意到孩子皮肤有咸味。囊性纤维化患者通常有慢性咳嗽，伴有痰液浓稠、喘息和呼吸困难。胰腺功能不全和糖尿病很常见，男性患者可能患有无精症。患者常伴有鼻息肉，杵状指也是十分典型的表现。

对于不明原因的慢性鼻窦疾病、支气管扩张症、胰腺炎、吸收不良或与输精管缺失相关的男性不育症患者，应考虑鉴别囊性纤维化。肺功能检查提示过度充气和阻塞性通气功能障碍，伴或不伴舒张试验阳性。胸部影像学提示过度充气、支气管壁增厚以及支气管扩张。

诊断和鉴别诊断

CF 诊断需要检测汗液氯化物浓度（汗液试验）。如果临床表现与 CF 一致，并且在得到认证的实验室中行氯浓度检测且至少分别两次超过 60 mmol/L，则可以确诊。如果在两个基因座等位基因中都发现了已知突变，基因分型也可以确诊，如果汗液检测结果不能明确诊断，则可以使用基因分型。

治疗

囊性纤维化治疗的重点是积极的气道清洁。典型的气道清洁程序包括一系列按以下顺序展开的治疗环节：首先，患者使用支气管扩张剂，如沙丁胺醇或异丙托溴铵。其次，采用高渗生理盐水雾化（7%）来水化和松解分泌物，接下来，使用雾化重组人脱氧核糖核酸酶Ⅰ（Domase alfa）以降低痰液黏度。然后，采用气道清洁手段，具体技术通常由患者的偏好决定。可选择振动背心、肺内叩击通气或人工胸部物理治疗。气道清洁技术的目标是诱导咳痰，以尽可能清除气道中的黏液。最后，可给予吸入性抗生素（如适用），如妥布霉素、黏菌素或氨曲南，接着使用丙酸氟替卡松或布地奈德等吸入用糖皮质激素。

吸入性抗生素仅适用于假单胞菌定植的患者。吸入用妥布霉素自 1997 年以来提供雾化剂型，自 2013 年以来提供干粉吸入剂型。吸入妥布霉素通常每间隔 1 个月处方 28 天疗程。最近已有可用的吸入性黏菌素和氨曲南，可以在妥布霉素的"非治疗月"期间使用。如果患者出现无法耐受的妥布霉素副作用，或者如果假单胞菌耐药谱导致需要更换药物，则吸入用黏菌素或氨曲南可以替代妥布霉素。此外，阿奇霉素的慢性抗炎治疗可能对某些囊性纤维化患者有益。

自 2012 年以来，由于 CFTR 调节剂的药物开发，CF 治疗取得了重大进展。截至 2019 年，有三种调节剂可用，依伐卡托（通用名 ivacaftor，商品名 Kalydeco®）、鲁玛卡托 / 依伐卡托（通用名 lumacaftor/ivacaftor，商品名 Orkambi®）和替扎卡托 / 依伐卡托（通用名 tezacaftor/ivacaftor，商品名 Symdeko®）。依伐卡托用于Ⅲ类基因突变患者，它结合 CFTR，使有缺陷的通道保持开放，从而实现氯离子转运。在一项大型临床试验中，依伐卡托将汗液氯化物减少了约 50%，将 FEV_1 增加了约 10%，并将肺病的急性加重发生率降低了一半。依伐卡托也可用于某些具有Ⅴ类突变的患者，通过增加有功能 CFTR 的氯离子转运，以弥补相关蛋白表达的降低。

鲁玛卡托有助于 CFTR 的正确折叠，并与依伐卡托联合用于治疗 ΔF508（Ⅱ类突变）纯合子患者。临床试验显示，鲁玛卡托 / 依伐卡托可改善 FEV_1、增加 BMI 并减少肺病的急性加重频率，其常见副作用是胸部不适。

替扎卡托也可用于因副作用而不能耐受鲁玛卡托 / 依伐卡托的 ΔF508 纯合子患者。此外，替扎卡托 / 依伐卡托也可用于 ΔF508 突变以外的某些Ⅱ类突变患者。

首款三联药物 Trikafta 的开发是通过在依伐卡托 / 替扎卡托中加入依来卡托（elexacaftor）而实现的。Trikafta 于 2019 年获得 FDA 批准，用于至少一种 ΔF508 突变的患者。在改善肺功能、生活质量、减少汗液氯浓度、降低急性加重频率方面，已被证明优于其他 CF 调节剂。与其他阻塞性肺疾病一样，囊性纤维化和终末期肺病患者的终极治疗方法是双侧肺移植。

预后

尽管囊性纤维化仍然是一种致命疾病，但治疗的重大进展已导致中位生存时间的显著改善。

widespread but variable airflow obstruction within the lung that is often reversible either spontaneously or with treatment."

The incidence of asthma is highest in children, but it affects all ages and occurs worldwide, with a preponderance of the disease in developed industrialized countries. Asthma affects millions of individuals worldwide. In the United States in 2017, 7.9% of the population (approximately 25,000,000 persons) were estimated to have asthma according to the Centers for Disease Control and Prevention. The prevalence of asthma has increased markedly over recent decades. Nevertheless, after rising in the late 20th century, the number of deaths from asthma has declined since 2000. Asthma death rates are higher in older age groups, females, and blacks.

Pathology

Underlying chronic airway inflammation is considered to be a major pathogenic feature of asthma. Patients with asthma have higher numbers of activated inflammatory cells within the airway wall, and the epithelium is typically infiltrated with eosinophils, mast cells, macrophages, and T lymphocytes, which produce multiple soluble mediators such as cytokines, leukotrienes, and bradykinins. Airway inflammation in asthma is typified by a type 2 helper T-cell (T_H2) response with predominantly eosinophilic inflammation, but some patients with severe asthma exhibit neutrophilic airway inflammation and cytokine production more characteristic of T_H1 inflammation.

The hallmark of asthma is airway hyperresponsiveness—a tendency of the airway smooth muscle to constrict in response to levels of inhaled allergens or irritants that would not typically elicit such a response in normal hosts. Inhaled allergens provoke airway mast cell degranulation by binding to and cross-linking IgE on the mast cell surface. Mast cell degranulation leads to the release of chemical mediators, which cause acute bronchoconstriction and thus increased airway resistance and wheezing as well as mucus hypersecretion. Disruption of the continuity of the ciliated columnar epithelium and increased vascularity and edema of the airway wall also follow antigen exposure. In addition to allergens, factors such as stimulation of irritant receptors, respiratory tract infections, and airway cooling can provoke bronchoconstriction in asthmatic individuals. Airway cooling appears to be responsible for exercise-induced bronchoconstriction as well as some wintertime asthma attacks.

Asthma is associated with airway wall remodeling, which is characterized by hyperplasia and hypertrophy of smooth muscle cells, edema, inflammatory infiltration, angiogenesis, and increased deposition of connective tissue components such as type I and type III collagen. This last effect leads not only to a thickening of the subepithelial lamina reticularis but also to an expansion of the entire airway wall. Airway remodeling may begin fairly early in the course of the disease. Whether inflammation leads to remodeling or whether these processes represent two independent manifestations of the disease is unknown. Pulmonary function does seem to decline at an accelerated rate in patients with asthma, and airway wall remodeling may play a role in this functional loss. Over time, airway wall remodeling may lead to irreversible airflow limitation, which can worsen the disease by rendering bronchodilator drugs less effective. In this way, airway wall remodeling may make the clinical distinction between asthma and COPD difficult.

The cause of asthma is unknown, but it is likely to be a polygenic disease influenced by environmental factors. Atopy is strongly linked to asthma. Exposure to indoor allergens such as dust mites, cockroaches, furry pets, and fungi is a significant factor; outdoor pollution and other irritants, including cigarette smoke, are also important.

Current concepts of asthma pathogenesis include a focus on impairment of the shift from a T_H2-predominant immunity to a T_H1

immune response early in life. Paradoxically, in the developed world, the perpetuation of T_H2 immune responses and the development of inappropriate allergic responses may be related to a relative lack of exposure of the immune system to appropriate infectious antigenic stimuli in childhood, the so-called hygiene hypothesis. Farming, for example, appears to be protective against the development of asthma and allergic disease, possibly in part because of the increased exposure to microbial antigens eliciting a T_H1 response. Increased exposure to other children (as in daycare settings) and less frequent use of antibiotics may also decrease asthma risk. On the other hand, asthma is common in poor urban settings in which there is heavy exposure to allergic antigens from dust mites and cockroaches. The timing and roles of particular environmental exposures in utero and in early life in the pathogenesis of asthma and allergic diseases remain to be fully elucidated, and there is no current theory that completely explains asthma pathogenesis or the recent increased incidence of asthma. The interplay of other aspects of modern life, such as changes in the microbiome, with regard to asthma propensity continues to be explored.

Several genetic polymorphisms have been associated with asthma, including variations in the β-adrenergic receptor leading to diminished responsiveness to β-agonists. Identification of other genetic polymorphisms that are important in asthma is a subject of ongoing research. Although asthma is more common in male children than in female children, the prevalence of asthma changes after puberty, and it is more common in adult women than in men. These facts, along with evidence of variation in asthma symptoms during the menstrual cycle and during pregnancy, suggest possible hormonal influences on asthma pathogenesis.

Asthma can be induced by workplace exposures in persons having no previous history of asthma (occupational asthma). Certain substances, such as isocyanates (used in spray paints) and Western red cedar wood dust, are provocative agents for the development of occupational asthma. Obesity has been linked to a higher incidence of asthma though the mechanisms by which obesity may influence asthma development remain unclear. Other potentiators of acute bronchospasm include viral infections, gastroesophageal reflux disease (GERD), and exposure to gases or fumes. These disorders may play a role in asthma development and may be targeted for therapy in some cases of asthma.

Clinical Presentation

Major symptoms of asthma are wheezing, episodic dyspnea, chest tightness, and cough. The clinical manifestations vary widely, from mild intermittent symptoms to catastrophic attacks resulting in asphyxiation and death. Although wheezing is not a pathognomonic feature of asthma, in the setting of a compatible clinical picture, asthma is the most common diagnosis. Often symptoms worsen at night or during the early hours of the morning. Other associated symptoms are sputum production and chest pain or tightness. Patients may exhibit only one or a combination of symptoms, such as chronic cough only (cough-variant asthma). Wheezing may occur several minutes after exercise (exercise-induced bronchoconstriction). Physical examination typically shows evidence of wheezing, although findings may be normal in between symptomatic periods. Rhinitis or nasal polyps may be present. In the case of an acute episode of bronchospasm or an exacerbation, the clinician may find that the patient has difficulty talking, is using accessory muscles of inspiration, has pulsus paradoxus, is diaphoretic, and has mental status changes ranging from agitation to somnolence. In patients with these findings, treatment should be immediate and aggressive.

哮喘

定义和流行病学

哮喘全球倡议（GINA）将哮喘描述为"一种慢性气道炎症性疾病"，许多细胞及细胞组分发挥作用。慢性炎症与气道高反应性有关，引起喘息、呼吸困难、胸闷和咳嗽等症状反复发作，尤其是在夜间或清晨。这些发作通常与肺内广泛而可变的气流阻塞有关，气流阻塞通常可自行逆转或给药后可逆。

哮喘的发病率在儿童中最高，但它影响到所有年龄段人群，并且在世界范围内发生，以发达的工业化国家占主导地位。哮喘影响着全世界数以百万计的人。根据美国疾病控制和预防中心（CDC）的数据，2017年美国估计有 7.9% 的人口（约 25 000 000 人）患哮喘。近几十年来，哮喘的患病率显著增加。哮喘死亡人数在 20 世纪后期先是上升，自 2000 年以来又有所下降。老年、女性和黑人的哮喘死亡率较高。

病理学

慢性气道炎症是哮喘的主要致病特征。哮喘患者气道壁内活化的炎症细胞数量较高，嗜酸性粒细胞、肥大细胞、巨噬细胞和 T 淋巴细胞浸润气道上皮，产生多种可溶性介质，如细胞因子、白三烯和缓激肽。哮喘的气道炎症的典型代表为 2 型辅助性 T 细胞（TH2）反应，主要表现为嗜酸性粒细胞炎症，但一些重度哮喘患者也表现出中性粒细胞性气道炎症和更具有 TH 1 型炎症特征的细胞因子谱。

哮喘的标志是气道高反应性，即气道平滑肌因吸入的一定量的过敏原或刺激物而收缩的倾向，而这些过敏原或刺激物通常不会在正常宿主中引起这种反应。吸入过敏原通过与肥大细胞表面的 IgE 结合并交联来引起气道肥大细胞脱颗粒。肥大细胞脱颗粒导致化学介质释放，引起急性支气管收缩，从而增加气道阻力并引起喘息，造成黏液高分泌。抗原暴露后，纤毛柱状上皮的连续性被破坏，气道壁的血管增多，水肿也随之而来。除过敏原外，刺激性受体接受刺激、呼吸道感染和气道遇冷等因素也会引起哮喘患者的支气管收缩。气道遇冷似乎是运动诱发支气管收缩以及一些冬季哮喘发作的原因。

哮喘与气道壁重塑有关，其特征是平滑肌细胞增生和肥大、水肿、炎症浸润、血管生成以及结缔组织成分（如 I 型和 III 型胶原）沉积增加。最后一种效应不仅导致上皮下网状层增厚，还导致整个气道壁的扩张。气道重塑可能在病程早期就启动了。尚不清楚炎症是否会导致重塑，抑或炎症与重塑是否代表了疾病的两种独立表现。哮喘患者的肺功能会加速下降，气道重塑可能在肺功能丧失中发挥作用。随时间推移，气道重塑可引起不可逆的气流受限，从而使支气管扩张剂的效果下降，进而使疾病恶化。因此，气道重塑可能会使哮喘和慢阻肺病二者不易鉴别。

哮喘病因尚不清楚，但它很可能是受环境因素影响的多基因疾病。特应性与哮喘密切相关。接触室内过敏原是一个重要因素，包括尘螨、蟑螂、带毛宠物和真菌；室外污染和其他刺激物也很重要，包括香烟烟雾。

目前哮喘发病机制所涉及概念包括生命早期从 TH2 主导免疫到 TH 1 免疫反应转变的损伤。矛盾的是，在发达国家，TH2 免疫反应的持续存在和不适当的过敏反应的发展可能与免疫系统在儿童时期相对缺乏暴露于适当的感染性抗原刺激有关，即所谓的卫生假说（hygiene hypothesis）。务农似乎可以防止哮喘和过敏性疾病的发展，部分原因可能是暴露于引起 TH 1 反应的微生物抗原的机会增加。增加与其他儿童的接触（如在日托环境中）和减少抗生素的使用频率也可能降低哮喘风险。另外，哮喘在贫穷的城市环境中很常见，在这些环境中，尘螨和蟑螂的过敏原大量暴露。尚不完全清楚子宫内和生命早期特定环境暴露的时机和作用如何参与了哮喘和过敏性疾病发病机制，目前尚无理论可以完全解释哮喘发病机制或近期哮喘发病率的增加。现代生活其他方面的相互作用亟待探索，例如微生物组的变化与哮喘倾向的相互作用。

几种遗传多态性与哮喘有关，包括 β 肾上腺素能受体的变异导致对 β 受体激动剂的反应减弱。目前有持续开展的研究旨在鉴定哮喘中其他重要的遗传多态性。虽然哮喘在男孩中比在女孩中更常见，但哮喘的患病率在青春期后发生变化，成年女性比男性更常见。这些事实，以及月经周期和怀孕期间哮喘症状变化的证据，表明激素可能对哮喘发病产生影响。

既往没有哮喘病史的人，如果发生工作场所暴露，可诱发哮喘（职业性哮喘）。某些物质，如异氰酸酯（用于喷漆）和西方红雪松木屑，可以诱发职业性哮喘。肥胖与哮喘发病率较高有关，但肥胖影响哮喘发展的机制尚不清楚。急性支气管痉挛的其他诱发因素包括病毒感染、胃食管反流病（GERD）以及气体或烟雾暴露。上述疾病可能在哮喘的发展中发挥作用，并可能在某些哮喘病例中成为治疗目标。

临床表现

哮喘主要症状是喘息、发作性呼吸困难、胸闷和咳嗽。临床表现差异很大，从轻微的间歇性症状到引起窒息和死亡的灾难性发作。虽然喘息并非哮喘所独有的临床表现，但若喘息在夜间或凌晨出现或加重，伴有咳嗽、胸闷或胸痛等症状，则哮喘是最常见的引起喘息的诊断。患者可能仅表现出一种或多种症状，例如仅有慢性咳嗽（咳嗽变异型哮喘），运动后几分钟出现喘息（运动诱发哮喘）。典型的体格检查异常表现为肺部哮鸣音，但在两次发作之间可以完全正常。可能合并鼻炎或鼻息肉。在支气管痉挛急性加重发作的情况下，临床医生可能发现患者说话困难、需要动用辅助吸气肌、出现奇脉、大汗淋漓，以及发生从躁动到嗜睡的精神状态改变。对于有上述表现的患者，应立即进行积极治疗。

Diagnosis and Differential Diagnosis

A diagnosis of asthma requires documentation of bronchial hyperreactivity and reversible airway obstruction. The history may provide sufficient documentation because most patients complain of characteristic periodic episodes of wheezing and other symptoms that respond to use of a bronchodilator. However, spirometry is recommended to assess formally for expiratory flow limitation, and reversibility is demonstrated by repeat spirometry after bronchodilator administration. At least 12% and 200 mL improvement in FEV_1 after bronchodilator use indicates reversibility. Because asthma is episodic, airflow limitation is variable and patients may exhibit symptoms at a time when spirometry cannot be performed. Peak expiratory flow measurements can be performed at home and may be helpful in establishing evidence of variability in expiratory flow.

Depending on the circumstances, formal testing for airway hyperactivity by bronchoprovocation challenge may be necessary. A stimulant with bronchoconstrictor activity, most commonly methacholine, is applied to the patient's airway. Methacholine, a synthetic form of acetylcholine, is preferred to histamine because there are fewer systemic side effects. Exercise can also be used to trigger an attack. Although most patients with or without asthma develop some degree of airflow limitation during bronchoprovocation testing, those with asthma develop airflow limitation at much lower doses. For a methacholine challenge, the concentration of methacholine required to produce a 20% decline in FEV_1 from baseline is reported. Although a positive bronchoprovocation challenge result is not by itself diagnostic of asthma, a negative result is helpful in ruling out asthma as a diagnosis.

Lung volume measurements may show hyperinflation during active disease, but the DLco is typically normal or even elevated. During acute exacerbations of asthma, analysis of arterial blood gases is useful to determine gas-exchange status. A chest radiograph should be obtained if a concern for pulmonary infection exists, but routine chest radiography is not necessary. Fleeting or migratory infiltrates on chest radiographs in a patient with difficult asthma should suggest the possibility of allergic bronchopulmonary aspergillosis. Blood tests in asthma might reveal eosinophilia and increased levels of IgE. Skin tests might be useful to identify household products or other antigens that could precipitate asthma attacks in a specific patient.

The differential diagnosis includes tracheal disorders, respiratory tract tumors and foreign bodies, COPD, and bronchiectasis. In patients whose primary presenting complaint is chronic cough, the differential diagnosis includes other causes of chronic cough, such as GERD and postnasal drip. A major differential consideration in patients not responding to typical asthma treatment is vocal cord dysfunction.

Treatment

Simple, inexpensive peak expiratory flow meters can be used at home to monitor airflow obstruction. A diary should be maintained, and a clear written plan should be in place for using symptoms and peak flow information to intervene early in exacerbations and to tailor long-term therapy for optimal control of symptoms. Short-acting β-agonists are used for acute relief of symptoms such as wheezing. However, the cornerstone of maintenance therapy in all but mild intermittent asthma is administration of inhaled corticosteroids, which are highly effective in improving asthma control. Long-acting β-agonists may be added for additional symptomatic control as needed. LABAs should not be used as a monotherapy for asthma control because they do not control airway inflammation and increased mortality has been demonstrated with this therapeutic approach. However, these medications may be added to inhaled corticosteroids to provide additional symptom control.

Alternatively, leukotriene modifiers can be used in maintenance therapy, although they appear to be somewhat less effective than inhaled corticosteroids (see Fig. 5.4). Theophylline preparations may have additional benefit in some patients, but the narrow therapeutic window and modest efficacy of this drug limits its value. Recent evidence suggests that use of long-acting anticholinergics in patients with poor control on LABAs and inhaled corticosteroids may increase the time to exacerbation and provide additional bronchodilation. Oral or intravenous corticosteroids are used during acute asthma exacerbations. Long-term use of oral corticosteroids should be avoided, if possible, given the various side effects associated with chronic glucocorticoid administration.

Patients with severe refractory asthma who frequently require systemic corticosteroids might benefit from a monoclonal antibody therapy. Targets of monoclonal antibodies include IgE (omalizumab), IL-5 (mepolizumab, reslizumab), and IL-4 (dupilumab). Patients with poorly controlled asthma are candidates for anti-IgE therapy if they have elevated total IgE levels and positive allergy skin or radioallergosorbent testing (RAST). Patients are candidates for anti-IL-5 or anti-IL-4 therapy if they have peripheral eosinophilia.

Allergen avoidance is a reasonable measure in asthma, although the effects of specific interventions, such as mattress barrier protection to reduce dust mite exposure, appear limited. Treatment of associated conditions that may exacerbate asthma, such as allergic rhinitis and GERD, may be clinically beneficial and may aid in achieving asthma control. Bronchial thermoplasty is a new endoscopic technique in which radiofrequency energy delivered in a series of treatments is used to destroy airway smooth muscle. It has been shown to reduce exacerbations and improve quality of life in the months following treatment.

Acute severe asthma, or status asthmaticus, is an attack of severe bronchospasm that is unresponsive to routine therapy. Such attacks may be sudden (hyperacute asthma) and can be rapidly fatal, often before medical care can be obtained. In most cases, however, patients have a history of progressive dyspnea over hours to days, with increasing bronchodilator use. Treatment of status asthmaticus should be aggressive, including administration of nebulized bronchodilators and intravenous steroids. Heliox can be used in severe causes of asthma, which is a mixture of oxygen and helium (typically 70% helium and 30% oxygen) that promotes laminar flow rather than turbulent flow of gas through the airways. Continuous monitoring of blood oxygen saturation by pulse oximetry should be performed, often supplemented by arterial blood gas analysis to evaluate for hypercarbia. A rising $Paco_2$ in a patient with asthma is an ominous sign and may portend need for ventilatory support. Noninvasive ventilation has been used successfully to decrease the work of breathing and avoid the need for endotracheal intubation in patients with exacerbations of asthma, but intubation and mechanical ventilation are necessary for the management of respiratory failure in status asthmaticus. Mechanical ventilation of the patient with status asthmaticus can be extremely challenging and may require the use of paralytic agents to control the breathing pattern or even use of inhaled general anesthesia to relieve bronchospasm. Lastly, if a patient is unable to maintain adequate oxygenation with maximal ventilator support, extracorporeal membrane oxygenation (ECMO) can be considered.

Prognosis

The prognosis in most patients with asthma is excellent. Although there is no cure, most patients can achieve appropriate control of their asthma.

诊断和鉴别诊断

哮喘的诊断需要气道高反应性和可逆性气流受限的证据。病史可能足够充分，因为大多数患者主诉为很有特点的发作性喘息以及其他对支气管扩张剂反应良好的症状。然而，仍然建议进行肺通气功能检查，正式评估呼气气流受限，并且在应用支气管扩张剂后重复检查肺通气功能来证明气流受限的可逆性。使用支气管扩张剂后，FEV_1 需至少改善 12% 比例且绝对值至少改变 200 ml，才表明可逆性。由于哮喘是发作性的，气流受限是可变的，患者可能在出现症状时无法行肺通气功能检测。因此采用居家呼气峰流速监测有助于证实呼气流量的可变性。

根据具体情况，可能需要通过支气管激发试验明确是否存在气道高反应性。试验要求让患者经气道吸入具有支气管收缩活性的刺激剂（最常见的是乙酰甲胆碱）。乙酰甲胆碱是乙酰胆碱的一种合成形式，较组胺更好，因其全身副作用较少。运动也可用于诱发哮喘发作。尽管大多数哮喘及非哮喘患者都会在支气管激发试验期间表现出一定程度的气流受限，但哮喘患者在低得多的剂量下就会出现气流受限。乙酰甲胆碱激发试验应当报告使 FEV_1 从基线下降 20% 所需的药物浓度。虽然支气管激发试验阳性结果本身并不能诊断哮喘，但阴性结果有助于除外哮喘。

在疾病活动期，肺容积检查可能提示过度充气，但 D_{LCO} 通常正常甚至升高。在哮喘急性加重期间，动脉血气分析有助于了解气体交换状态。如存在肺部感染问题，应行胸部 X 线片检查，但不需要常规进行。难治性哮喘患者胸部 X 线片上的短暂或游走性浸润影提示变应性支气管肺曲霉病。哮喘患者的血液检查可能提示嗜酸性粒细胞增多和 IgE 水平升高。皮肤点刺试验可用来识别诱发患者哮喘的日用品或其他抗原。

鉴别诊断包括气管疾病、呼吸道肿瘤和异物、慢阻肺病和支气管扩张症。对于主诉为慢性咳嗽的患者，鉴别诊断包括慢性咳嗽的其他原因，包括胃食管反流病、鼻后滴漏。对经典哮喘治疗无反应的患者而言，重点鉴别声带功能障碍。

治疗

简易、经济的呼气峰流速计可以用于居家监测气流阻塞。哮喘患者要写日记，并应制订明确的书面计划，利用症状记录和呼气峰流速数据，在哮喘急性加重的早期进行干预，并调整长期治疗以最佳地控制症状。短效 β 受体激动剂用于紧急缓解喘息等症状。然而，除轻度间歇性哮喘外，维持治疗必须给予 ICS，这在改善哮喘控制方面非常有效。可根据需要加用长效 β 受体激动剂以进一步控制症状。LABA 不应成为哮喘控制的单药方案，因为 LABA 不能控制气道炎症，并且 LABA 单药治疗已被证明会增加哮喘患者死亡率。

不过 LABA 可以和 ICS 联用，以更好地控制症状。

此外，白三烯调节剂也可用于维持治疗，尽管不如 ICS 有效（见图 5.4）。茶碱制剂可助于某些患者额外获益，但其因治疗窗窄和效果一般而不太有价值。最新研究表明，在 LABA/ICS 控制不佳的患者中应用 LAMA 可推迟急性加重发作，并进一步扩张支气管。哮喘急性发作可采用口服或静脉注射糖皮质激素。但因长期给药存在各种副作用，应尽量避免长期使用口服糖皮质激素。

频繁需要全身应用糖皮质激素的重度难治性哮喘患者可受益于单克隆抗体治疗。单克隆抗体的靶点包括 IgE（奥马珠单抗）、IL-5（美泊利单抗、瑞利珠单抗）和 IL-4（度普利尤单抗）。哮喘控制不佳的患者如果总 IgE 水平升高，伴有皮肤过敏试验或放射性变应吸附试验（RAST）阳性，则适合抗 IgE 单抗治疗。如果患者有外周血嗜酸性粒细胞增多症，则适合抗 IL-5 或抗 IL-4 单抗治疗。

避开过敏原是治疗哮喘的合理手段，但特定干预措施（如床垫屏障保护以减少尘螨暴露）的效果十分有限。针对可能加重哮喘的共病开展治疗，例如过敏性鼻炎和胃食管反流病，将产生临床获益并可能有助于实现哮喘控制。支气管热成形术是一种新的内镜介入技术，射频能量可以破坏气道平滑肌，有证据表明它可以减少治疗后几个月的急性加重并改善生活质量。

急性重度哮喘或哮喘持续状态是一种对常规治疗无反应的严重支气管痉挛状态。这种发作可能是突然的（超急性哮喘），并且可能在得到医疗救治前已迅速致命。然而，在大多数情况下，患者会有持续数小时或数日的进行性呼吸困难，不断增加支气管扩张剂的用量。对于哮喘持续状态应积极治疗，包括雾化支气管扩张剂和静脉注射糖皮质激素。氦氧混合气可用于治疗重度哮喘，氦氧混合气是氦气和氧气（通常为 70% 氦气和 30% 氧气的混合物），可促进气体以层流而不是湍流的方式通过气道。应持续监测血氧饱和度，采用动脉血气分析以评估高碳酸血症。哮喘患者出现 $PaCO_2$ 升高是一种不祥的征兆，提示需要通气支持。在哮喘急性加重患者中，无创通气已成功用于减少呼吸功并避免气管插管，但气管插管和机械通气对于哮喘持续状态呼吸衰竭的治疗仍然是必要的。哮喘持续状态患者的机械通气会很有难度，可能需要用到肌松剂来控制呼吸模式，甚至要用到吸入全身麻醉来缓解支气管痉挛。最后，如果患者无法在最大条件的呼吸机支持下维持足够氧合，可以考虑采用体外膜肺氧合（ECMO）。

预后

大多数哮喘患者的预后良好。虽然无法治愈，但大多数患者可以良好控制哮喘。

❖   For a deeper discussion on this topic, please see Chapter 81 ("Asthma"), Chapter 82 ("Chronic Obstructive Pulmonary Disease"), Chapter 83 ("Cystic Fibrosis"), and Chapter 84 ("Bronchiectasis, Atelectasis, Cysts, and Localized Lung Disorders") in *Goldman-Cecil Medicine*, 26th Edition.

SUGGESTED READINGS

Buist AS, McBurnie MA, Vollmer WM, et al: On behalf of the BOLD Collaborative Research Group: International variation in the prevalence of COPD (the BOLD Study): a population-based prevalence study, Lancet 370:741–750, 2007.

Burgel P-R, Bergeron A, de Blic J, et al: Small airways diseases, excluding asthma and COPD: an overview, Eur Respir Rev 22:131–147, 2013.

Decramer M, Janssens W, Miravitlles M: Chronic obstructive pulmonary disease, Lancet 379:1341–1351, 2012.

Global Initiative for Asthma: GINA report: global strategy for asthma management and prevention (updated 2012), Available at: http://www.ginasthma.org. Accessed August 29, 2014.

Global Initiative for Chronic Obstructive Lung Disease: Global strategy for the diagnosis, management, and prevention of chronic obstructive pulmonary disease (updated 2013), Available at: http://www.goldcopd.org. Accessed August 29, 2014.

Kim V, Criner GJ: Chronic bronchitis and chronic obstructive pulmonary disease, Am J Respir Crit Care Med 187:228–237, 2013.

King PT: The pathophysiology of bronchiectasis, Int J COPD 4:411–419, 2009.

McDonough JE, Yuan R, Suzuki M, et al: Small-airway obstruction and emphysema in chronic obstructive pulmonary disease, N Engl J Med 365:1567–1575, 2011.

Mogayzel PJ, Naureckas ET, Robinson KA, et al, and the Pulmonary Clinical Practice Guidelines Committee: Cystic fibrosis pulmonary guidelines: chronic medications for maintenance of lung health, Am J Respir Crit Care Med 187:680–689, 2013.

Pasteur MC, Bilton D, Hill AT: On behalf of the British Thoracic Society Bronchiectasis (Non-CF) Guideline Group: British Thoracic Society guideline for non-CF bronchiectasis, Thorax 65:i1–i58, 2010.

Ren CL, Morgan RL, Oermann C, et al: Cystic fibrosis pulmonary guidelines: use of cftr modulator therapy in patients with cystic fibrosis, Ann Am Thorac Soc, 2018.

❖ 有关此专题的深入讨论，请参阅 *Goldman-Cecil Medicine* 第 26 版第 81 章（"哮喘"），第 82 章（"慢性阻塞性肺疾病"），第 83 章（"囊性纤维化"）和第 84 章（"支气管扩张、肺不张、囊肿和局限性肺病"）。

推荐阅读

Buist AS, McBurnie MA, Vollmer WM, et al: On behalf of the BOLD Collaborative Research Group: International variation in the prevalence of COPD (the BOLD Study): a population-based prevalence study, Lancet 370:741–750, 2007.

Burgel P-R, Bergeron A, de Blic J, et al: Small airways diseases, excluding asthma and COPD: an overview, Eur Respir Rev 22:131–147, 2013.

Decramer M, Janssens W, Miravitlles M: Chronic obstructive pulmonary disease, Lancet 379:1341–1351, 2012.

Global Initiative for Asthma: GINA report: global strategy for asthma management and prevention (updated 2012), Available at: http://www.ginasthma.org. Accessed August 29, 2014.

Global Initiative for Chronic Obstructive Lung Disease: Global strategy for the diagnosis, management, and prevention of chronic obstructive pulmonary disease (updated 2013), Available at: http://www.goldcopd.org. Accessed August 29, 2014.

Kim V, Criner GJ: Chronic bronchitis and chronic obstructive pulmonary disease, Am J Respir Crit Care Med 187:228–237, 2013.

King PT: The pathophysiology of bronchiectasis, Int J COPD 4:411–419, 2009.

McDonough JE, Yuan R, Suzuki M, et al: Small-airway obstruction and emphysema in chronic obstructive pulmonary disease, N Engl J Med 365:1567–1575, 2011.

Mogayzel PJ, Naureckas ET, Robinson KA, et al, and the Pulmonary Clinical Practice Guidelines Committee: Cystic fibrosis pulmonary guidelines: chronic medications for maintenance of lung health, Am J Respir Crit Care Med 187:680–689, 2013.

Pasteur MC, Bilton D, Hill AT: On behalf of the British Thoracic Society Bronchiectasis (Non-CF) Guideline Group: British Thoracic Society guideline for non-CF bronchiectasis, Thorax 65:i1–i58, 2010.

Ren CL, Morgan RL, Oermann C, et al: Cystic fibrosis pulmonary guidelines: use of cftr modulator therapy in patients with cystic fibrosis, Ann Am Thorac Soc, 2018.

6

Interstitial Lung Diseases

Abhinav Kumar Misra, Matthew D. Jankowich, Barry S. Shea

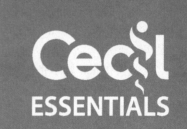

OVERVIEW

The interstitial lung diseases (ILDs) are a heterogenous group of non-malignant and noninfectious lung diseases characterized by varying amounts of inflammation and/or fibrosis (scarring) of the lung parenchyma. The lung involvement in these disorders is often diffuse but can occur in a wide array of patterns. The disease process can involve any part of the anatomic lung interstitium, including that within the alveolar walls, the intra- and interlobular septa, and the airways. However, it can also involve the air spaces and airway lumens themselves, and therefore the term *interstitial* lung disease is somewhat misleading. *Diffuse parenchymal* lung disease (DPLD) is the more accurate name for this collection of disorders, but for the sake of convention, we will refer to them as ILDs throughout this chapter.

Well over 100 distinct ILDs have been described, and there is no universally accepted classification system. One useful way of approaching ILDs is to consider them as all belonging to one of three broad categories: (1) exposure-related ILDs, (2) ILDs attributable to systemic diseases, and (3) idiopathic ILDs (Table 6.1). Exposure-related ILDs can be broadly thought of as those ILDs caused by environmental and occupational exposures (e.g., hypersensitivity pneumonitis, pneumoconiosis), iatrogenic exposures (e.g., drug-induced ILD, radiation pneumonitis or fibrosis), or intentional exposures (e.g., cigarette smoking, inhalational drug use). The most common systemic diseases known to cause ILD are the connective tissue diseases (e.g., rheumatoid arthritis, systemic sclerosis, and polymyositis/dermatomyositis), but there are many others, including the vasculitides, amyloidosis, sarcoidosis, and a variety of genetic conditions (e.g., lysosomal storage diseases). Idiopathic ILDs are those for which a specific cause is unknown or not identified. Most of the idiopathic ILDs fall into a group of clinicopathologic entities known as the idiopathic interstitial pneumonias (IIPs), but there are some additional isolated ILDs that are also idiopathic (e.g., eosinophilic PNA, pulmonary alveolar proteinosis).

TABLE 6.1 Categories of Interstitial Lung Diseases		
Idiopathic ILDs	**Exposure-Related ILDs**	**Systemic Disease-Associated ILDs**
Idiopathic interstitial pneumonias	Environmental and occupational exposures	Connective tissue diseases
Idiopathic pulmonary fibrosis (IPF)	Hypersensitivity pneumonitis (see Table 6.3)	Rheumatoid arthritis
Idiopathic nonspecific interstitial pneumonia (NSIP)	Pneumoconioses	Systemic sclerosis
Acute interstitial pneumonia (AIP)	Silicosis	Polymyositis and dermatomyositis
Cryptogenic organizing pneumonia (COP)	Asbestosis	Sjögren syndrome
Respiratory bronchiolitis–interstitial lung disease (RB-ILD)	Coal-worker's pneumoconiosis	Systemic lupus erythematosus
Desquamative interstitial pneumonia (DIP)	Berylliosis	Mixed connective tissue disease
Idiopathic lymphoid interstitial pneumonia (LIP)	Talc pneumoconiosis	Vasculitides
Idiopathic pleuroparenchymal fibroelastosis (IPPFE)	Hard metal pneumoconiosis	Granulomatosis with polyangiitis (GPA)
Eosinophilic pneumonia (acute and chronic)	Iatrogenic exposures	Microscopic polyangiitis (MPA)
Pulmonary alveolar proteinosis	Radiation-induced lung injury	Eosinophilic granulomatosis with polyangiitis (EGPA)
	Drug-induced lung injury (see Table 6.4)	Anti-glomerular basement membrane (anti-GBM) disease
	Antineoplastic therapies	Pauci-immune pulmonary capillaritis
	Biological agents	Sarcoidosis
	Cardiovascular drugs	Amyloidosis
	Antimicrobials	Lymphangioleiomyomatosis (LAM)
	Anti-inflammatory agents	Neurofibromatosis
	Intentional exposures	Hermansky-Pudlak syndrome
	Cigarette smoking	Inborn errors of metabolism
	Pulmonary Langerhans cell histiocytosis (PLCH)	Niemann-Pick disease
	Vaping associated pulmonary illness (VAPI)	Gaucher's disease
	Illicit drug use	
	"Crack lung"	
	Foreign body granulomatosis	
	Inhalational talcosis	

间质性肺疾病

黄慧 译 徐作军 代华平 审校 王辰 通审

概述

间质性肺疾病（ILD）是一组以肺实质不同程度的炎症和（或）纤维化（瘢痕形成）为主要表现的非肿瘤性和非感染性的异质性肺疾病。ILD 的肺部受累一般呈弥漫性分布，但可以有多种不同的表现；病变可累及包括肺泡壁、小叶内间质和小叶间隔以及气道在内的所有肺间质结构，此外还可累及肺泡和气腔，故在某种意义上"间质性肺疾病"这一称谓有一定的误导性，而弥漫性实质性肺疾病（DPLD）则更为准确，但为了方便起见，我们在本章中仍将其统称为 ILD。

虽然目前已命名了上百种 ILD，但尚无公认的分

类标准。其中较为实用的一种分类方法是将 ILD 分为三大类：①暴露相关 ILD；②系统性疾病相关 ILD；③特发性 ILD（表 6.1）。广义上，暴露相关 ILD 是指环境和职业暴露（如过敏性肺炎、尘肺病），医源性暴露（如药物相关性 ILD、放射性肺炎或纤维化）或有意暴露（如吸烟、吸入毒品）引起的 ILD。最常见的系统性疾病相关 ILD 是结缔组织病（如类风湿关节炎、系统性硬化症和多发性肌炎 / 皮肌炎），此外，还包括血管炎、淀粉样变性、结节病和遗传性疾病（如溶酶体贮积病）。特发性 ILD 是指其病因未明或未确定的 ILD，大多数特发性 ILD 属于特发性间质性肺炎（IIP），除此之外，还有一些其他特发性 ILD（如嗜酸粒细胞性肺炎、肺泡蛋白沉积症）。

表 6.1 间质性肺疾病分类

特发性 ILD	暴露相关 ILD	系统性疾病相关 ILD
特发性间质性肺炎	环境和职业暴露	结缔组织病
特发性肺纤维化（IPF）	过敏性肺炎（见表 6.3）	类风湿关节炎
非特异性间质性肺炎（NSIP）	肺尘埃沉着病	系统性硬化症
急性间质性肺炎（AIP）	硅沉着病	多发性肌炎及皮肌炎
隐源性机化性肺炎（COP）	石棉沉着病	干燥综合征
呼吸性细支气管炎相关间质性肺疾病（RB-ILD）	煤工肺尘埃沉着病	系统性红斑狼疮
脱屑性间质性肺炎（DIP）	铂肺	混合性结缔组织病
淋巴细胞性间质性肺炎（LIP）	滑石尘肺	血管炎
特发性胸膜肺实质弹力纤维增生症（iPPFE）	硬金属尘肺	肉芽肿性多血管炎（GPA）
嗜酸粒细胞性肺炎（急性和慢性）	医源性暴露	显微镜下多血管炎（MPA）
肺泡蛋白沉积症	放射相关性肺炎	嗜酸性肉芽肿性多血管炎（EGPA）
	药物相关性 ILD（见表 6.4）	抗肾小球基底膜（抗 GBM）病
	抗肿瘤药物	寡免疫性肺毛细血管炎
	生物制剂	结节病
	心血管类药物	淀粉样变性
	抗生素	肺淋巴管平滑肌瘤病（LAM）
	消炎药	神经纤维瘤病
	有意暴露	赫曼斯基-普德拉克综合征
	吸烟	遗传代谢病
	肺朗格汉斯细胞组织细胞增生症（PLCH）	尼曼-匹克病
	电子烟相关肺损伤（VAPI）	戈谢病
	违禁药物使用	
	"快克肺"	
	异物肉芽肿	
	吸入性滑石肺	

Because ILDs comprise a broad spectrum of disorders, the symptoms, exam findings, and physiologic, radiographic, and histologic abnormalities associated with them can vary greatly. Dyspnea on exertion and chronic cough are the two most common symptoms encountered in ILD patients, although these are nonspecific. These symptoms can often be insidious and progressive, and in many cases they can be present for months to years before a diagnosis is made. Exertional dyspnea can lead to exercise limitation, and in many cases patients, family members, and providers attribute such limitations to other factors, including aging, weight gain, and deconditioning. The presence of unexplained and gradually progressive dyspnea on exertion, with or without a persistent dry cough, should alert the clinician to the possibility of ILD. Other symptoms, such as wheezing, chest pain, hemoptysis, or constitutional symptoms are less common but can occur, and when present these symptoms may be clues to a specific diagnosis or class of ILDs. Most forms of ILD are chronic and progressive, but others can have more acute or subacute presentations and can be difficult to distinguish from infectious pneumonia. Waxing and waning symptoms can occur and are often associated with ILD caused by intermittent exposures. Some patients are asymptomatic and are diagnosed with ILD as an incidental finding on chest imaging done for other reasons (e.g., lung cancer screening).

Basic demographic factors such as age, sex, and race can provide some clues in determining potential causes of ILD. For example, idiopathic pulmonary fibrosis (IPF) is more common in men than in women and its incidence increases with age; it is only very rarely diagnosed in individuals under the age of 50 years. In contrast, connective tissue disease–associated ILD (CTD-ILD) tends to be more common in women and can occur often in young adults and even in the pediatric population. Inherited forms of ILD (Gaucher disease, Neiman-Pick disease) are also more likely in younger patients. Sporadic lymphangiomyomatosis (LAM) occurs almost exclusively in premenopausal women, sarcoidosis occurs more frequently in African Americans, and pulmonary Langerhans cell histiocytosis (LCH) is more common in young or middle-aged male smokers.

The history can further narrow the differential diagnosis for suspected ILD. Important factors to specifically query include rash, skin thickening, arthritis, myalgias or proximal muscle weakness, dysphagia, and Raynaud's phenomenon, any of which may suggest an underlying connective tissue disease. If a patient with ILD carries a known diagnosis of connective tissue disease, the work-up may be limited if imaging findings are typical of the pulmonary manifestations of that disease. A history of severe or poorly controlled asthma for a patient with radiographic infiltrates and constitutional symptoms should lead to consideration of eosinophilic granulomatosis with polyangiitis (EGPA), whereas a history of severe sinus disease should raise the possibility of granulomatosis with polyangiitis (GPA).

A detailed exposure history, including both domestic and occupational environmental exposures, is also important when evaluating a patient with ILD. For example, routine exposure to domestic birds, hot tubs, molds, or farming environments may suggest hypersensitivity pneumonitis. Home visits can also be informative here. Although the pneumoconioses due to asbestos and silica exposure are becoming much less common with modern safeguards and restrictions, these diseases continue to manifest long after exposure. High-technology manufacturing has particular hazards, such as beryllium exposure leading to berylliosis in susceptible individuals.

A medication exposure history is also important, and drug-induced ILD should be considered for all patients with diffuse lung disease seen on imaging. Smoking history is important because several ILDs are seen almost exclusively in cigarette smokers, including respiratory bronchiolitis–associated interstitial lung disease, desquamative interstitial pneumonia, and pulmonary LCH. Cigarette smoking and inorganic dust exposure also appear to be risk factors for the development of IPF. Acute and subacute ILD has also been described as a consequence of smoking or inhaling a variety of substances, including marijuana, synthetic cannabinoids, "crack" cocaine, and more recently electronic cigarettes.

Physical exam findings can also vary greatly. The most common finding is the presence of inspiratory crackles on lung exam, often most pronounced in the lung bases. Wheezing can be heard and can be a clue towards specific diagnoses (e.g., hypersensitivity pneumonitis), or it can be a sign of concomitant asthma or COPD. Some patients exhibit digital clubbing, focal enlargement of the terminal aspects of the fingers and/or toes with an unclear pathogenesis. Although this finding should prompt the clinician to suspect the presence of ILD, it can also be seen in other conditions, and it is of unknown significance. Exam findings of pulmonary hypertension with cor pulmonale (peripheral edema, loud P_2) can be seen in more advanced disease or can suggest the presence of a disorder known to cause both ILD and pulmonary vascular disease (e.g., systemic sclerosis). Similarly, extrapulmonary exam findings, such as synovitis, sclerodactyly, telangiectasias, mechanic's hands, muscle weakness, or lymphadenopathy can also provide important clues to a potential cause of ILD. In some cases the physical exam, including lung auscultation, can be entirely normal.

Pulmonary function testing (PFT) in ILDs generally reflects the pattern and severity of the disease process. Since most ILDs involve some combination of alveolar wall thickening and loss of functional air spaces, impaired gas exchange (reduced diffusion capacity for carbon monoxide, D_{LCO}) and evidence of restriction (reduced total lung capacity, TLC) are the most common abnormalities seen. The ratio of forced expiratory volume in 1 second to forced vital capacity (FEV_1/FVC) is generally preserved (i.e., no obstruction to airflow), although obstruction can also be seen when there is prominent airways involvement, such as with hypersensitivity pneumonitis, sarcoidosis, and lymphangioleiomyomatosis. An isolated reduction in the D_{LCO} may be the only obvious PFT abnormality in early or mild disease. In these cases the oxygen saturation may be normal at rest, but exercise oximetry may reveal the presence of exertional hypoxemia. Routine laboratory testing is often normal but some abnormalities, if present, can provide important clues to a specific diagnosis (e.g., peripheral eosinophilia, elevated serum creatinine). Detailed serologic testing to look for evidence of an underlying autoimmune or other systemic disease known to cause ILD is often performed.

Plain radiographs of the chest can provide evidence suggesting the presence of ILD, and in some cases can also help to establish a more definitive diagnosis, but high-resolution computed tomography (HRCT) of the chest provides much more detailed information and is almost always indicated in these cases. A variety of abnormalities can be seen on HRCT in ILD, including reticular, ground-glass, nodular, and consolidative opacities, mosaic attenuation, and honeycombing, and specific combinations and distributions of these abnormalities can often provide useful information when trying to determine a specific diagnosis. Certain HRCT patterns can often allow the diagnostic considerations to be significantly narrowed, and in some cases the HRCT pattern can be essentially pathognomonic for a particular disease. For example, a finding of bilateral, upper lung zone predominant peribronchovascular opacities with perifissural nodules and mediastinal and hilar lymphadenopathy would be highly suggestive of ILD due to sarcoidosis. Hypersensitivity pneumonitis (HP), pneumoconiosis, and lymphangioleiomyomatosis also tend to be upper lung zone predominant ILDs. Pulmonary LCH has a characteristic pattern of irregular nodules and thick-walled cysts in the mid to upper lung zones bilaterally, that when seen in a young-to-middle-aged active cigarette

　　由于 ILD 是一组疾病，所以患者的症状、体征、呼吸生理异常、胸部影像和肺组织病理表现的差异性变化很大。劳力性呼吸困难和慢性咳嗽是 ILD 最常见的、非特异性的临床表现；一般起病隐匿，可以在诊断 ILD 前数月甚至数年出现，但可呈进行性加重。劳力性呼吸困难可使患者活动受限，但患者、家属及照护者常会将此表现归咎于衰老、体重增加及失能等其他因素。所以，在患者出现不明原因的、逐渐加重的劳力性呼吸困难时，不论是否伴有干咳，临床医生均应警惕 ILD 的可能。喘息、胸痛、咯血或全身症状不常见，不过，一旦出现则常常是某些特殊类型 ILD 的提示。虽然大多数 ILD 呈现慢性、进行性加重的病程，但也有些 ILD 可表现为急性或亚急性病程，此时很难与肺部感染鉴别。部分患者症状波动，可见于间歇性暴露引起的 ILD；还有部分患者并无症状，是因其他原因（如肺癌筛查）行胸部影像学检查时偶然发现 ILD。

　　包括年龄、性别、种族等在内的基线流行病学史，对 ILD 的病因诊断有一定的提示意义。例如，特发性肺纤维化（IPF）男性多见，且随着年龄的增长发病率增加；50 岁以下人群少见。相反，结缔组织病相关 ILD（CTD-ILD）多见于女性、青年甚或儿童。遗传性 ILD（戈谢病、尼曼-匹克病）则多见于更小年龄的人群。散发性肺淋巴管平滑肌瘤病（LAM）几乎均见于绝经前女性，结节病多见于非裔美国人，而肺朗格汉斯细胞组织细胞增生症（LCH）则以吸烟的青中年男性多见。

　　病史询问有助于缩小 ILD 的鉴别诊断范围；对于 ILD 患者，需要注重包括皮疹、皮肤增厚、关节炎、肌痛或近端肌无力、吞咽困难及雷诺现象等表现的问询，因为任一上述表现均可能提示某些潜在的结缔组织病。对于已知病种的结缔组织病相关 ILD 患者，若胸部影像学呈现典型表现时，可以酌情减少进一步的辅助检查项目。难治性或控制不佳的哮喘患者，若同时有肺部浸润影及全身症状时需考虑嗜酸性肉芽肿性多血管炎（EGPA），但若有严重鼻窦炎的病史，则肉芽肿性多血管炎（GPA）的可能性更大。

　　在接诊 ILD 患者时，详细询问包括家庭居住环境和职业环境暴露在内的病史也很重要。例如，养鸟、热浴、霉菌或农作环境暴露等提示可能患过敏性肺炎。访视患者的居住环境也可能提示诊断。随着职业防护措施水平的提高，石棉和二氧化硅暴露导致的肺尘埃沉着病的患者明显减少，但此类疾病也可在暴露后很长一段时间后才发生。某些高科技材料暴露史也可为致 ILD 的危险因素，如某些敏感个体接触铍后会引起铍肺。

　　询问用药史也很重要，所有弥漫性肺疾病的患者均应常规排查药物相关性间质性肺疾病的可能。此外，询问吸烟史也很重要：某些 ILD，如呼吸性细支气管炎相关间质性肺疾病（RB-ILD）、脱屑性间质性肺炎

（DIP）及肺 LCH 几乎仅见于吸烟者（译者注：临床上少数 DIP、肺 LCH 患者可无吸烟史）；吸烟和无机粉尘暴露也可能是引起 IPF 的危险因素。吸烟、吸入某些物品（包括大麻、合成类大麻素、"快克"可卡因以及近年来的电子烟）可能引起急性和亚急性 ILD。

　　虽然肺底、吸气末爆裂音是最常见的体征，但不同 ILD 患者的体征也可以有很大差异：喘鸣音提示某些特殊疾病（如过敏性肺炎）或提示合并哮喘或慢阻肺病；一些患者可伴有杵状指，表现为发病机制不明的手指或足趾末端膨大。不过，虽然上述体征提示 ILD，但这些表现并非 ILD 患者所特有，也可出现在其他疾病中。P2 亢进及肢端水肿等肺动脉高压、肺源性心脏病的体征可见于终末期 ILD 患者，也可见于可以同时导致 ILD 和肺血管病变的疾病（如系统性硬化症）。滑膜炎、肢端硬化、毛细血管扩张、技工手、肌无力或淋巴结肿大等肺外表现也对诊断某些 ILD 有提示意义。不过，对于部分 ILD 患者而言，包括肺部听诊在内的体格检查结果可能完全正常。

　　ILD 患者的肺功能检测（PFT）常可以提示疾病的类型和严重程度。由于大多数 ILD 患者存在肺泡壁增厚和肺泡功能丧失，因此气体交换受损［一氧化碳弥散量（D_{LCO}）下降］和限制性通气功能障碍［肺总量（TLC）减少］是 ILD 患者最常见的肺功能受损表现。一般情况下，ILD 患者的一秒率（FEV_1/FVC）正常（即，无气流受限）；但在患者气道受累明显时，如过敏性肺炎、结节病和肺淋巴管平滑肌瘤病，也可能出现阻塞性通气功能障碍。早期或轻度 ILD 患者可仅仅表现为孤立性 D_{LCO} 减低，这些患者静息状态下氧饱和度可以正常，但运动时存在劳力性低氧血症。常规的化验检查一般无异常，但如果指标异常可为某些特殊疾病提供重要线索（如外周血嗜酸性粒细胞增多、血清肌酐升高等）。所以对 ILD 患者要常规安排详尽的血清学化验，以期明确可能导致 ILD 的自身免疫性疾病或其他系统性疾病。

　　虽然胸部 X 线片可提示患者可能存在 ILD，某些情况也可协助确诊，但胸部高分辨率 CT（HRCT）能提供更多、更详细的影像学信息。ILD 患者在胸部 HRCT 上可以有多种表现，包括网格影、磨玻璃影、结节影、实变影、马赛克征和蜂窝影；上述阴影的特定组合和分布特征可提示某些特定的 ILD 诊断。某些特定的 HRCT 表型可显著缩小 ILD 的鉴别诊断范围：例如，双上肺野为主的沿着支气管血管束分布的斑片影、叶间裂结节及肺门、纵隔淋巴结肿大提示结节病。此外，过敏性肺炎（HP）、肺尘埃沉着病、淋巴管肌瘤病的病变也往往以上肺分布为主。双侧中上肺野分布为著的不规则结节和厚壁囊腔影是肺 LCH 的特征性表现，故吸烟的青中年患者出现上述胸部 HRCT 表现时基本可以确诊肺 LCH。其他的 ILD，肺

smoker can be viewed as confirmatory of the diagnosis. Other forms of ILD are often more pronounced in the lower lung zones, and there can be other features that suggest different diagnoses (e.g., honeycombing with IPF and subpleural sparing with NSIP). The presence of bilateral calcified pleural plaques can be strongly suggestive of asbestosis as the cause of ILD.

In many cases of ILD, a definitive diagnosis can be made on the basis of the medical history, physical exam, laboratory and physiological testing, and HRCT, often in the context of a multidisciplinary approach. However, in some cases this information is insufficient, and a lung biopsy is needed to obtain a lung tissue sample for histologic evaluation. Surgical lung biopsy (SLB), typically using a thoracoscopic approach, is the preferred method for evaluating most forms of ILD. Bronchoscopic transbronchial lung biopsy (TBLB) is less invasive but yields much smaller fragments of tissue, typically too small to allow appropriate examination of the lung architecture. TBLB is not recommended for the assessment of suspected IPF and many other forms of chronic fibrosing ILD, but it can be useful for diagnosing certain ILDs, most notably sarcoidosis and HP. Transbronchial lung cryobiopsy, which is less invasive than SLB but provides larger samples of lung tissue than those obtained with TBLB, is currently in use in many centers, but its exact role in tissue diagnosis of ILD remains unclear.

The lung's response to injury is relatively stereotyped, and particular biopsy patterns of injury, such as usual interstitial pneumonia or granulomatous inflammation, are seen in a variety of disorders. Interpretation of lung biopsy results must be done in the appropriate context and with incorporation of clinical and imaging data. For example, a biopsy result of usual interstitial pneumonia may carry a different prognosis in the setting of rheumatoid arthritis–associated ILD than in the setting of IPF.

Management of ILD depends on the specific disease, and treatments appropriate to specific entities are discussed throughout this chapter. Historically, pharmacologic therapy has largely consisted of glucocorticoids and other immunosuppressive agents, an approach that seems to be effective for those ILDs with a significant inflammatory component but is of unclear benefit when fibrosis predominates. More recently, antifibrotics have been developed that appear to be effective at slowing the progression of IPF and some other chronic fibrotic ILDs. Other key aspects of ILD management include exposure avoidance (particularly for exposure-related ILDs, such as HP, smoking-related ILD, and drug-induced ILD), supplemental oxygen, and pulmonary rehabilitation. Lung transplantation can be performed in patients who have advanced disease that is expected to severely limit life expectancy, but unfortunately many patients are not candidates for lung transplant due to age or other comorbidities. Even then there is a scarcity of suitable donor lungs available such that every year many patients die while on lung transplant waiting lists.

The remainder of this chapter is organized around the three broad categories of ILDs described above: idiopathic ILDs, exposure-related ILD, and ILDs due to systemic diseases.

IDIOPATHIC INTERSTITIAL LUNG DISEASES

Idiopathic Interstitial Pneumonias

The idiopathic interstitial pneumonias (IIPs) are a group of ILDs of unknown origin, each of which has distinct clinicopathologic features. For several decades, these conditions were generally considered to be different variations of idiopathic pulmonary fibrosis (IPF). However, with growing appreciation that the different radiographic and histologic patterns of disease had distinct clinical presentations, natural histories, and responses to treatment, they were formally reclassified as IIPs by the American Thoracic Society (ATS) and European Respiratory

TABLE 6.2 Idiopathic Interstitial Pneumonias (IIPs)

Major IIPs	
Chronic fibrosing	Idiopathic pulmonary fibrosis (IPF)
	Idiopathic nonspecific interstitial pneumonia (NSIP)
Acute/Subacute	Cryptogenic organizing pneumonia (COP)
	Acute interstitial pneumonia (AIP)
Smoking-related	Respiratory bronchiolitis–interstitial lung disease (RB-ILD)
	Desquamative interstitial pneumonia (DIP)
Rare IIPs	Idiopathic lymphoid interstitial pneumonia (LIP)
	Idiopathic pleuroparenchymal fibroelastosis (IPPFE)
Unclassifiable IIP	

Society (ERS) in 2002. This classification scheme was updated in 2013, at which time these entities were divided into major IIPs, rare IIPs, and unclassifiable IIPs (Table 6.2). The 6 major IIPs are IPF, idiopathic nonspecific interstitial pneumonia (NSIP), respiratory bronchiolitis–associated interstitial lung disease (RB-ILD), desquamative interstitial pneumonia (DIP), cryptogenic organizing pneumonia (COP), and acute interstitial pneumonia (AIP), and these can be further characterized as chronic fibrosing IPs (IPF and NSIP), smoking-related IPs (RB-ILD and DIP), and acute/subacute IPs (COP and AIP) (see Table 6.2). Rare IIPs include idiopathic lymphoid interstitial pneumonia (LIP) and idiopathic pleuroparenchymal fibroelastosis (PPFE). Some patients have idiopathic interstitial lung disease that does not meet criteria for any of these entities, and they are considered to have unclassifiable IIP.

Idiopathic Pulmonary Fibrosis

Definition, epidemiology, and pathogenesis. IPF has been defined in a consensus statement as a "specific form of chronic, progressive fibrosing interstitial pneumonia of unknown cause, occurring primarily in older adults, limited to the lungs, and associated with the histopathologic and/or radiologic pattern of usual interstitial pneumonia (UIP)." It is the most common of the IIPs, with an estimated incidence of 16.3 per 100,000 person years and prevalence of 42.7 per 100,000 people in the United States as of 2000, which translates to an estimated 89,000 individuals in the United States living with IPF at that time. The incidence of IPF appears to be increasing worldwide. There are likely many factors contributing to this increasing incidence, and one factor may be the overall aging of the world's population. Age is the single biggest risk factor for IPF, as many studies have shown that the incidence and prevalence increases steadily during each decade of life. It is only rarely diagnosed before the age of 50 years. Cigarette smoking has also been strongly associated with the development of IPF, as up to two thirds of IPF patients are current or former smokers. Other potential risk factors include exposure to inorganic and organic dusts and gastroesophageal reflux disease (GERD), the latter of which may lead to repetitive lung injury from recurrent microaspiration.

There is growing understanding of the role that genetics plays in IPF. Numerous genetic polymorphisms have been found to increase the risk of developing IPF. Most notably, a common polymorphism in the promoter region of the *MUC5B* gene has been found to confer a 5-fold and 18-fold increased risk of developing IPF when one or two copies of the risk allele are present, respectively. The fact that a family history of pulmonary fibrosis has also been increasingly recognized as

内病变一般以下肺野分布为著，而一些特征性表现也有一定的提示诊断作用：如 IPF 的蜂窝影，非特异性间质性肺炎（NSIP）病灶远离胸膜，双侧钙化的胸膜斑提示石棉肺。

　　多数 ILD 患者，通过基于临床病史、体格检查、实验室和肺功能检查、胸部 HRCT 的多学科讨论后可以确诊。然而，凭借这些资料，有部分患者仍不能确诊，此时需要借助于肺活检来获取肺组织病理以协助诊断。胸腔镜下外科肺活检（SLB）为多数 ILD 获取肺组织病理的最佳方法。经支气管镜透壁肺活检（TBLB）虽创伤较小，但由于获取的组织标本过小而难以很好地评价肺内病变结构。因此不推荐 TBLB 用于可疑 IPF 或其他慢性纤维化性 ILD 的辅助诊断，但可用于诊断结节病、过敏性肺炎等这些特殊的 ILD。经支气管冷冻肺活检比 SLB 创伤小，还可以获取较 TBLB 更大的肺标本，目前在许多医疗中心已用于 ILD 的诊断；但冷冻肺活检在 ILD 诊断中的确切价值尚不明确，还有待进一步评价。

　　肺损伤的表现形式相对一致，特定的肺损伤如普通型间质性肺炎或肉芽肿性炎症可见于多种类型的疾病。肺组织活检的结果必须结合临床及影像学资料才能得出正确的解读。例如，类风湿关节炎相关的 ILD 及 IPF 的肺病理均可表现为普通型间质性肺炎，但两者的预后不同。

　　ILD 的治疗措施因病种不同而不同，不同 ILD 的治疗策略详见本章相应的部分。糖皮质激素和其他免疫抑制剂是 ILD 的主要治疗药物，它们可在炎症为主的 ILD 中起效，而在纤维化性病变为主的 ILD 中疗效不明确。近年来问世的抗纤维化药物可有效减缓 IPF 和其他慢性纤维化性 ILD 的进展。其他关键的 ILD 治疗措施包括脱离相关暴露因素（特别是暴露相关 ILD，如 HP、吸烟相关性 ILD 和药物相关性 ILD）、氧疗及肺康复。肺移植可用于预期寿命很有限的终末期 ILD 患者，但遗憾的是许多患者由于年龄限制或合并某些并发症而不适合肺移植；另外，可用的合适供体肺数量也很少，因此每年都有许多患者在肺移植等待期间死亡。

　　接下来，本章将主要介绍以下三大类 ILD：特发性 ILD、暴露相关 ILD 和系统性疾病相关 ILD。

特发性间质性肺疾病
特发性间质性肺炎

　　特发性间质性肺炎（IIP）是一组病因不明但具有特征性临床病理特征的 ILD。在过去的数十年里，IIP 往往被认同是特发性肺纤维化（IPF），后来随着对这组疾病的进一步认识，发现它包括了一系列有着不同的胸部影像学、组织病理学以及临床表现，且自然病程和治疗反应也不同的多种疾病，一直到 2002 年，美国胸科学会（ATS）及欧洲呼吸病学会（ERS）首次正

表 6.2　特发性间质性肺炎

主要 IIP	
慢性纤维化性	特发性肺纤维化（IPF）
	特发性非特异性间质性肺炎（NSIP）
急性 / 亚急性	隐源性机化性肺炎（COP）
	急性间质性肺炎（AIP）
吸烟相关	呼吸性细支气管炎相关间质性肺疾病（RB-ILD）
	脱屑性间质性肺炎（DIP）
罕见 IIP	特发性淋巴细胞性间质性肺炎（LIP）
	特发性胸膜肺实质弹力纤维增生症（iPPFE）
未能分类的 IIP	

式把这类 ILD 命名为 IIP，且在 2013 年又更新了 IIP 相关内容，并将 IIP 分为主要 IIP、罕见 IIP 和不能分类的 IIP（表 6.2）。主要 IIP 可以分为 3 类、6 种不同 ILD：IPF、特发性非特异性间质性肺炎（NSIP）、呼吸性细支气管炎相关间质性肺疾病（RB-ILD）、脱屑性间质性肺炎（DIP）、隐源性机化性肺炎（COP）和急性间质性肺炎（AIP）；其中，IPF 和 NSIP 属于慢性纤维化性 IIP，RB-ILD 和 DIP 属于吸烟相关 IIP、COP 和 AIP 属于急性 / 亚急性 IIP（见表 6.2）。罕见 IIP 包括特发性淋巴细胞性间质性肺炎（LIP）及特发性胸膜肺实质弹力纤维增生症（PPFE）。那些不符合上述任何一类疾病的诊断标准的特发性间质性肺炎被称为未能分类的 IIP。

特发性肺纤维化

　　定义、流行病学和发病机制　共识中把 IPF 定义为：一种病因不明的、慢性、进行性、纤维化性间质性肺炎，好发于老年人，病变局限于肺部、组织病理学及影像学表现为普通型间质性肺炎（UIP）。IPF 为 IIP 中最常见的，2000 年，美国人群中 IPF 发病率约为 16.3/100 000 人年、患病率约为 42.7/100 000 人，推测当时在美国有 89 000 例 IPF 患者。世界范围内 IPF 发病率都呈现上升趋势，这可能与多种因素有关，如世界人口整体老龄化、吸烟。年龄是 IPF 的最大风险因素，多项研究表明，年龄每增长 10 岁 IPF 的发病率和患病率都稳步上升；而 50 岁之前的 IPF 罕见。吸烟也与 IPF 发生、发展密切相关，高达 2/3 的 IPF 患者还在吸烟或有既往吸烟史。其他潜在的致 IPF 风险因素包括接触无机和有机粉尘，以及胃食管反流病（GERD），后者可能与反复微吸入引起的反复肺损伤有关。

　　目前越来越认识到遗传学在 IPF 发病中的作用，已发现很多遗传多态性会增加 IPF 的风险。最值得注意的是，当存在一个或两个拷贝的风险等位基因时，*MUC5B* 基因启动子区的常见多态性会使患 IPF 的风险分别增加 5 倍和 18 倍。肺纤维化的家族史也是患 IPF 的危险因素，这也凸显了遗传学在 IPF 发生发展中的重要作用。

an important risk factor for IPF also underscores the important genetic contribution to the disease. Some studies have suggested that up to 20% of cases may be familial (i.e., occurring in two or more first-degree relatives). The nomenclature of the familial form(s) of the disease is evolving; it has been referred to as familial IPF, familial pulmonary fibrosis (FPF), and familial interstitial pneumonia (FIP), the latter term reflecting the fact that in some cases the radiographic and/or histologic pattern of disease can be more suggestive of one of the other types of IIP rather than IPF. The familial form of the disease is often inherited in mendelian fashion, and specific causative mutations have been identified in 20% to 30% of these families, most commonly in the telomerase complex genes but also in the surfactant protein genes.

The pathogenesis of IPF is complex. Although it was for many years thought of as a disease driven by chronic inflammation, the paucity of inflammation seen on histologic sample from IPF lungs and the lack of response to aggressive anti-inflammatory therapy challenged this notion. It is now thought instead to be a disease characterized by aberrant or dysregulated wound-healing responses to repetitive lung injury. This current paradigm of IPF pathogenesis suggests that a complex interaction between host susceptibility (aging, genetics) and environmental factors (cigarette smoking, inhaled particulates, etc.) is ultimately what leads to the development of IPF. This shift in the understanding of IPF as being driven by aberrant wound-healing rather than chronic inflammation has also been important in leading to the discovery of effective therapies for this disease, as discussed below.

Pathology. The underlying histopathologic pattern found in the lungs of patients with IPF is called *usual interstitial pneumonia* (UIP). The characteristic histologic features of UIP include scar tissue deposition that is predominantly peripheral and patchy, with areas of fibrosis interspersed with areas with relatively normal lung (Fig. 6.1), along with fibroblastic foci, which are areas of active fibroblast proliferation and are thought to be the "leading edge" of fibrosis development. There is generally a paucity of inflammation, and in areas of more advanced fibrosis, microscopic honeycombing is often seen. Importantly, this UIP pattern can be seen in other disorders (e.g., connective tissue disease–related ILD and asbestosis), and therefore the diagnosis of IPF depends on not only identifying UIP, but also ruling out known causes of that histologic pattern (i.e., IPF is *idiopathic* UIP).

Clinical presentation. IPF is characterized by progressive accumulation of scar tissue in the lungs. As a consequence, patients typically present with insidious, gradually worsening dyspnea on exertion and a nonproductive cough. Symptoms are frequently present for 1 to 2 years before a diagnosis is made, although in some cases they can progress more slowly or more rapidly. Some patients with IPF are asymptomatic, and the disease is discovered because of abnormal physical exam findings or as an incidental finding on chest imaging studies done for other reasons (e.g., lung cancer screening).

Physical examination often reveals inspiratory crackles in the bases of both lungs, indicating the predominant site of scarring. Clubbing may exist, but extrapulmonary findings are generally absent. With increased scar deposition, the lungs become stiffer, as evidenced by decreased compliance. Pulmonary function tests show decreased lung volumes consistent with a restrictive process, and the DLco is generally reduced. Impaired oxygenation in IPF, initially with exercise and later at rest, often requires long-term oxygen supplementation.

The chest radiograph shows reticular opacities that are most predominant at the bases and the periphery of the lungs. HRCT allows better visualization of the lung and is useful in evaluating the extent and pattern of disease. The classic HRCT findings of IPF are bilateral, subpleural reticular opacities that are more pronounced in the lower lung zones, along with areas of radiographic honeycombing and traction bronchiectasis and bronchiolectasis (Fig. 6.2) in the absence of

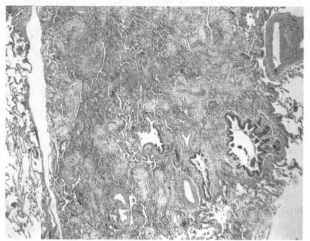

Fig. 6.1 Pulmonary fibrosis in idiopathic pulmonary fibrosis with usual interstitial pneumonia pathology that is adjacent to normal lung parenchyma. (Courtesy Dr. Charles Kuhn.)

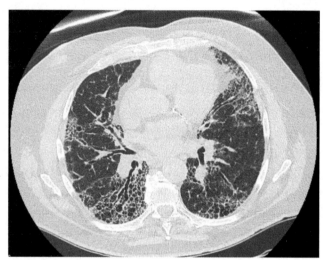

Fig. 6.2 Typical usual interstitial pneumonia (UIP) pattern of abnormality seen on chest computed tomography (CT) of a patient with IPF, demonstrating patchy, bilateral areas of subpleural reticulation, traction bronchiectasis and bronchiolectasis, and honeycombing.

significant ground-glass opacification, nodules, consolidation, or other features that suggest an alternative diagnosis. When these features are present on an HRCT in the absence of other abnormalities that suggest an alternative diagnosis (e.g., extensive ground-glass opacification, diffuse nodules or areas of consolidation), then a confident diagnosis of a UIP pattern can often be made without the need for a lung biopsy. In other cases when the HRCT pattern is not as definitive, a lung biopsy may be required to help distinguish UIP/IPF from other types of ILD.

Diagnosis and differential diagnosis. IPF is diagnosed on the basis of typical clinical, radiographic (HRCT), and if available, pathologic features (i.e., biopsy showing a UIP pattern). Other potential causes of ILD, such as connective tissue disease, hypersensitivity pneumonitis, and asbestosis, must be ruled out as best as possible by the history, examination, and selected laboratory testing. When an HRCT scan shows the typical UIP pattern described above (lower lung zone predominant, subpleural reticular opacities with areas of honeycombing) and no feature to suggest an alterative diagnosis, a diagnosis of IPF can be made without the need for a surgical lung biopsy. If honeycombing is

有研究表明，高达 20% 的病例可能是家族性的（即发生在两个或两个以上的一级亲属中）。该疾病家族性形式的命名正在演变：包括家族性 IPF、家族性肺纤维化（FPF）和家族性间质性肺炎（FIP），后者反映了这样一个事实，即在某些情况下，疾病的放射学和（或）组织学模式可能更提示其他类型的 IIP，而不是 IPF。这种疾病的家族形式通常是以孟德尔方式遗传的，这些特殊的基因突变发生于 20% ～ 30% 的家族成员中，以编码端粒酶复合体基因和编码表面活性蛋白基因突变最常见。

IPF 的发病机制复杂，虽然多年来都认为慢性炎症是引起 IPF 的始动因素，但 IPF 患者肺组织中炎症表现并不明显，抗炎类药物并未起到很好的疗效，使得这一观点备受挑战。反而，目前认为肺泡上皮反复损伤后异常修复是 IPF 的主要特征。所以，宿主易感性（衰老、遗传）和环境因素（吸烟、吸入颗粒物等）之间复杂的相互作用是最终导致 IPF 发生发展的可能机制。意识到反复损伤后的异常修复而并非慢性炎症是导致 IPF 的机制，这一转变将更有助于探索 IPF 的有效治疗措施。

病理学　IPF 对应的组织病理学表现为 UIP。其组织学特征为：外周分布为著的斑片状瘢痕和成纤维细胞灶，穿插着相对正常的肺结构（图 6.1）；成纤维细胞灶处是活动性的成纤维细胞所在处，也是纤维化发展的"前沿地带"。肺内炎症不明显、纤维化程度较高的区域即为组织病理学中的蜂窝。值得关注的是，UIP 型 ILD 也可见于其他疾病（如结缔组织病相关 ILD 及石棉沉着病）；因此诊断 IPF 除组织病理学表现为 UIP 外，还需除外其他已知病因的 ILD（即，IPF 是特发性 UIP）。

临床表现　IPF 特征性表现为肺内进行性进展的瘢痕组织沉积，故而，这类患者的典型表现是隐匿性、逐渐加重的劳力性呼吸困难和干咳。上述症状一般早于 IPF 诊断 1 ～ 2 年出现，虽然一些患者病情进展可能较慢或较快。一些 IPF 患者可以无症状，而是通过查体发现或因其他原因筛查胸部影像学时偶然发现（如肺癌筛查）。

IPF 患者体格检查时常常可在双肺基底部闻及吸气相爆裂音，这对应着显著的纤维化区域。部分患者可伴有杵状指，但一般无其他肺外异常体征。随着瘢痕化进一步加重，肺硬度增加，顺应性下降。肺功能检查提示肺容积减少的限制性通气功能障碍，常常伴有 D_{LCO} 下降。IPF 患者的氧合能力下降，早期仅在运动时出现，随病情进展，在静息状态下也会出现低氧并需要长期氧疗。

IPF 患者的胸部 X 线片主要表现为下肺基底部、肺外带的网格影，HRCT 可更好地显示肺内病变，并有助于评估病变范围及严重程度。IPF 的典型 HRCT 表现为双下肺、近胸膜分布的网格影、蜂窝影及牵拉性支气管扩张及细支气管扩张（图 6.2），并缺乏明显的

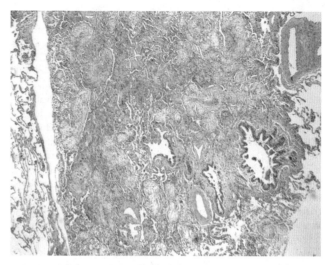

图 6.1　特发性肺纤维化的组织病理表现为普通型间质性肺炎，肺纤维化与正常肺组织毗邻（经 Dr. Charles Kuhn. 授权）

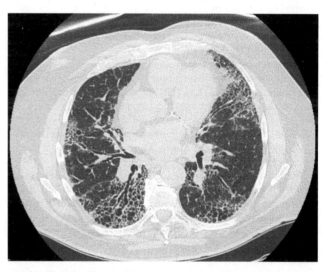

图 6.2　IPF 患者胸部 CT 异常所见：典型的普通型间质性肺炎（UIP）改变，表现为双肺、斑片状分布的胸膜下网格影、牵拉性支气管扩张和细支气管扩张及蜂窝影

磨玻璃影、结节影、实变或提示其他诊断的肺部阴影。当患者的胸部 HRCT 呈现上述典型表现且没有提示其他诊断的表现（如大量磨玻璃影、弥漫性结节或实变）时，即可诊断确定 UIP 型，而不必安排肺活检。若患者的胸部 HRCT 并非确定 UIP 型，则可能需要通过肺活检来鉴别 UIP/IPF 和其他类型 ILD。

诊断及鉴别诊断　诊断 IPF 有赖于典型的临床表现、影像学（HRCT）表现及组织病理学特点（即，肺活检表现为 UIP），还需结合病史、体格检查及必要的实验室检查来尽可能地除外可能导致 ILD 的潜在病因，如结缔组织病、过敏性肺炎及石棉沉着病。若胸部 HRCT 呈现 UIP 型（下肺、胸膜下分布为著的网格影、蜂窝影），且无提示其他诊断的表现时，无需进行肺活检即可诊断 IPF。若 HRCT 中无蜂窝影，或伴有非

absent on HRCT or atypical features such as ground-glass infiltrates, consolidation, diffuse nodules, or extensive air trapping are found, the radiographic diagnosis becomes less certain. In these cases, a lung biopsy may be indicated, and incorporation of the clinical, HRCT, and histologic information are then needed to make a diagnosis of IPF. Multidisciplinary discussion during the diagnostic process, with input from experienced clinicians, radiologists, and pathologists, is ideal.

Treatment. For decades there were no pharmacologic therapies that were proven to be helpful at slowing the progression of IPF. However, with improved understanding of IPF pathogenesis (described above), many novel therapies that target aberrant wound-healing responses have been studied in IPF. Two such therapies, pirfenidone (multiple mechanisms of action) and nintedanib (inhibits intracellular signaling of fibroblasts), have been shown in large randomized controlled trials to slow IPF progression by approximately 50%. In 2014, these drugs became the first ever to be approved by the US Food and Drug Administration (FDA) for treatment of IPF. Importantly, neither nintedanib or pirfenidone reverses established fibrosis or even completely stops the progression of the disease. Therefore, these treatments do not cure IPF, nor do they alleviate the symptoms of breathlessness or coughing, both of which can be debilitating. As such, the search for other potentially effective therapies for IPF is an area of intense ongoing investigation.

Because IPF is a progressive disease, even despite the availability of effective antifibrotic therapies, lung transplantation should be considered for patients with IPF. Many patients with IPF are not candidates for lung transplantation because of age, comorbidities, or other factors, but for those who are candidates, lung transplant may offer a chance at prolonged survival and improved quality of life. The median survival rate after lung transplant is only about 5.8 years, but this is steadily improving and still compares favorably to the expected survival of IPF patients at or near the top of lung transplant waiting lists, which is likely only weeks to months. Because of the unpredictable nature of disease progression in IPF, early referral for transplantation evaluation should be considered.

Prognosis. IPF is a progressive disease, and historically it has carried a poor prognosis. Median survival is often reported to be 2 to 3 years from the time of diagnosis. It is likely that the median survival will be prolonged in the era of antifibrotic therapy, but as stated, these therapies still do not cure the disease. There is considerable heterogeneity in the pace of progression in IPF, as the rate of lung function decline varies greatly between different individuals with the disease and even within any given patient over time. Furthermore, some patients with IPF experience acute or subacute respiratory deterioration in the absence of any clinically apparent superimposed cause (e.g., heart failure, pulmonary embolism, pneumonia). These episodes of acute deterioration are referred to as acute exacerbations of IPF and are associated with a very poor prognosis. HRCT findings include new ground-glass opacities and/or consolidation superimposed on the background of pulmonary fibrosis. Histologically, evidence of acute lung injury (i.e., diffuse alveolar damage) can be found on the background of UIP. These patients are often treated with high doses of steroids and/or other immunosuppressant medications, although data supporting such approaches are lacking. Mortality for IPF patients hospitalized with acute exacerbations is very high (50% to 90%).

Other Idiopathic Interstitial Pneumonias

The other major chronic fibrosing IIP is idiopathic nonspecific interstitial pneumonia (NSIP). This condition exhibits a histologic picture that is distinct from that of UIP/IPF and is characterized by diffuse, uniform infiltration of the lung interstitium with varying amounts of chronic (lymphoplasmacytic) inflammation and fibrosis, in contrast to the patchy, heterogenous pattern seen in UIP. It is sometimes characterized

as either cellular NSIP or fibrotic NSIP depending on the predominance of either inflammation or fibrosis, although it is not clear if these are truly distinct entities. As a clinical entity, idiopathic NSIP is not as well defined as IPF, and as a result it is not as well studied either. As with IPF, patients with idiopathic NSIP usually present with progressive dyspnea and cough, and HRCT typically reveals diffuse, bilateral, peripheral reticular opacities, although ground-glass opacities are often more prominent with NSIP and honeycombing is generally absent. In many instances, distinguishing between IPF and idiopathic NSIP by HRCT alone can be difficult. The prognosis for NSIP is much better than for IPF, with a 5-year survival rate of greater than 82% in one series. It may be responsive to immunosuppressive therapy, and although data are lacking, a trial period with such agents can be considered. Lung transplantation should be considered in these patients if they exhibit progressive disease. Importantly, the same NSIP histologic pattern may occur in other conditions, most notably connective tissue disorders (e.g., systemic lupus erythematosus, rheumatoid arthritis, polymyositis), and therefore the identification of a histologic pattern of NSIP should prompt a detailed search for these conditions, which occasionally can otherwise be occult.

Cryptogenic organizing pneumonia (COP) and acute interstitial pneumonia (AIP) are classified as acute/subacute IIPs. Patients with COP exhibit subacute onset of dyspnea and/or cough, often with associated constitutional symptoms. Radiographically, patients with COP typically have areas of air space consolidation, often multifocal and bilateral, that mimic infectious pneumonia. Concomitant ground-glass opacities are also common. Histologically, COP is characterized by patchy areas of organizing pneumonia, which is accumulation of granulation tissue (a loose collection of fibrin, fibroblasts, collagen, and inflammatory cells) within the distal air spaces (alveoli and alveolar ducts), with or without extension into the respiratory and terminal bronchioles (bronchiolitis obliterans). COP is generally very responsive to corticosteroid therapy, often with complete resolution, but it can also relapse when steroids are stopped. The histologic pattern of organizing pneumonia (OP) can be seen in a variety of conditions, specifically connective tissue diseases, acute/subacute hypersensitivity pneumonitis, inhalational exposures, and drug-induced ILD, so as with NSIP, a histologic finding of OP should prompt a thorough evaluation for known causes before it is classified as an idiopathic process.

Acute interstitial pneumonia (AIP) is an IIP that is characterized by the rapid onset and progression of dyspnea and hypoxemia. Symptoms and radiographic opacities develop over days to a few weeks, invariably leading to respiratory failure. Many patients report a prior illness suggesting an upper respiratory infection with constitutional symptoms. The histologic pattern shows diffuse alveolar damage with hyaline membrane formation with or without organization. These patients can therefore be thought of as having acute respiratory distress syndrome (ARDS) of unknown cause. Although a trial of high-dose steroids with or without additional immunosuppressants is generally recommended, data indicating efficacy for this approach are lacking. Mortality rates for AIP are high at approximately 50%. Most survivors have a good long-term prognosis, although in some instances they experience persistent severe lung fibrosis. Occult connective tissue disease—most notably polymyositis/dermatomyositis—can present with an acute respiratory illness that mimics AIP, and this association may account for the fact that some patients clearly improve with aggressive treatment.

Desquamative interstitial pneumonia (DIP) is a rare idiopathic pneumonia usually seen in younger individuals. It is associated in most cases with a history of cigarette smoking. Patients exhibit a progressive shortness of breath and bilateral infiltrates on chest radiographs. The HRCT pattern shows extensive ground-glass infiltrates, and a biopsy is often required for diagnosis. Tissue histologic findings show the accumulation of so-called smoker's macrophages, which contain

典型 UIP 型 ILD 的影像学表现时，如磨玻璃影、实变影、弥漫性结节影或气体陷闭征象时，胸部影像学表现依据不足以诊断 UIP 型 ILD；此时可能需要肺活检，并结合临床特点、HRCT 表现和肺组织病理表现后方可诊断为 IPF。由具有丰富经验的临床医生、影像科医生及病理学家组成的多学科讨论是诊断 IPF 的理想模式。

　　治疗　数十年来，尚无药物治疗可减缓 IPF 进展。不过，随着对 IPF 发病机制（如上所述）进一步认识，开展了许多针对损伤异常修复的新型治疗探索。已有两种药物，吡非尼酮（多种作用机制）和尼达尼布（抑制成纤维细胞的细胞内信号通路）在大型的随机对照试验中显示出可延缓 50%IPF 进展的疗效。并在 2014 年被美国食品药物监督管理局批准作为首批 IPF 治疗药物。不过，尼达尼布或吡非尼酮均不能逆转已发生的肺纤维化，也不能完全阻止 IPF 进展。由于这些药物尚不能治愈 IPF，也不能改善呼吸困难或咳嗽等困扰患者的症状，因此，尚需积极探索其他更有效的 IPF 治疗措施。

　　IPF 患者即便接受抗纤维化药物治疗仍呈现进行性进展，故而尚需考虑肺移植治疗。虽然许多 IPF 患者由于年龄、合并症或其他因素而不适合肺移植，但对于那些符合肺移植适应证的患者，肺移植手术可延长生存期、改善生活质量。目前肺移植后的中位生存率为 5.8 年左右，肺移植治疗 IPF 的有效率还在逐渐提高中；尤其是明显改善了肺移植候选名单上排名靠前 IPF 患者的预期生存率，因为这些患者的预期寿命可能只有几周到几个月。由于 IPF 患者的疾病进展不可预测性，应考虑早期转诊接受肺移植评估。

　　预后　IPF 是进展性疾病，预后较差：自诊断后其中位生存期一般仅有 2～3 年。抗纤维化药物治疗可能延长 IPF 患者中位生存期，但是仍不能治愈 IPF。IPF 患者的进展速度有很大的异质性，不同患者间，甚至同一患者随时间推移肺功能下降的速度差异也很大。此外，一些 IPF 患者可在无任何诱因（如心功能不全、肺栓塞、肺炎）的情况下出现急性或亚急性呼吸功能恶化，即 IPF 急性加重，预后极差。此时，HRCT 表现为在肺纤维化背景下新发磨玻璃浸润影和（或）实变影；组织学表现为 UIP 基础上的急性肺损伤（即弥漫性肺泡损伤）。虽然尚无客观依据来支持，但一般用大剂量糖皮质激素和（或）其他免疫抑制剂治疗 IPF 急性加重；IPF 急性加重住院的患者死亡率高达 50%～90%。

其他类型的间质性肺炎

　　另一种主要的慢性纤维化性 IIP 是特发性非特异性间质性肺炎（NSIP），其组织病理学表现与 UIP/IPF 不同，特征性地表现为弥漫性均匀一致的肺间质内不同程度的慢性（淋巴浆细胞）炎症浸润和纤维化，这与 UIP 型 ILD 中多种病变呈斑片状分布大相径庭。根据炎症或纤维化的程度不同，NSIP 可分为富细胞型或纤维化型 NSIP；但其实目前也不明确这两型之间是否确实存在本质差异。此外，对于特发性 NSIP 的认识远没有对于 IPF 的认识充分，迄今也未能深入探究特发性 NSIP。不过，与 IPF 患者相似，进行性呼吸困难和咳嗽也是特发性 NSIP 患者的常见临床表现；胸部 HRCT 特征性表现为双肺弥漫性外带分布为著的网格影；相较于 IPF，NSIP 患者的磨玻璃影更为明显，一般没有蜂窝影。大多数情况下，仅凭借 HRCT 表现难以鉴别 IPF 和特发性 NSIP。NSIP 患者的预后优于 IPF，曾有研究报道 NSIP 的 5 年生存率高于 82%。免疫抑制剂可能使 NSIP 患者获益，因此，虽然缺乏客观证据支持，但仍可尝试应用免疫抑制剂治疗 NSIP；对于进展期患者可以考虑肺移植。值得关注的是，NSIP 型的组织病理学表现也可见于其他疾病如结缔组织病（系统性红斑狼疮、类风湿关节炎及多发性肌炎）。鉴于往往上述疾病的表现隐匿，对于肺病理为 NSIP 型的 ILD 患者要详尽地筛查上述疾病。

　　急性 / 亚急性 IIP 包括隐源性机化性肺炎（COP）和急性间质性肺炎（AIP）；COP 患者呈现亚急性病程，临床上表现为呼吸困难和（或）咳嗽，常伴有全身症状。其典型影像学特点为两肺、多灶性肺内实变影，很像肺部感染性疾病。COP 的病理学特点为片状机化性肺炎，即远端气腔（肺泡、肺泡管）内肉芽组织（纤维蛋白、成纤维细胞、胶原蛋白及炎性细胞聚集）填充，上述病变可累及呼吸性终末细支气管（即闭塞性细支气管炎）。大部分 COP 患者对糖皮质激素反应很好，常可完全缓解，但也可在停药后复发。机化性肺炎（OP）的病理组织类型可见于多种疾病，尤其是结缔组织病、急性 / 亚急性过敏性肺炎、暴露相关 ILD 和药物相关 ILD，因此，与 NSIP 相同，病理表现为 OP 后，需要尽快全面筛查继发性因素后方可诊断 COP。

　　急性间质性肺炎是以急性起病后、快速进展的呼吸困难和低氧血症为特征的一类 IIP。症状及肺阴影可于数天至数周内进行性加重，最终导致呼吸衰竭。一些 AIP 患者在发病前有过上呼吸道感染以及全身症状。其肺组织学表现为弥漫性肺泡损伤伴透明膜形成，伴或不伴机化。所以 AIP 也可认为是原因不明的急性呼吸窘迫综合征（ARDS）。虽然尚无客观数据支持，但这类患者一般都会给予大剂量糖皮质激素和（或）免疫抑制剂治疗。AIP 死亡率高达 50%，虽然一些患者可能遗留严重的肺纤维化，但大部分幸存者长期预后良好。某些隐匿的结缔组织病——特别是多发性肌炎 / 皮肌炎，可以出现类似 AIP 的急性呼吸疾病；这也解释了部分 AIP 患者在积极救治后病情明显改善的现象。

　　脱屑性间质性肺炎（DIP）是罕见的特发性间质性肺炎，年轻人多见。绝大部分患者与吸烟史密切相关。患者常表现为进行性加重的呼吸困难及两肺浸润影。HRCT 表现为弥漫磨玻璃影，该病一般需要通过肺活检来诊断。组织病理学可见肺泡内大量烟尘细胞聚集，即内含棕黄色色

yellow-brown pigment and fill the alveolar spaces, and some degree of interstitial inflammation and fibrosis.

Respiratory-bronchiolitis interstitial lung disease (RB-ILD) and DIP are classified as smoking-related IPs. Although these are classified as "idiopathic" ILDs, all cases of RB-ILD and the vast majority of cases of DIP are seen in cigarette smokers. RB-ILD and DIP are thought to represent a spectrum of illness, as both are characterized by abnormal accumulation of pigment-laden macrophages. The histologic finding of RB-ILD—accumulation of these macrophages in the lumens of the respiratory bronchioles—is considered a universal finding in active smokers and considered an asymptomatic/subclinical process. When the extent of macrophage accumulation becomes more extensive, involves the peribronchiolar air spaces, and/or causes symptoms or radiographic findings, it is referred to as RB-ILD. When the macrophage accumulation is even more extensive and involves the air spaces more diffusely, it is referred to as DIP. The prognosis for RB-ILD is generally excellent, with complete resolution occurring with smoking cessation alone. For DIP, the prognosis is more variable. Smoking cessation is still the mainstay of treatment, but many patients often also require treatment with corticosteroids. Some patients unfortunately develop progressive pulmonary fibrosis despite this approach. Very rare cases of DIP have been described in nonsmoking adults, although secondhand cigarette smoke and other inhalational exposures have been implicated.

Idiopathic lymphoid interstitial pneumonia (LIP) and idiopathic pleuroparenchymal fibroelastosis (PPFE) are classified as rare IIPs. LIP is characterized by extensive, relatively homogenous lymphoid infiltration of the interstitium, often with numerous lymphoid follicles. On HRCT, LIP is characterized by the combination of diffuse ground-glass opacity and frequently numerous thin-walled cysts. In many instances, LIP may be part of a spectrum of pulmonary lymphoproliferative disorders or true lymphoma. The vast majority of histologic LIP cases are associated with other conditions (e.g., connective tissue disease, HIV) and therefore are not truly idiopathic. Idiopathic pleuroparenchymal fibroelastosis (PPFE) is a relatively recently described entity characterized by dense, elastotic fibrosis of the pleura and subpleural lung parenchyma. HRCT typically shows patchy areas of subpleural, dense, plaque-like consolidation, often predominantly in the upper lung zones. Spontaneous pneumothorax is common. It is typically progressive and unresponsive to steroids or other immunosuppressive treatments. Idiopathic PPFE is still poorly understood, and the PPFE pattern has been described in a variety of conditions, including as a complication of both stem cell transplant and lung transplant. Additional rare histologic patterns of ILD have been described, such as acute fibrinous organizing pneumonia (AFOP) and bronchiolocentric pulmonary fibrosis and inflammation, but whether or not these represent distinct IIPs is still unclear. AFOP may exist along a clinical spectrum that includes AIP and COP, and bronchiolocentric patterns of ILD may be predominantly exposure-related. Lastly, there are some cases of IIP that, despite multidisciplinary discussion and review of clinical, HRCT, and histologic findings, do not fit into any of the clinicopathologic entities described above, and these are often referred to as unclassifiable IIP.

Other Idiopathic ILDs
Eosinophilic Pneumonia

Acute eosinophilic pneumonia (AEP) and chronic eosinophilic pneumonia (CEP) are two clinically distinct idiopathic forms of ILD characterized by eosinophilic infiltration of the lung parenchyma. AEP is typically characterized by fever, a nonproductive cough, and dyspnea that progresses over several days to weeks, often leading to acute respiratory failure. This disease typically affects male smokers between the ages of 20 and 40 years who are otherwise healthy. Chest imaging

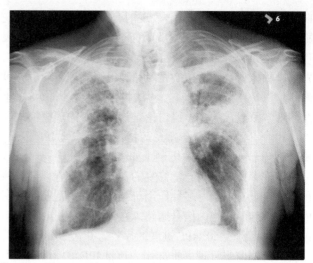

Fig. 6.3 Photographic negative of pulmonary edema in chronic eosinophilic pneumonia.

reveals diffuse bilateral pulmonary infiltrates. Eosinophilia is often not found in the peripheral blood initially but may occur 7 to 30 days after onset. Abundant eosinophils can be found in BAL fluid, and a level of greater than 25% of all nucleated cells is helpful in making the correct diagnosis. Although lung biopsy is typically not required to make the diagnosis, it can show eosinophilic infiltration with acute and organizing diffuse alveolar damage. Treatment with corticosteroids typically offers rapid and complete clinical and radiographic resolution without recurrence or residual sequelae.

Chronic eosinophilic pneumonia is an idiopathic disease predominantly of middle-aged women with a history of asthma. Also called *prolonged pulmonary eosinophilia*, this illness is characterized by a productive cough, dyspnea, malaise, weight loss, night sweats, and fever associated with progressive peripheral lung infiltrates that have been described as resembling the photographic negative of pulmonary edema on chest radiographs (Fig. 6.3). On presentation, most patients with chronic eosinophilic pneumonia have a peripheral eosinophilia of greater than 30% and BAL fluid eosinophilia. Histologic examination shows eosinophils and histiocytes in the lung parenchyma and interstitium, but minimal fibrosis. There is often histologic overlap with organizing pneumonia (OP). Spontaneous remissions have been reported, but respiratory failure can develop. Typically, treatment with corticosteroids is rapidly effective, but unlike AEP relapses are common and therefore prolonged therapy is often required.

Both AEP and CEP are diagnoses of exclusion, and other causes of eosinophilic lung infiltration must be ruled out, including fungal and parasitic infections, drug-induced ILD, connective tissue disease–ILD, EGPA, and hypereosinophilic syndrome (HES).

Pulmonary Alveolar Proteinosis

Pulmonary alveolar proteinosis (PAP) is a rare disorder in which lipoproteinaceous material accumulates within the alveoli due to impaired surfactant metabolism by alveolar macrophages. There are a variety of forms of PAP, which occurs more frequently in middle-aged patients and in current or former smokers. Primary PAP is due to impaired granulocyte-macrophage colony-stimulating factor (GM-CSF) signaling and can occur as an autoimmune disease due to neutralizing antibodies against GM-CSF, or as a hereditary disease due to mutations in GM-CSF receptor mutations. Secondary PAP occurs in conditions in which there is a functional impairment or decrease in the number of alveolar macrophages, as seen in various hematologic malignancies

素小粒的巨噬细胞，可伴一定程度的间质炎症或纤维化。

吸烟相关 IIP 包括呼吸性细支气管炎相关间质性肺疾病（RB-ILD）和 DIP。虽然它们属于"特发性"ILD，但几乎所有 RB-ILD 和大部分 DIP 患者均有吸烟史。RB-ILD 和 DIP 是同一类疾病，其肺内均有色素沉着的巨噬细胞（烟尘细胞）的异常积聚。RB-ILD 患者的肺组织中可见呼吸性细支气管内巨噬细胞积聚，这是活动性吸烟者的普遍表现，此时一般无症状 / 呈现亚临床过程。但当巨噬细胞积聚的程度变得更加广泛，累及细支气管周围的肺泡腔和（或）引起临床症状或影像学异常表现时，称为 RB-ILD。当巨噬细胞积聚更加广泛，累及更多的细支气管周围的肺泡腔时，被称为 DIP。一般来说，RB-ILD 患者预后良好，可在戒烟后完全缓解。DIP 患者的预后呈多样性。戒烟仍然是主要治疗措施，但多数患者常需要糖皮质激素治疗。不幸的是，一些患者仍会出现进行性肺纤维化。很少一部分 DIP 患者无明确的吸烟史，但不排除有二手烟和其他吸入性物质接触史。

罕见 IIP 包括特发性淋巴细胞性间质性肺炎（LIP）和特发性胸膜肺实质弹力纤维增生症（PPFE）。LIP 特征为肺间质广泛、均一的淋巴细胞浸润，常伴大量淋巴滤泡形成。HRCT 表现为弥漫性磨玻璃影及大量薄壁囊腔。多数情况下 LIP 常有潜在病因，可能是肺淋巴增殖性疾病或淋巴瘤。大部分肺组织病理 LIP 型的 ILD 并非真正的特发性，常有基础病（如结缔组织病、HIV 感染）。特发性 PPFE 是一种较新的疾病类型，其特征是胸膜和胸膜下肺实质中致密的弹力纤维增生。HRCT 通常显示胸膜下致密斑块样实变，主要集中在上肺。自发性气胸很常见。PPFE 是进展性疾病，对糖皮质激素或其他免疫抑制剂无效。人们对特发性 PPFE 仍然知之甚少，PPFE 可继发于一系列疾病，包括造血干细胞移植或肺移植。还有一些其他罕见的 ILD 的病理组织学类型，如急性纤维素性机化性肺炎（AFOP）和细支气管中心性炎症伴纤维化，但尚不明确这些病理表现是否代表着不同的 IIP 亚型。AFOP 的病理学表现可见于 AIP 和 COP 患者，细支气管中心性 ILD 可能与暴露相关因素有关。最后，虽然基于临床、HRCT 及病理组织学的评估开展了多学科讨论，仍有一些患者不能归为上述任一临床病理类型，此时常常被诊断为未能分类的 IIP。

其他特发性 ILD

嗜酸粒细胞性肺炎

急性嗜酸粒细胞性肺炎（AEP）和慢性嗜酸粒细胞性肺炎（CEP）是以肺实质嗜酸性粒细胞浸润为特征的两种不同临床表现形式的特发性 ILD。AEP 特征性表现为发热、干咳及呼吸困难，持续时间数日至数周，常导致急性呼吸衰竭。本病好发于 20 ~ 40 岁、既往体健的男性吸烟患者。胸部 X 线片上表现为双肺弥漫

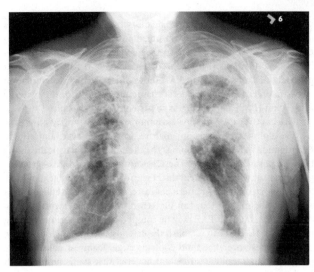

图 6.3　慢性嗜酸粒细胞性肺炎的反肺水肿征

浸润影。起病初期外周血嗜酸性粒细胞不高，但起病后 7 ~ 30 天可出现外周血嗜酸粒细胞升高。支气管肺泡灌洗液中有大量嗜酸性粒细胞，嗜酸性粒细胞占有核细胞总数的 25% 以上时有助于诊断。肺活检并非诊断急性嗜酸性粒细胞性肺炎所必需，其组织病理表现为嗜酸性粒细胞浸润伴急性机化性弥漫肺泡损伤。糖皮质激素治疗可快速消除临床表现和肺部阴影，且不复发或遗留后遗症。

慢性嗜酸粒细胞性肺炎（CEP）多见于有哮喘病史的中年女性，也称为迁延性肺嗜酸性粒细胞浸润症。该病表现为咳嗽、咳痰、呼吸困难、全身不适、体重下降、盗汗和发热，并因肺外周嗜酸性粒细胞浸润而使胸部 X 线片出现"反肺水肿征"（图 6.3）。大多数慢性嗜酸粒细胞性肺炎患者的外周血嗜酸性粒细胞比例大于 30%，其支气管肺泡灌洗液中嗜酸性粒细胞增多。组织病理学表现为肺实质和间质嗜酸性粒细胞及组织细胞浸润，但纤维化少见，常伴有机化性肺炎（organizing pneumonia, OP）。部分患者可自发缓解，但部分患者可进展为呼吸衰竭。糖皮质激素治疗可快速起效，但与 AEP 不同，CEP 常常会复发而往往需要延长激素疗程。

AEP 和 CEP 都是排除性诊断，均须排除嗜酸性粒细胞浸润的其他原因，包括真菌和寄生虫感染、药物相关 ILD、结缔组织病相关 ILD、EGPA 和嗜酸性粒细胞增多综合征（HES）。

肺泡蛋白沉积症

肺泡蛋白沉积症（PAP）是一种由于肺泡巨噬细胞内表面活性物质代谢异常后导致的肺泡腔内脂蛋白样物质沉积所致的罕见病。有好几种不同类型的 PAP，但以有吸烟史的中年患者多见。原发性 PAP 是由于粒细胞-巨噬细胞集落刺激因子（GM-CSF）信号转导异常所致，包括由于体内产生抗 GM-CSF 中和抗体所致的自身免疫性疾病和由于编码 GM-CSF 受体的基因突变而引起的遗传性 PAP。继发性 PAP 是由于肺泡巨噬

(e.g., leukemia), inhalation of toxic dusts (e.g., silica, aluminum), or after allogeneic bone marrow transplantation. PAP also has congenital forms that typically present in the neonatal period and are caused by various mutations that lead to dysregulated or defective surfactant production. Lung biopsy in PAP shows intra-alveolar accumulation of eosinophilic, acellular material staining positive with the periodic acid–Schiff (PAS) stain, which is consistent with surfactant.

Patients with PAP may be asymptomatic, or they may have progressive dyspnea on exertion, malaise, low-grade fever, and cough. Examination may reveal clubbing. The chest radiograph typically shows bilateral perihilar opacities. The CT scan may show diffuse ground-glass opacities with prominent thickening of the intralobular and interlobular septa, creating a pattern called "crazy paving," although this is a nonspecific finding that can be seen in many other forms or lung disease. The course of PAP may be complicated by opportunistic lung infection. BAL fluid can establish the diagnosis because it has a milky, opaque appearance. The fluid contains large, foamy alveolar macrophages and extracellular surfactant material that stains positive with PAS. Surgical or transbronchial lung biopsy may also be performed to establish the diagnosis if the BAL is nondiagnostic.

Asymptomatic patients with PAP and those with mild symptoms require no immediate treatment. Sequential whole lung lavage with warmed saline is indicated for patients with hypoxemia or severe dyspnea, and in up to 40% of patients it may be required only one time. Limited lobar lavage may be performed in milder disease. GM-CSF administration in patients with acquired PAP may be beneficial. Rituximab has been used in refractory PAP. The prognosis of autoimmune PAP is good, with excellent survival since the introduction of whole lung lavage.

EXPOSURE-RELATED ILDS

Environmental and Occupational Interstitial Lung Disease

Several environmental and occupational exposures may cause ILD, and these are generally classified as hypersensitivity pneumonitis (HP) and the pneumoconioses. Pneumoconioses are lung diseases resulting from the inhalation of mineral dusts, including silica, coal dust, or asbestos. HP is typically caused by the inhalation of organic dusts.

Hypersensitivity Pneumonitis

Definition and epidemiology. HP (also called *extrinsic allergic alveolitis*) is a relatively common ILD resulting from an abnormal immune response in the lungs to various inhaled agents, typically organic antigens. This immune response consists of both humoral and cellular components and causes a pattern of airway-centered inflammation and/or fibrosis. Potential antigens are diverse, ranging from bacterial, fungal, and animal proteins to low-molecular-weight chemicals that can act as haptens (Table 6.3). Host susceptibility seems to play an important role, because the vast majority of individuals subject to a particular exposure do not develop HP. The mechanisms contributing to host susceptibility are unclear but likely include genetic, environmental, and epigenetic factors. Although evocative descriptions have been given to occupational forms of this disease (e.g., paprika splitter's lung resulting from sensitivity to inhaled paprika dust contaminated with *Mucor stolonifer*), more routine exposures may occur in everyday life, such as hot tub water contaminated by mycobacterium avium complex (MAC), antigens from pet birds, or even common mold spores. The incidence and prevalence of HP are not well known and vary considerably based on many factors, such as geographic conditions, prevalent industries, and host mix. There is likely significant underdiagnosis of HP. For reasons that are unclear,

TABLE 6.3 **Hypersensitivity Pneumonitis: Partial List of Common Etiologic Agents**

Antigen	Source	Diseases
Bacteria	Moldy hay Sugar cane Compost Contaminated water	Farmer's lung, bagassosis, mushroom-worker's lung, humidifier lung, summer-type HP, composter's lung
Fungi	Moldy hay, cork, bark, cheese or wood dust Grains Compost Contaminated water or ventilation systems	Farmer's lung, suberosis, malt-worker's lung, maple bark-splitter's lung, humidifier lung, summer-type HP, composter's lung, sequoiosis, wood pulp-worker's disease, miller's lung
Mycobacteria	Contaminated water Metal cutting fluid	Hot tub lung, humidifier lung, swimming pool lung, machine-worker's lung
Animal proteins	Bird droppings, serum proteins, and feathers Pituitary powder Rat urine or serum proteins Fish meal	Pigeon breeder's lung, bird fancier's lung, feather duvet lung, duck fever, poultry-worker's lung, pituitary snuff-taker's lung, laboratory-worker's lung, fish meal-worker's lung
Chemicals	Isocyanates Anhydrides Bordeaux mixture	Chemical worker's lung, epoxy resin lung, vineyard-sprayer's lung

active cigarette smoking has been associated with a decreased risk of developing HP.

Pathology. Typical lung biopsy findings in HP demonstrate an airway-centered (i.e., bronchiolocentric) chronic inflammatory process involving the interstitium and air spaces, along with poorly formed granulomas containing multinucleated giant cells (Fig. 6.4). These findings are classically associated with the subacute form of the disease. In chronic HP there is generally considerable fibrosis and often features of fibrosing NSIP or UIP patterns in addition to areas of granulomatous and airway-centered inflammation. It is rare that lung biopsies are obtained in the acute form of HP, as it often resolves quickly, but histologic findings more associated with acute lung injury (along the diffuse alveolar damage organizing pneumonia (DAD-OP) spectrum) have been described in that setting.

Clinical presentation. HP can be classified as acute, subacute or chronic, although there can be considerable overlap between these forms. Acute HP usually presents with cough and dyspnea within hours after an intense exposure to a provocative antigen, often with prominent constitutional symptoms (e.g., fever, chills, malaise), and symptoms last for up to 24 hours. At the time of presentation, acute HP can be difficult to differentiate from bacterial or viral infection. Subacute HP is characterized by the gradual onset of cough and dyspnea, often with fatigue, anorexia, and weight loss, in response to prolonged lower level or intermittent antigen exposure. With intermittent exposure, symptoms of subacute HP may wax and wane. Chronic HP develops even more slowly than the subacute form, typically with insidious and gradually progressive cough and dyspnea and less variation in symptoms over time. Chronic HP is also thought to occur in response to sustained lower level antigen exposure, but it remains unclear if it represents the progression of prolonged, untreated subacute HP, or if subacute and chronic HP represent different host responses (inflammatory vs. fibrotic) to antigen-triggered immune-mediated lung injury.

细胞功能缺陷或数量减少所致，可见于多种血液系统恶性肿瘤（如白血病）、吸入有毒物质（如二氧化硅、铝）或同种异体骨髓移植后。先天性 PAP 多于新生儿期起病，可因多种基因突变引起肺泡表面活性物质代谢异常所致。PAP 的组织病理学表现为肺泡腔内存在嗜酸性、无细胞结构、过碘酸-希夫（PAS）染色呈阳性的物质（即肺表面活性物质）聚积。

　　PAP 患者可无临床症状，也可出现逐渐进展的劳力性呼吸困难、乏力、低热及咳嗽；体格检查可见杵状指。典型胸部 X 线片特征表现为双肺门周围浸润影，CT 表现为弥漫性磨玻璃影、小叶内间隔和小叶间隔增厚，呈现"铺路石征"；不过该征象并非 PAP 特有，也可见于其他多种肺病。PAP 病程中可伴有机会性肺部感染。PAP 患者特征性的支气管肺泡灌洗液表现为牛奶样浑浊的液体，具有 PAP 诊断意义。支气管肺泡灌洗液中含有大个的泡沫样肺泡巨噬细胞及 PAS 染色阳性的表面活性物质。若无上述特征性的支气管肺泡灌洗液，可经外科肺活检或经支气管镜透壁肺活检来诊断 PAP。

　　无症状或症状较轻的 PAP 患者可不必治疗。存在低氧血症或重度呼吸困难的患者可用温盐水行序贯全肺灌洗治疗，40% 以上 PAP 患者仅需一次灌洗。对于轻症患者，也可行局部肺叶灌洗。GM-CSF 可有效治疗获得性 PAP。利妥昔单抗适用于反复复发性 PAP。自身免疫性 PAP 患者预后好，全肺灌洗可显著提高其生存率。

暴露相关 ILD

环境和职业相关性间质性肺疾病

　　一些环境和职业暴露可能导致 ILD，包括过敏性肺炎（HP）及肺尘埃沉着病。肺尘埃沉着病是由于吸入矿物粉尘导致的肺病，包括二氧化硅、煤尘或石棉。HP 则是由于吸入有机粉尘导致。

过敏性肺炎

　　定义和流行病学　过敏性肺炎（又称为外源过敏性肺泡炎），一般是由于吸入有机抗原引起的肺内异常免疫反应而导致的一类常见的 ILD。这类免疫反应包括体液免疫和细胞免疫反应导致的以气道为中心的炎症和（或）纤维化。可能致敏的抗原成分多种多样，包括细菌、真菌、动物蛋白及作为半抗原的小分子化学物质等（表 6.3）。宿主易感性可能起着重要作用，因为大多数接触这些物质的人并不会患 HP。导致宿主易感性的机制尚不清楚，可能包括遗传、环境和表观遗传因素。虽然某些特征性物质吸入后引起的 HP 划归为职业相关性 ILD（如吸入被匍枝状毛霉菌污染的辣椒粉引起的辣椒粉碎工肺），但其实日常生活中经常被暴露于一些潜在变应原，如被鸟分枝杆菌复合菌群污染的热浴盆水、宠物鸟，甚至常见的霉菌孢子等。HP 的发

表 6.3　过敏性肺炎部分常见变应原

变应原	来源	疾病
细菌	霉干草 甘蔗 堆肥 污染的水源	农民肺、蔗尘肺、采蘑菇者肺、湿化器肺病、夏季型过敏性肺炎、堆肥肺
真菌	发霉的干草、软木、树皮、奶酪或木屑 谷物 堆肥 污染的水源或通风系统	农民肺、软木尘肺、收割大麦工人肺、剥枫树皮者肺、湿化器肺病、夏季型过敏性肺炎、堆肥肺、红杉尘肺、木浆工人肺、磨坊工人肺
分枝杆菌	污染的水源 金属切屑液	热浴盆肺病、湿化器肺病、泳池肺、机械工肺
动物蛋白	鸟排泄物、血清蛋白和羽毛 垂体后叶粉 大鼠尿液或血清蛋白 鱼粉	养鸽者肺、养鸟者肺、羽绒被肺、鸭瘟、家禽饲养者肺、垂体后叶粉吸入病、实验员过敏性肺炎、鱼粉工人肺
化学制剂	异氰酸酯 酐 波尔多液	化学工人肺、环氧树脂肺、葡萄园喷雾工人肺

病率及患病率尚不明确，因地理特征、主流行业和宿主等不同而异。HP 常常被忽视。吸烟可降低患 HP 的风险，但具体原因未明。

　　病理学　HP 的肺组织病理特征性地表现为气道中心性（以细支气管为中心的）慢性炎症反应，可累及肺间质及肺泡，伴有分化不良的多核巨细胞肉芽肿（图 6.4）。上述表现见于亚急性 HP。慢性 HP 可见明显的肺纤维化，除肉芽肿性病变及气道中心炎症外，其余部分呈现 UIP 或纤维化性 NSIP 型 ILD 的表现。由于急性 HP 可迅速消退，很少进行肺组织活检，但其组织学表现多与急性肺损伤相似（呈现弥漫性肺泡损伤-机化性肺炎特征）。

　　临床表现　HP 按病程可分为急性、亚急性或慢性 HP，这些类型之间可交叉存在。急性 HP 表现为暴露于大量致敏原后数小时内出现的咳嗽及呼吸困难，常常伴有明显的全身症状（如发热、寒战、全身不适），上述症状可持续 24 h 以上。急性 HP 患者起病时的症状很难与细菌或病毒感染鉴别。亚急性 HP 是由于长期低水平接触或间歇性接触致敏原所致，临床上表现为逐渐出现的呼吸困难和咳嗽。间歇性暴露于致敏原时，HP 相关的症状会波动。慢性 HP 的进展速度比亚急性 HP 更慢，一般起病隐匿，常表现为逐渐进展的咳嗽和呼吸困难，病程中上述表现一般无明显波动。慢性 HP 也是因持续、长期接触低水平的致敏原所致，但尚不明确是否由长期、未治疗的亚急性 HP 进展而来，也不明确亚急性和慢性 HP 是否代表宿主对致敏原触发的免疫介导的肺损伤的不同应答类型（炎症和纤维化）。

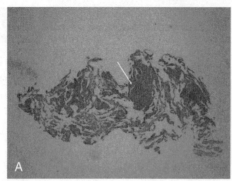
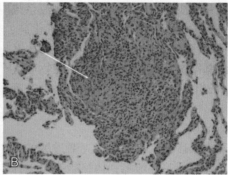

Fig. 6.4 (A) Poorly formed granulomas *(arrow)* in a patient with hypersensitivity reaction to a chemotherapy drug (low magnification). (B) Poorly formed granuloma *(arrow)* in a patient with a hypersensitivity reaction to a chemotherapy drug (high magnification).

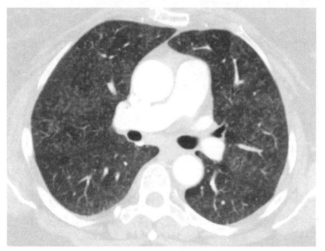

Fig. 6.5 CT image from a patient with hypersensitivity pneumonitis demonstrating diffuse, poorly formed, centrilobular nodules.

Tachypnea, hypoxemia, and diffuse inspiratory crackles are common physical exam findings in acute and subacute HP. Diffuse wheezes may also be present. Inspiratory crackles are also common in chronic HP, and these patients may also have digital clubbing. Hypoxemia with exertion may occur in earlier stages of chronic HP, with resting hypoxemia developing as the disease progresses. Pulmonary function tests usually show a restrictive pattern with abnormal gas exchange in subacute and chronic HP, although obstructive or mixed patterns are sometimes seen.

Chest radiographs in HP are characterized by nonspecific infiltrates, often in the middle and upper lung fields, although plain radiography may be normal in acute HP due to the fleeting nature of the disease. HRCT scanning is more sensitive than chest radiography and typically reveals ground-glass opacities, poorly formed centrilobular nodules (Fig. 6.5), and mosaic attenuation and air trapping patterns resulting from airway obstruction. Chronic HP may have architectural distortion with traction bronchiectasis and honeycombing and may be difficult to differentiate from IPF.

BAL findings are nonspecific but may demonstrate a lymphocytic alveolitis with a low CD4:CD8 ratio, although these findings seem to be less sensitive and specific for chronic compared to subacute disease. Patients with HP may have circulating IgG antibodies (serum precipitins) to the offending antigen, but these are not sufficiently sensitive nor specific for the diagnosis. The specific antigen may not be known or may not be tested for with standard test panels.

Diagnosis. An appropriate exposure, clinical history, BAL, and HRCT imaging findings can suggest the diagnosis, but a lung biopsy may be necessary for confirmation in some cases. Transbronchial biopsy has a relatively high yield for diagnosing subacute HP, but surgical lung biopsy is often required to differentiate chronic HP from other chronic fibrosing ILDs, such as IPF and NSIP.

Treatment and prognosis. For acute and subacute HP, clinical improvement often occurs with separation from the offending exposure, if it is identified. A typical clinical course of acute/subacute HP is improvement in the hospital setting (often with empiric antibiotics for presumed infection), followed by relapse when the patient returns to her or his prehospitalization environment. This waxing and waning pattern of illness can often be an important clue to the diagnosis of HP. The prognosis for acute and subacute HP is favorable, particularly if the offending antigen can be identified and the exposure eliminated. Corticosteroids can help relieve symptoms and accelerate recovery in subacute HP or in more severe cases of acute disease. Corticosteroids and/or other immunosuppressants are also often administered to patients with chronic HP, but data indicating efficacy are lacking. Even with aggressive immunosuppressive therapy, many patients with chronic HP continue to experience gradual worsening of their disease. The presence of fibrosis in HP is a poor prognostic indicator. In fact, chronic (fibrotic) HP often behaves similarly to IPF, with many patients progressing to lung transplantation or death from pulmonary fibrosis. As a result, there is great interest in the potential role of antifibrotic therapy for chronic HP. Identification of the offending antigen is of critical importance in HP, but even then antigen avoidance can be financially or psychologically challenging for patients in the setting of occupational, pet, or residential exposures.

Pneumoconioses

The pneumoconioses are fibroinflammatory lung diseases that result from the inhalation and accumulation of inorganic and mineral dusts in the lungs. The risk and extent of these diseases are related to the intensity and cumulative amount of exposure over time. Prevention of the pneumoconioses through occupational safeguards or, in the case of asbestos, legislative bans on use, is important because there are no effective treatments for these diseases.

Silicosis is caused by exposure to crystalline silica (silicon dioxide), which results in an inflammatory and fibrotic reaction and the formation of the characteristic silicotic nodule. Crystalline silica is abundant in nature, most commonly in the form of quartz, and is present in stone, sand, and concrete. Occupations with a higher likelihood of

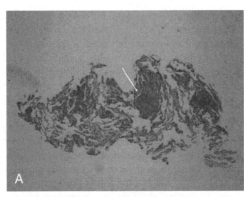
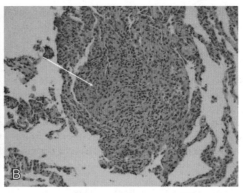

图 6.4　对化疗药物出现过敏反应的患者肺内分化不良的肉芽肿（箭头所示）：（**A**）低倍放大，（**B**）高倍放大

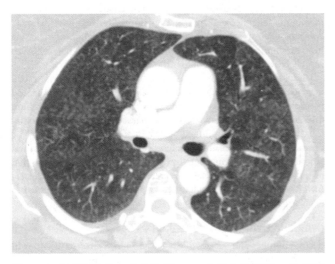

图 6.5　过敏性肺炎患者的胸部 CT，表现为弥漫性、边界模糊的小叶中心结节影

呼吸急促、低氧血症及弥漫性吸气相爆裂音是急性和亚急性 HP 的常见体征，也可闻及双肺弥漫性哮鸣音。吸气相爆裂音在慢性 HP 中也很常见，并可出现杵状指。活动后低氧血症是慢性 HP 的早期表现，到了晚期可进展为静息状态时也有低氧血症。亚急性及慢性 HP 的肺功能检查常呈限制性通气功能障碍和弥散功能障碍，有时也可出现阻塞性或混合性通气功能障碍。

HP 患者的胸部 X 线片特征性表现为非特异性中上肺野浸润影，不过，由于急性 HP 可短期内好转，部分患者的胸部 X 线片可正常。HRCT 较胸部 X 线片能更好地显示肺部病变，可特征性表现为磨玻璃影、边界模糊的小叶中心结节影（图 6.5）、气道阻塞引起的马赛克征及气体陷闭征。慢性 HP 可表现为肺结构受损伴牵拉性支气管扩张及蜂窝形成，可能难以与 IPF 鉴别。

BALF 结果无特异性，可表现为 $CD4^+/CD8^+$ T 淋巴细胞比值降低的淋巴细胞性肺泡炎；相较于亚急性 HP，这一特征在慢性 HP 中的敏感性和特异性更差。HP 患者可存在致敏原特异性的循环 IgG 抗体（血清沉淀素），但对于诊断 HP 来说，这些抗体的检测结果尚不具足够的敏感性及特异性。特异性抗原可能未知或还没有可供检测的标准试剂盒。

诊断　基于暴露史、临床表现、支气管肺泡灌洗液分析及 HRCT 影像学表现可能提示 HP 的诊断，但对于一些患者来说还是需要通过肺活检来诊断 HP。经气管镜透壁肺活检对亚急性 HP 的诊断率较高，但往往需要通过外科肺活检来鉴别诊断慢性 HP 与其他慢性纤维化性 ILD，如 IPF、NSIP。

治疗及预后　对于急性和亚急性 HP，若能明确致敏原，则去除致敏原暴露后临床症状即可缓解；急性和亚急性 HP 患者的典型临床表现在住院、离开致敏环境后好转（因疑诊感染常常给予经验性抗生素治疗），出院回到其住院前的环境后再次患病。这一波动性的临床特征是诊断 HP 的重要线索。急性和亚急性 HP 的预后好，尤其是若能确定致敏原且能脱离致敏环境时。糖皮质激素可缓解临床症状，并促进亚急性 HP 或严重急性 HP 患者康复。糖皮质激素和（或）其他免疫抑制剂也常用于治疗慢性 HP 患者，但其疗效尚无相关客观证据支持。即使接受了积极的免疫抑制治疗，许多慢性 HP 患者病情仍逐渐恶化。肺纤维化是 HP 患者预后不良的指标。实际上，慢性（纤维化性）HP 的表现与 IPF 相似，多数患者可进展为终末期肺纤维化，最终需肺移植或导致死亡。因此，大家对抗纤维化药物治疗慢性 HP 的潜在作用很感兴趣。寻找 HP 的致敏原至关重要，但避免接触职业环境、宠物或居住环境中存在的致敏原，对于这些患者来说，无疑在其经济收入和心理负担层面带来挑战。

肺尘埃沉着病

肺尘埃沉着病是吸入的无机粉尘和矿物粉尘在肺内沉积后导致的纤维化和炎症性疾病。本病的发生及其严重程度与上述粉尘的暴露强度、累积暴露量有关。迄今尚无有效的治疗措施，职业防护或立法禁用某些高致病性矿材（如石棉）就尤为重要。

硅沉着病（硅肺）是接触游离晶体硅（二氧化硅）后，引起肺部炎症及纤维化反应、特征性的矽结节形成。游离晶体硅广泛存在于自然界中，最常见的是石英，也可存在于石头、沙子和混凝土中。很容易暴露

exposure to silica include mining, stone cutting, carving, polishing, foundry work, and abrasive clearing (e.g., sandblasting). Although exposure is usually chronic (over years), accelerated and acute disease manifestations have been described in the setting of heavier short-term exposures.

Acute silicosis is rare and the consequence of high-level silica exposure over a relatively short period of time. It is characterized by alveolar filling with silica dust and surfactant material, causing a pattern of disease that closely resembles pulmonary alveolar proteinosis (described above). Chronic silicosis results in simple nodular silicosis, and progressive massive fibrosis, which is characterized by extensive bilateral apical fibrosis resulting from the confluence of many silicotic nodules.

Patients with silicosis may have dyspnea or may be relatively asymptomatic but require further evaluation of an abnormal chest radiograph. Chest radiographs in uncomplicated silicosis show upper lobe nodular opacities, which may be subtle, whereas progressive massive fibrosis results in marked architectural distortion of the upper lobes (Fig. 6.6). Hilar node enlargement may be accompanied by "eggshell" nodal calcification. Pulmonary function tests in simple nodular silicosis may be normal or show a mixed obstructive or restrictive pattern, whereas progressive massive fibrosis is typically associated with severe restriction and hypoxemia. Patients with silicosis are at elevated risk for tuberculosis and should be screened for latent tuberculosis infection; there is also an association between silicosis and rheumatoid arthritis.

Coal worker's pneumoconiosis is an uncommon cause of pulmonary fibrosis, occurring in workers exposed to coal dust and graphite. Usually, the patients are exposed while working in underground mines. Coal worker's pneumoconiosis results in the formation of pigmented lesions in the lung surrounded by emphysema, called *coal macules*. Progressive massive fibrosis may subsequently occur. Most patients have chronic cough, which is usually productive, resulting from bronchitis related to coal exposure or to tobacco. The chest radiograph shows diffuse, small, rounded opacities. As with silicosis, there is an association with rheumatoid arthritis. Caplan's syndrome is the occurrence of multiple, large, sometimes cavitary lung nodules in association with rheumatoid arthritis after coal dust exposure.

Asbestosis results from chronic exposure to asbestos, which is a fibrous silicate used for insulation, for friction-bearing surfaces, and to strengthen materials. The inhaled asbestos fibers are deposited in the lungs, where the small fibers may be phagocytosed and cleared through lymphatics to the pleural space, but the longer fibers are often retained. Asbestos exposure typically leads to pleural disease characterized by pleural plaques, effusion, and fibrosis, but it does not necessarily affect the lung parenchyma. If it does, it is called *asbestosis*, with interstitial lung fibrosis resulting from asbestos exposure.

Asbestosis is characterized by a gradual onset of dyspnea. As with other pneumoconioses, the risk and severity of disease are related to the extent and duration of exposure. Asbestosis is often diagnosed after exposure has ceased, and disease progression may continue in the absence of ongoing exposure because of the reaction to retained asbestos fibers in the lung. The clinical presentation, pulmonary function tests, and imaging studies are similar to those for restrictive lung diseases such as IPF. However, the detection of significant pleural disease is useful in distinguishing this illness from other ILDs.

The diagnosis of asbestosis is made from the history of exposure and demonstration of concomitant pleural plaques and lower lobe predominant fibrotic changes on the chest radiograph or CT scan. In uncertain cases, the demonstration of asbestos in tissue specimens may be necessary. Asbestos bodies are the characteristic finding and consist of asbestos fibers coated by iron-containing (ferruginous) material. Asbestos exposure increases the incidence of malignancy, including lung carcinoma and mesothelioma, especially among people who also smoke. No specific treatment for asbestosis exists.

Berylliosis results from exposure to beryllium, a rare metal useful in modern, high-technology industries. Exposure to beryllium can lead to an acute chemical bronchitis and pneumonitis or chronic beryllium disease. Chronic beryllium disease is characterized by a granulomatous pneumonitis that is difficult to distinguish from sarcoidosis. The diagnosis is made by history of exposure, histologic examination, and laboratory confirmation using the beryllium lymphocyte proliferation test that is available at specialized centers. Corticosteroids may be useful in the treatment of berylliosis, but patients should avoid further exposure to beryllium.

Drug and Radiation-Induced ILD

A large number and variety of drugs can induce adverse reactions in the lung, often in the form of ILD (Table 6.4). These reactions vary in severity from self-limited hypersensitivity reactions to acute respiratory distress syndrome (ARDS) resulting in respiratory failure and even death. Together, this group of illnesses is often referred to as drug-induced lung injury (DILI). A high index of suspicion is needed to make the association between a drug and a pulmonary reaction, and a careful review of medications and other pharmacologic substances used by a patient is necessary in the setting of diffuse lung disease.

The clinical presentation of a drug-induced ILD is often nonspecific, with cough and dyspnea accompanied by radiographic

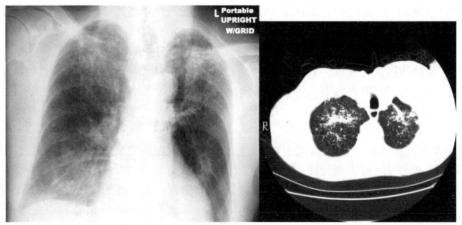

Fig. 6.6 Architectural distortion of the upper lobes in a patient with silicosis.

于硅的职业包括从事硅开采、石材切割、雕刻、抛光、铸造、磨料清理（如喷砂）等。虽然往往是持续数年的慢性暴露后引起硅肺，但也有报道在短期内暴露于大量二氧化硅导致的速发型急性硅肺。

急性硅沉着病是一种罕见疾病，是短期内暴露在高浓度二氧化硅环境中所致。其特征性的表现为肺泡腔内二氧化硅粉尘和表面活性物质沉积，这种表现与之前提到的肺泡蛋白沉积症很相似。而慢性硅沉着病多表现为单纯性矽结节形成和进行性大块肺纤维化，其特征为大量二氧化硅结节融合后导致广泛的双肺尖纤维化。

硅沉着病患者可以出现呼吸困难，也可以无明显临床症状，但若出现了胸部 X 线片异常后均需进一步评价。非复杂性硅沉着病的胸部 X 线片表现为上肺分布的、边界不清的结节影，但进展性大块肺纤维化时表现为肺上叶结构的严重破坏（图 6.6）。肺门淋巴结肿大可伴"蛋壳样"钙化。单纯性矽结节患者的肺功能检查结果可正常，或出现混合性通气功能障碍，或限制性通气功能障碍，但进展性大块肺纤维化患者则表现为严重限制性通气功能障碍及低氧血症。硅沉着病患者患结核病的风险高于常人，故而应注意筛查潜在的结核感染；此外，硅沉着病与类风湿关节炎也相关。

煤工肺尘埃沉着病（煤工尘肺）是导致肺纤维化的少见病因，发生在有煤及石墨暴露史的工人。患者多在地下煤矿开采时暴露于此种物质。煤工尘肺患者肺气肿围绕着的肺内色素斑即煤斑，出现后可继发快速进展的大块纤维化。暴露于煤尘或烟草引起支气管炎后，大部分煤工尘肺患者会出现慢性咳嗽、咳痰。胸部 X 线片表现为弥漫性、小圆结节。与硅沉着病一样，煤工尘肺患者也与类风湿关节炎有关。Caplan 综合征是指煤尘暴露后的类风湿关节炎患者出现的肺内多发大结节，部分可出现空洞。

石棉沉着病是慢性石棉暴露后引起的，石棉是一种用于绝缘、摩擦轴承表面并具加固作用的纤维硅酸盐材料。吸入的石棉纤维在肺内沉积后，其中较小的石棉纤维可被肺泡内巨噬细胞吞噬并通过淋巴管到达

胸膜腔，但较长的石棉纤维无法被清除。石棉暴露常可导致胸膜病变，其特征性的表现为胸膜斑、胸腔积液及纤维化，但并不一定会累及肺实质。若病变累及肺实质出现肺间质纤维化则称为石棉沉着病。

石棉沉着病在临床上表现为逐渐加重的呼吸困难，与其他肺尘埃沉着病一样，其发病与否及严重程度取决于暴露的持续时间及暴露量。石棉沉着病常在停止石棉暴露后才出现，且因石棉纤维持续存在于肺内，即便停止石棉暴露，肺纤维化仍在进展。石棉沉着病的临床表现、肺功能及影像学特点与 IPF 等其他限制性肺疾病类似。伴有显著的胸膜病变有助于鉴别石棉沉着病和其他疾病。

诊断石棉沉着病要基于职业暴露史、并存的胸膜斑及影像学上出现的以肺下叶受累为主的肺纤维化。对一些表现不典型的患者，有必要进行病变部位的活检以证实石棉沉积。石棉小体由被覆含铁物质的石棉纤维组成，是该病特征性的组织病理学表现。石棉暴露会增加恶性肿瘤发生的风险，包括肺癌及肺间皮瘤，尤其是有吸烟史的患者。目前尚无有效治疗石棉沉着病的措施。

铍肺是暴露于铍引起的，铍是一种罕见的金属，用于现代化高科技工业中。铍暴露会导致急性化学性支气管肺炎或慢性铍病。慢性铍病表现为肉芽肿性肺炎，与结节病很难鉴别。铍病的诊断需结合暴露史、病理学检查及铍淋巴细胞增殖实验（仅能在特定中心检测）。糖皮质激素治疗可能有效，但务必脱离铍接触。

药物和放射相关性 ILD

很多类药物可产生肺毒性，常表现为 ILD（表 6.4）。这些疾病的严重程度差异很大，从自限性的高敏反应至导致严重呼吸衰竭甚至死亡的急性呼吸窘迫综合征均可出现。这组疾病统称药物相关性肺损伤（DILI）。对弥漫性肺病的患者，需要常规疑诊用药史与肺病的相关性，详细问询患者的用药史及其他可能有药物相互作用的物质的使用情况。

药物相关性 ILD 并无特异性临床表现，可出现咳嗽、呼吸困难伴肺部浸润影。可伴有发热，部分伴有

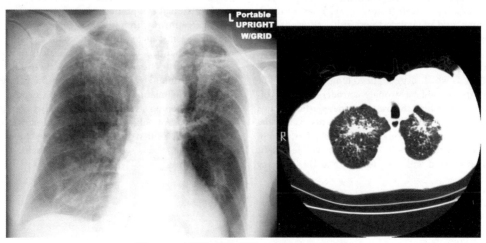

图 6.6　硅沉着病患者肺上叶结构扭曲变形

TABLE 6.4	Common Medications Associated With Drug-Induced Interstitial Lung Disease		
Class	**Drug**	**Class**	**Drug**
Antineoplastic			Osimertinib
Cytotoxic agents	Bleomycin		Panitumumab
	Bortezomib		Rituximab
	Busulfan		Trametinib
	Carmustine		Trastuzumab
	Chlorambucil	Immune checkpoint inhibitors	Atezolizumab
	Cyclophosphamide		Avelumab
	Cytarabine		Durvalumab
	Docetaxel		Ipilimumab
	Doxorubicin		Nivolumab
	Etoposide		Pembrolizumab
	Fludarabine		
	Gemcitabine	Other Biologic Agents	Adalimumab
	Hydroxyurea		Anakinra
	Ifosfamide		Etanercept
	Irinotecan		Infliximab
	Lomustine		Tocilizumab
	Melphalan	Cardiovascular	Amiodarone
	Methotrexate		Captopril
	Mitomycin-C		Flecainide
	Oxaliplatin		Hydralazine
	Paclitaxel		Procainamide
	Pemetrexed		Quinidine
	Procarbazine		Statins
	Temozolomide		Sotalol
	Thalidomide		Tocainide
	Vinblastine		
Molecularly targeted agents	Bevacizumab	Antimicrobial	Daptomycin
	Brigatinib		Nitrofurantoin
	Erlotinib		Sulfasalazine
	Ceritinib	Anti-inflammatory	Cyclophosphamide
	Cetuximab		Gold
	Crizotinib		Leflunomide
	Dasatinib		Methotrexate
	Gefitinib		Sulfasalazine
	Imatinib		

opacities. Fevers can be present, and peripheral eosinophilia is sometimes found. Pulmonary function tests, if performed, usually reveal decreases in diffusion capacity and often show a restrictive pattern. ILD caused by medications usually does not produce a unique radiographic or histologic pattern of lung injury but may result in a variety of nonspecific reactions, including eosinophilic pneumonia, a hypersensitivity pneumonitis-type pattern, organizing pneumonia (OP), diffuse alveolar damage (DAD), nonspecific interstitial pneumonia (NSIP), and pulmonary fibrosis. Drug-induced systemic lupus erythematosus (SLE) can result in an acute pneumonitis, and pleural and pericardial effusions may also be present. Because the clinical presentation of patients with drug-induced ILDs lacks specificity, these are typically diagnoses of exclusion.

There are settings in which drug-induced lung disease may be especially relevant and should be strongly considered in the differential diagnosis. They include the use of antineoplastic therapy, patients with an acute SLE-like illness, and patients using specific agents known to induce pulmonary toxicity, such as methotrexate, amiodarone or nitrofurantoin. All types of antineoplastic therapy have been associated with lung toxicity and ILD, ranging from classic cytotoxic agents (e.g., bleomycin, gemcitabine, taxanes), molecularly targeted therapies (e.g., tyrosine kinase inhibitors, EGFR inhibitors), and more recently immune checkpoint inhibitors (ICIs, e.g., nivolumab, pembrolizumab, ipilimumab). It has been estimated that up to 20% of patients receiving antineoplastic therapy develop some form of lung toxicity. Diagnosis of drug-induced ILD and identification of the offending medication can be challenging in patients receiving antineoplastic therapy because infection and chemotherapy-induced heart failure may result in similar symptoms and radiographic findings, and combination treatment with multiple agents (and radiation) is common. Biologic agents, such as tumor necrosis alpha (TNF-alpha) inhibitors and rituximab, have also rarely been associated with the development of drug-induced ILD. Because these drugs are often used to treat autoimmune conditions that are themselves associated with ILD (e.g., rheumatoid arthritis), in many cases it can be difficult to definitively assign a causal relationship between the drug exposure and the ILD. An online reference website (http://www.pneumotox.com) is available that tabulates the reported pulmonary toxicities of various drugs and is searchable by drug name and pattern of lung involvement.

表 6.4　引起药物相关性间质性肺疾病的常见药物

分类	药物	分类	药物
抗肿瘤药物			奥希替尼
细胞毒性药物	博来霉素		帕尼单抗
	硼替佐米		利妥昔单抗
	白消安		曲美替尼
	卡莫斯汀		曲妥珠单抗
	苯丁酸氮芥	免疫检查点抑制剂	阿特珠单抗
	环磷酰胺		阿维鲁单抗
	阿糖胞苷		德瓦鲁单抗
	多西他赛		伊匹木单抗
	多柔比星		纳武利尤单抗
	依托泊苷		帕博利珠单抗
	氟达拉滨	其他生物制剂	阿达木单抗
	吉西他滨		阿那白滞素
	羟基脲		依那西普
	异环磷酰胺		英夫利昔单抗
	伊立替康		托珠单抗
	洛莫司汀	心血管药物	胺碘酮
	美法仑		卡托普利
	甲氨蝶呤		氟卡尼
	丝裂霉素 -C		肼屈嗪
	奥沙利铂		普鲁卡因胺
	紫杉醇		奎尼丁
	培美曲塞		他汀类药物
	甲基苄胺		索他洛尔
	替莫唑胺		妥卡尼
	沙利度胺	抗生素	达托霉素
	长春碱		呋喃妥因
分子靶向药物	贝伐珠单抗		柳氮磺吡啶
	布加替尼	抗炎药	环磷酰胺
	厄洛替尼		姜黄素
	赛瑞替尼		来氟米特
	西妥昔单抗		甲氨蝶呤
	克唑替尼		柳氮磺吡啶
	达沙替尼		
	吉非替尼		
	伊马替尼		

外周血嗜酸性粒细胞增多。肺功能检查常提示弥散功能障碍伴限制性通气功能障碍。药物相关性 ILD 的影像学并无特异性，组织病理学有肺损伤，可伴有一系列非特异性反应，包括嗜酸粒细胞性肺炎、过敏性肺炎样表现、机化性肺炎、弥漫性肺泡损伤、非特异性间质性肺炎和肺纤维化。药物性系统性红斑狼疮（SLE）可出现急性肺炎，也可伴有胸腔积液和心包积液。药物相关性 ILD 的临床表现并无特异性，往往是排除性诊断。

　　某些药物相关性 ILD 与药物使用密切相关，临床用药时要尤其关注；在出现相关表现时的鉴别诊断过程中需重点考虑，如抗肿瘤药物使用史、患者出现急性狼疮样表现、肺毒性药物（如甲氨蝶呤、胺碘酮或呋喃妥因）使用史。所有抗肿瘤药物都可有肺毒性，都可能导致药物相关性 ILD，包括传统的细胞毒性药物（如

博来霉素、吉西他滨、紫杉烷）、分子靶向药物（如酪氨酸激酶抑制剂、EGFR 抑制剂）和最近使用的免疫检查点抑制剂（ICI，如纳武利尤单抗、帕博利珠单抗、伊匹木单抗）。据统计，高达 20% 的患者在抗肿瘤药物治疗中会出现肺毒性。由于肺部感染和化疗所致的心功能不全的临床症状及影像学表现均与药物相关性 ILD 类似，且肿瘤患者经常接受多种药物（和放射治疗）的联用，故而对这类患者来说药物相关性 ILD 的诊断和致病药物的确定很有挑战性。生物制剂，如肿瘤坏死因子 - α（TNF- α）抑制剂和利妥昔单抗，导致药物相关性 ILD 罕见。但此类药物常用于治疗可能导致 ILD 的自身免疫性疾病（如类风湿关节炎），对多数患者来说很难确定药物暴露与 ILD 之间的因果关系。网站（http://www.pneumotox.com）列举了目前已报道的具有肺毒性的药品，可按药品及肺受累的类型进行查询。

Drug-induced ILD may be dose dependent, as with bleomycin, for which the risk of lung toxicity increases with cumulative doses exceeding 450 U. Amiodarone lung disease typically occurs with dosages greater than 400 mg per day. In other cases (e.g., with biologic or molecularly targeted therapies or immune checkpoint inhibitors) these reactions can be idiosyncratic and can occur either early or late in the treatment course. Synergistic lung toxicities may occur. For example, exposure to high levels of inspired oxygen may precipitate bleomycin lung injury and should be avoided if possible in exposed patients. Treatment of drug-induced ILD consists of discontinuation of the offending agent, glucocorticoids, and supportive care.

ILD can also be caused by ionizing radiation and is referred to as radiation-induced lung injury (RILI). There are two distinct types of RILI, radiation pneumonitis and radiation fibrosis, and these can occur in any patient undergoing thoracic irradiation for treatment of malignancy (e.g., lung or breast cancer, thoracic lymphoma). The main risk factors are the total dose of radiation delivered to the lung and volume of lung irradiated. Concurrent chemotherapy, particularly those that are known to sensitize tumors to radiation therapy, can also increase the risk of RILI. Interestingly, preexisting ILD also seems to confer an increased risk of RILI, suggesting that there may be host factors (e.g., genetics, prior environmental exposures) that predispose an individual to developing inflammatory or fibrotic reactions to a variety of insults to the lung.

Radiation pneumonitis usually develops within the first 3 months following irradiation, whereas radiation fibrosis typically presents much later (greater than 6 months). Symptoms are nonspecific and included dyspnea and a dry cough. Constitutional symptoms (fevers, malaise) may also be present. The physical exam typically reveals inspiratory crackles. Chest radiographs typically show hazy opacities in acute pneumonitis or reticulonodular opacities when fibrosis is present. HRCT imaging is generally done and provides more detailed information, demonstrating ground-glass opacities and areas of consolidation in radiation pneumonitis and reticular opacities, traction changes, and architectural distortion in the setting of radiation fibrosis. Although not always present, a "straight line effect"—the presence of radiographic or CT opacity that terminates abruptly, with a demarcation border that does not respect normal anatomic boundaries (Fig. 6.7)—is virtually pathognomonic for RILI. There are reports of RILI

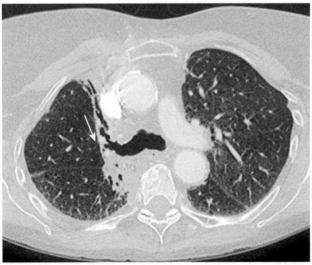

Fig. 6.7 CT image from a patient with lung fibrosis due to prior mediastinal radiation. There is a sharp demarcation between the fibrotic and normal lung *(arrow)* that crosses the major fissure, representing the "straight-line" effect.

occurring outside of the radiation field, but the mechanisms for more widespread lung injury after radiation are unknown. Bronchoscopy with BAL and/or lung biopsy can be helpful for ruling out infection or other processes (e.g., progression of cancer), but otherwise these modalities have little role in the diagnosis of RILI since the BAL fluid characteristics and histologic features are nonspecific.

Treatment of symptomatic, moderate-to-severe radiation pneumonitis typically consists of an extended course (4-6 weeks) of high-dose glucocorticoids, followed by gradual tapering. There can often be significant improvement in symptoms, lung function, and radiographic abnormalities in the subacute setting. However, those patients who develop radiation lung fibrosis generally do not improve, and corticosteroids (or other treatments) are generally ineffective.

Intentional Exposures
Cigarette Smoking

Cigarette smoking is well known to be the primary cause of chronic bronchitis and emphysema, collectively referred to as chronic obstructive pulmonary disease (COPD). It is also a risk factor for idiopathic pulmonary fibrosis (IPF), as described above. Although much less common than COPD, several types of ILD can also be directly caused by cigarette smoking, specifically respiratory bronchiolitis–interstitial lung disease (RB-ILD), desquamative interstitial pneumonia (DIP), and pulmonary Langerhans cell histiocytosis (PLCH). These are sometimes collectively referred to as smoking-related interstitial lung disease, and in many cases radiographic and histologic features of two of these entities can coexist. Despite their causal association with cigarette smoking, RB-ILD and DIP are also classified as idiopathic interstitial pneumonias (IIPs) and are discussed earlier in this chapter. Therefore, we will limit our discussion here to PLCH.

Pulmonary Langerhans cell histiocytosis

Definition and epidemiology. Pulmonary Langerhans cell histiocytosis (PLCH), formerly called *eosinophilic granuloma* or *pulmonary histiocytosis X,* is a rare ILD that is most common in middle-aged adults and seen almost exclusively in cigarette smokers. It is characterized by an abnormal infiltration of Langerhans cells, which are specific types of dendritic cells, into the lung parenchyma. Although a multisystem Langerhans cell disease related to clonal proliferation of Langerhans cells occurs in children, isolated pulmonary LCH in adult smokers does not appear to be a clonal neoplastic disorder.

Pathology. Pulmonary LCH results in the formation of cysts and nodules in the lungs. The accumulation of activated Langerhans cells results in stellate nodular infiltrates around the small airways, with eventual destruction and dilation of the airway walls, resulting in cystic changes in the lung parenchyma. Smoking may alter local immune signaling, attracting the Langerhans cells to the lungs, or it may cause local proliferation and increased survival of Langerhans cells in the lungs. Biopsy of the lung demonstrates multiple stellate lung nodules that may be cellular or fibrotic, containing Langerhans cells that stain for Cd1a and S100. Electron microscopy may reveal Birbeck granules, distinctive racquet-shaped structures in the Langerhans cells.

Clinical presentation. Patients may be asymptomatic or may exhibit constitutional symptoms, dyspnea on exertion, and cough, possibly with hemoptysis. Spontaneous pneumothorax may also occur. Pulmonary function tests show impaired diffusion capacity, and an obstructive or restrictive pattern may be seen. Chest imaging shows nodules that may be cavitary and cysts that predominate in the middle and upper lung zones. Classic HRCT findings are bilateral, mid and upper lung zone predominant, irregular nodules and "bizarre," thick-walled cysts (Fig. 6.8).

药物相关性 ILD 可以呈现剂量依赖性，如当博来霉素的累积剂量超过 450 U 后，其肺毒性风险增加。胺碘酮肺病多发生于日剂量 400 mg 以上时。然而，对于其他一些药物（如生物制剂、分子靶向治疗药物或免疫检查点抑制剂），肺毒性则变化莫测，可在用药早期或晚期发生。此外，多种肺毒性因素联用时可能有协同作用。例如，高浓度氧疗可能加重博来霉素肺损伤，因此使用博来霉素的患者应尽量避免高浓度氧疗。药物相关性 ILD 的治疗包括停药、糖皮质激素和支持治疗。

由电离辐射引起的 ILD 称为放射性肺损伤（RILI）。有两种不同类型的 RILI——放射性肺炎和放射性肺纤维化，均可在任何接受胸部放疗的恶性肿瘤（如肺癌、乳腺癌、胸部淋巴瘤）患者中发生。RILI 的主要危险因素是肺部总辐射剂量和照射肺野的体积。联合化疗，即便是放疗的增敏化疗，也可能增加致 RILI 的风险。基线有 ILD 的肿瘤患者也会增加致 RILI 的风险，表明某些宿主因素（如遗传、环境暴露）会使这些患者易于在肺损伤后发生肺内炎症或纤维化反应。

放射性肺炎常发生在放疗后的前 3 个月内，而放射性肺纤维化则晚一些出现（大于 6 个月）。RILI 临床表现无特异性，常表现为呼吸困难和干咳。还可出现全身症状（发热、乏力）。体格检查常闻及吸气相爆裂音。胸部 X 线片上，在急性肺炎期表现为模糊的斑片渗出影，在纤维化期表现为网状结节影。HRCT 则能更全面地反映肺内病变：放射性肺炎期表现为磨玻璃影、局灶实变影；放射性纤维化期表现为网格影、牵拉性支气管扩张和肺结构扭曲变形。有时可见放射野和正常肺之间形成锐利的"刀切征"，不受肺叶的解剖学结构限制（图 6.7），这也是 RILI 的特征性影像学表现。RILI 也可发生在放射肺野之外的肺部，但

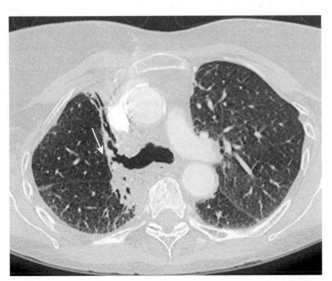

图 6.7　CT 示纵隔放疗后肺纤维化。在纤维化区域和正常肺组织间边界清晰，跨越叶间裂，呈现"刀切征"（箭头所示）

致放疗后大范围的肺损伤机制尚不明确。支气管镜下的 BALF 和（或）肺活检有助于排除感染或其他病因（如肿瘤进展），不过，RILI 的 BALF 和肺组织病理学并无特异性表现。

有症状的、中重度放射性肺炎的治疗往往推荐延长疗程（4 ~ 6 周）的大剂量糖皮质激素后再逐渐减量。对于亚急性放射性肺炎患者，经上述治疗后，临床症状、肺功能和影像学表现均会显著改善。不过，放射性肺纤维化的患者一般糖皮质激素治疗无效。

有意暴露
吸烟

众所周知，吸烟是慢性支气管炎、肺气肿、慢性阻塞性肺疾病（慢阻肺病，COPD）的主要病因。前面的章节中提到过，吸烟也是 IPF 的危险因素。虽然不如在慢阻肺病中这样常见，但有些类型的 ILD 也可以由吸烟直接导致，尤其是 RB-ILD、DIP 和肺朗格汉斯细胞组织细胞增生症（PLCH）。这些疾病可以统称为吸烟相关性间质性肺疾病，对于许多患者来说，可以同时存在上述两种疾病的影像学、病理组织学表现。不过，虽然 RB-ILD 和 DIP 与吸烟相关，但其已经被归类到 IIP 中，这些已在本章前面的章节描述，此处不再复述。因此，本部分仅讨论 PLCH。

肺朗格汉斯细胞组织细胞增生症

定义和流行病学　肺朗格汉斯细胞组织细胞增生症（PLCH），既往称为嗜酸性肉芽肿或肺组织细胞增生症 X，属于罕见 ILD，好发于中年患者，几乎仅见于吸烟人群。其特征是肺实质内朗格汉斯细胞（一种特殊的树突状细胞）异常浸润。虽然儿童患者可出现朗格汉斯细胞克隆性增生导致的多系统受累的朗格汉斯细胞疾病，但吸烟的成年患者的孤立性 PLCH 并无朗格汉斯细胞克隆性增生的生物学行为。

病理学　PLCH 的肺组织内出现多发囊泡及结节。活化的朗格汉斯细胞在小气道周围浸润形成星状结节，最终引起气道破坏及扩张导致肺实质内多发囊性病变。吸烟可改变局部免疫信号转导途径，趋化大量朗格汉斯细胞至肺，这或许会导致肺内朗格汉斯细胞增生或寿命延长。肺组织活检见肺内形成细胞性或纤维化性星状结节，包含 CD1a 及 S100 染色阳性的朗格汉斯细胞。电镜下可见 Birbeck 颗粒，这是朗格汉斯细胞特征性的"球拍样"结构。

临床表现　PLCH 患者可无症状，也可出现全身症状及劳力性呼吸困难、咳嗽，部分可见咯血；还可以发生自发性气胸。肺功能提示弥散功能减低，也可见阻塞性或限制性通气功能障碍。胸部 HRCT 可见双侧中上肺野分布为著的不规则结节影及奇形怪状的厚壁囊泡影（图 6.8）。

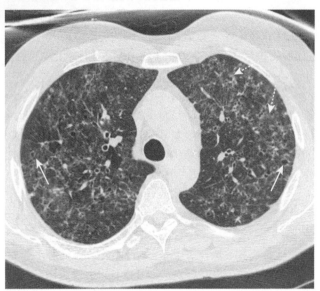

Fig. 6.8 CT image from a patient with pulmonary Langerhans cell histiocytosis (PLCH) demonstrating numerous thick-walled cysts *(solid arrows)* and irregularly shaped nodules *(dashed arrows)*.

Diagnosis and differential diagnosis. When the classic CT pattern described above is seen in a middle-aged cigarette smoker, PLCH can generally be diagnosed without the need for a lung biopsy. The differential diagnosis includes other cystic lung diseases, such as lymphangioleiomyomatosis (LAM), lymphocytic interstitial pneumonia (LIP), and Birt-Hogg Dubé syndrome, sarcoidosis, emphysema, and other smoking-related ILDs. The presence of coexisting emphysema or other smoking-related ILD (e.g., DIP) can sometimes confound the diagnosis on imaging alone.

Treatment and prognosis. The main treatment is tobacco cessation. Corticosteroids and cytotoxic agents are sometimes employed as adjunctive therapy. Lung transplantation may be considered in cases of advanced disease. In contrast to systemic LCH, pulmonary LCH is not a neoplastic disorder, and spontaneous regression may occur with smoking cessation. Although some patients have a benign course, others develop progressive disease or complications such as pulmonary hypertension, which may be fatal.

Other Exposures

Illicit drugs such as heroin and cocaine commonly produce adverse pulmonary reactions. Substances such as talc may be injected or inhaled inadvertently during the use of illicit drugs, resulting in pulmonary vascular or interstitial disease. Heroin use typically results in pulmonary edema or aspiration injury rather than ILD. Cocaine use can produce a variety of pulmonary effects, including organizing pneumonia, alveolar hemorrhage, and diffuse alveolar damage. "Crack lung" is a clinical diagnosis typified by dyspnea, hemoptysis, and pulmonary infiltrates occurring in the setting of crack cocaine use. Recently, the United States has seen an outbreak of acute ILD in the setting of electronic cigarette use or vaping, termed vaping-associated pulmonary illness (VAPI) or e-cigarette associated lung injury (EVALI). These cases have typically occurred in younger individuals and seem to be more common with the use of THC-containing e-cigarettes. A variety of patterns of lung injury have been seen, and many cases have been severe, with progression to ARDS and even death. The specific cause(s) of lung injury from e-cigarette use are currently unknown, but some cases have been linked to chemical additives (such as vitamin E acetate) in some e-cigarette products.

ILD DUE TO SYSTEMIC DISEASES

Interstitial lung disease can be a manifestation of a wide variety of systemic diseases (see Table 6.1), but by far the most common are the connective tissue disease (CTDs). Several vasculitides, which like CTDs are characterized by autoimmunity, also can cause ILD. Sarcoidosis is commonly thought of as a lung disorder, but it is in fact a multisystem disease that frequently involves the lung in a variety of different ways. In this chapter, we will discuss ILD associated with CTDs, the vasculitides, sarcoidosis, and lastly a more rare condition, lymphangioleiomyomatosis (LAM).

Connective Tissue Diseases

CTDs (also known as collagen vascular diseases, systemic rheumatic diseases) are a group of multisystem disorders characterized by dysregulation of the immune system (i.e., "autoimmunity") leading to inflammation and/or fibrosis of many different organ systems. ILD is a common manifestation of many CTDs, most notably systemic sclerosis (SSc), rheumatoid arthritis (RA), the idiopathic inflammatory myopathies (polymyositis/dermatomyositis; PM/DM), Sjögren's syndrome (SS), and mixed connective tissue disease (MCTD) (Table 6.5). Lung disease is a major cause of morbidity and mortality in these conditions. Chronic ILD is relatively uncommon in systemic lupus erythematosus (SLE), which usually is complicated by acute pneumonitis or diffuse alveolar hemorrhage. A finding of chronic ILD in a patient with SLE should prompt evaluation for MCTD or overlap syndromes (e.g., RA-SLE overlap).

Some patients presenting with ILD already have established CTD diagnoses, or the presence of CTD-ILD is discovered as a result of screening these high-risk patient populations. In other cases, a thorough history and physical examination may reveal abnormalities that strongly suggest an underlying CTD, such as inflammatory arthritis or joint deformities, myalgias or muscle weakness, sicca symptoms, esophageal dysmotility, Raynaud's phenomenon, rashes or other skin changes. In some cases, however, it appears that ILD can be the first sign of an otherwise occult CTD, with other manifestations of the disease not developing until months or even years later. This phenomenon of ILD preceding other CTD symptoms or signs is best described in RA and PM/DM, and the presence of an evolving CTD may be suspected based on the presence of circulating autoantibodies in the setting of ILD. For this reason, the evaluation of patients with newly diagnosed ILD typically involves routine serologic testing aimed at identifying evidence of occult CTD. Lastly, there are some patients with ILD who have circulating autoantibodies and/or clinical features that suggest a possible autoimmune process but do not meet criteria for any defined CTD. Terms that have been used to describe these entities include "lung-dominant" CTD, form fruste of CTD, or autoimmune-featured ILD. Recently, the term interstitial

TABLE 6.5 Frequency of Interstitial Lung Disease in Connective Tissue Diseases	
Connective Tissue Disease	**Incidence of ILD**
Systemic sclerosis	50-60%
Rheumatoid arthritis	10-15%
Polymyositis/dermatomyositis	20-80%
Mixed connective tissue disease	50-60%
Sjögren's syndrome	10-20%
Systemic lupus erythematosus	5-10%

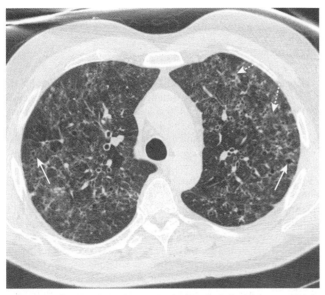

图 6.8　肺朗格汉斯细胞组织细胞增生症患者胸部 CT 可见大量厚壁囊腔（实线箭头所示）及形态不规则的结节影（虚线箭头所示）

诊断和鉴别诊断　当中年吸烟者出现典型 CT 表现时，可无需肺活检即可诊断为 PLCH。鉴别诊断包括其他肺部囊性病变，如 LAM、LIP 和 Birt-Hogg Dubé 综合征、结节病、肺气肿和其他吸烟相关性 ILD。合并肺气肿或其他吸烟相关性 ILD（如 DIP）时，很难仅凭影像学表现诊断为 PLCH。

治疗和预后　戒烟为 PLCH 最主要的治疗，糖皮质激素及细胞毒性药物有时可作为辅助治疗，晚期患者可考虑行肺移植。与系统性 LCH 不同，PLCH 并非为肿瘤性疾病，部分患者戒烟后可自发缓解。虽然某些患者预后良好，但部分患者病变可能进展或发生肺动脉高压等并发症，这可能致死。

其他暴露因素

海洛因和可卡因等违禁毒品常会引起肺部不良反应。滑石粉等物质可在静脉或刺入毒品时进入体内，引起肺血管疾病或间质性肺疾病。吸食海洛因常会引起肺水肿或吸入性损伤，并非 ILD。可卡因会产生多种肺部病变，包括机化性肺炎、肺泡出血和弥漫性肺泡损伤。用快克可卡因后可出现呼吸困难、咯血和肺部浸润影等"快克肺"的特异性表现。最近，美国暴发了电子烟或水烟吸入后导致的急性 ILD，分别称为水烟相关性肺疾病（VAPI）或电子烟相关性肺损伤（EVALI）。这类疾病好发于年轻人，使用含有四氢大麻酚的电子烟时更常见，可以出现多种类型的肺损伤，部分可进展为 ARDS，甚至死亡。电子烟引起的肺损伤的具体机制不明，不过，有些可能与电子烟产品中的化学添加剂（如维生素 E 醋酸酯）有关。

系统性疾病相关 ILD

间质性肺疾病可以是多种系统性疾病的表现（见表 6.1），但迄今为止最常见的是结缔组织病（CTD）。像 CTD 一样以自身免疫为特征的几种血管炎也可以引起 ILD。结节病往往被认为是肺病，但实际上它是一种多系统受累的疾病，且肺部受累的表现也多种多样。在本章中，我们将讨论与 CTD、血管炎、肉芽肿病相关的 ILD，最后还会提及一种较罕见的疾病，即肺淋巴管平滑肌瘤病（LAM）。

结缔组织病

结缔组织病（CTD，也称为胶原血管病、系统性风湿病）是一组由于免疫系统失调（即"自身免疫"）引起的多个不同器官系统的炎症和（或）纤维化的多系统疾病。ILD 是许多 CTD 的常见表现，尤其是系统性硬化症（SSc）、类风湿关节炎（RA）、特发性炎性肌病 [多发性肌炎（PM）/皮肌炎（DM）]、干燥综合征（SS）和混合性结缔组织病（MCTD）（表 6.5）。肺病是这些疾病发病和致死的主要原因。在系统性红斑狼疮（SLE）患者中，慢性 ILD 相对不多见，而急性肺炎或弥漫性肺泡出血更为常见。所以，在 SLE 患者出现慢性 ILD 时，应及时开展相关评价以明确是否存在 MCTD 或重叠综合征（例如 RA-SLE 重叠）。

有些患者在诊断 CTD 后出现 ILD 的表现，或在 ILD 高发的 CTD 患者中筛查时发现 CTD-ILD。另外，详细的病史和体格检查可能高度提示存在潜在 CTD，如炎性关节炎或关节畸形、肌痛或肌肉无力、干燥征的症状（口干、眼干等）、食管运动障碍、雷诺现象、皮疹或其他皮肤病变。此外，在某些情况下，ILD 似乎可能是某些 CTD 相关表现不明显患者的首发表现，而 CTD 的相关表现在 ILD 后数月甚至数年后才出现。这种情况常出现在 RA 和 PM/DM 患者中，一般因 ILD 患者出现上述疾病的特征性抗体时才被考虑到潜在 CTD 的可能。故而，对新发的 ILD 患者的初始临床评价中要常规包括潜在 CTD 的血清学筛查。最后，还有些 ILD 患者，虽然有某些血清自身抗体阳性和（或）CTD 相关的临床表现，但这些特征又不足以诊断某一确定的 CTD。有多个不同的术语来描述这些疾病，包括"肺部受累为主"的 CTD、顿挫型 CTD 或具有自身免疫特征的 ILD。最近，

表 6.5　结缔组织病中间质性肺疾病的发生率

结缔组织病	ILD 发生率
系统性硬化症	50% ~ 60%
类风湿关节炎	10% ~ 15%
多发性肌炎 / 皮肌炎	20% ~ 80%
混合性结缔组织病	50% ~ 60%
干燥综合征	10% ~ 20%
系统性红斑狼疮	5% ~ 10%

pneumonia with autoimmune features (IPAF) has been proposed, along with specific classification criteria, to better study and define this patient population. It remains to be seen whether the clinical course of those who could be classified as having IPAF more closely mimics that of defined CTD-ILD or that of the idiopathic interstitial pneumonias described above.

Lung biopsy is not typically indicated for the diagnosis of ILD in the setting of an established CTD, but when performed, the histologic patterns of ILD are similar to those seen with the IIPs. Nonspecific interstitial pneumonia (NSIP) is overall the most common histology associated with CTD-ILD, but usual interstitial pneumonia (UIP) and organizing pneumonia (OP) are also not uncommon. In some cases, there is a mix of histologic patterns (e.g. NSIP-OP overlap). HRCT patterns typically correspond to the histologic pattern.

Clinical manifestations of CTD-ILD are nonspecific but generally include exertional dyspnea and dry cough. CTD-ILD may be relatively asymptomatic, manifesting as an incidental finding on imaging or only detected as a consequence of aggressive screening with HRCT. Lung examination in patients with CTD-ILD may reveal bibasilar crackles, and pulmonary function tests often show a restrictive pattern with decreased diffusion capacity. If obstruction is identified on pulmonary function testing, airway manifestations of the connective tissue disorder, such as obliterative bronchiolitis in the setting of rheumatoid arthritis, must be considered. In the majority of cases of CTD-ILD, particularly with SSc and RA, the symptoms are chronic and slowly progressive, and this typically correlates with NSIP and/or UIP histologic and HRCT patterns of abnormality. More subacute symptoms can be seen with OP-like manifestations of CTD-ILD (often in RA or PM/DM). Importantly, acute fulminant presentations of CTD-ILD can also be seen, often with rapid progression to respiratory failure/ARDS. This is most often seen in PM/DM, where the histologic and HRCT patterns are often suggestive of diffuse alveolar damage (DAD) or a combination of DAD and OP, or in SLE, where DAD or capillaritis with DAH can be seen.

Other non-ILD forms of lung involvement can occur in CTD and may sometimes provide clues to the underlying diagnosis. The presence of pulmonary hypertension that does not seem to be attributable to the ILD itself is suggestive of SSc or MCTD, and the presence of pleural effusions suggests the possibility of SLE. Severe respiratory muscle weakness can occur in PM/DM and can contribute to dyspnea, PFT abnormalities, and respiratory failure. Lastly, pharyngeal muscle weakness (PM/DM) and/or esophageal dysfunction (SSc) can lead to recurrent aspiration.

Corticosteroids and other immunosuppressive drugs targeting the underlying disease process are generally considered the mainstay of treatment for CTD-ILD, although in most cases data from large, randomized controlled trials are lacking. Cyclophosphamide and mycophenolate have both been shown to be beneficial at slowing the progression of SSc-ILD, and smaller studies have suggested benefit to other treatment strategies in SSc and other CTDs (e.g., rituximab, azathioprine, calcineurin inhibitors, etc). In general, the likelihood of a response to immunosuppressive therapy seems to be somewhat determined by the pattern of ILD, similar to that seen in the IIPs (OP > cellular NSIP > fibrotic NSIP > UIP). As a group, CTD-ILDs are felt to be more responsive to treatment than IPF. However, because in many cases CTD-ILD can be predominantly a fibrotic process that is chronic and progressive (e.g., SSc-ILD and RA-ILD with a UIP pattern), there is a great deal of interest in using the newer antifibrotic agents developed for IPF in these patients, too. Indeed, a recent randomized controlled trial demonstrated that the antifibrotic drug nintedanib was able to successfully slow the progression of SSc-ILD.

Vasculitides

The vasculitides represent a group of entities characterized by inflammation of blood vessel walls, leading to loss of vascular integrity, bleeding, and tissue ischemia. They include GPA, microscopic polyangiitis (MPA), EGPA, pauci-immune pulmonary capillaritis, anti–glomerular basement membrane (anti-GBM) disease, and CTD-associated vasculitis. Many of the vasculitides that affect the lungs are associated with circulating autoantibodies directed against neutrophil cytoplasmic antigens (i.e., antineutrophil cytoplasmic antibodies [ANCA]). Two major immunofluorescent patterns can be seen in ANCA testing: diffuse staining throughout the cytoplasm (cANCA) or perinuclear staining (pANCA). Specific antigens that ANCAs are directed against include proteinase 3 (PR3), typically causing the cANCA pattern, and myeloperoxidase (MPO), which typically causes the pANCA pattern.

GPA is a systemic necrotizing granulomatous vasculitis that often involves the small and medium-sized vessels of the upper airway, the lower respiratory tract, and the kidney. Although this triad is not always seen at initial presentation because only 40% of those affected have renal disease at that time, 80% to 90% of patients eventually develop glomerulonephritis. The most frequent manifestations of this illness are pulmonary, as highlighted by cough, chest pain, hemoptysis, and dyspnea. Constitutional symptoms such as fever and weight loss and symptoms due to involvement of the skin, eye, heart, nervous system, and musculoskeletal system are also common.

Chest imaging may show bilateral disease and infiltrates that evolve over the course of the illness. Lung nodules are common and may cavitate. Effusions and adenopathy are uncommon. Sinus films or CT scans can diagnose upper airway involvement. The diagnosis of GPA is supported by clinical findings and by circulating ANCAs, which are seen in 90% of patients. The remaining 10% of patients are ANCA negative. In ANCA-positive patients, antibodies are usually in a cANCA pattern and are directed against PR3; however, 10% to 20% may have pANCA patterns with anti-MPO antibodies.

Tissue biopsy at a site of active disease is usually needed to confirm a diagnosis of GPA. A renal biopsy is preferred because it is easier to perform and more often diagnostic. In the absence of renal involvement, a lung biopsy should be considered. Pathologically, GPA is characterized by small and medium-sized vessel necrotizing vasculitis and granulomatous inflammation. Special stains and cultures should be performed to exclude infections that can produce similar findings.

MPA is a form of systemic necrotizing small vessel vasculitis that universally affects the kidneys, whereas pulmonary involvement occurs in only 10% to 30% of patients. This rare condition has a prevalence of 1 to 3 cases per 100,000 people, but it is the most common cause of pulmonary-renal syndrome. MPA often is heralded by a long prodromal phase, characterized by constitutional symptoms followed by the development of rapidly progressive glomerulonephritis. In patients who develop lung involvement, diffuse alveolar hemorrhage (DAH) due to capillaritis is the most common manifestation. Joint, skin, peripheral nervous system, and gastrointestinal involvement also can be seen.

Seventy percent of patients with MPA are ANCA positive, and most are in a pANCA pattern with anti-MPO antibodies. Because pANCA/anti-MPO and cANCA/anti-PR3 antibodies can occur in MPA and GPA, these diseases cannot be distinguished based on their ANCA pattern. However, they can be distinguished pathologically because MPA is characterized by a focal, segmental necrotizing vasculitis affecting venules, capillaries, arterioles, and small arteries without clinical or pathologic evidence of necrotizing granulomatous inflammation. The absence or paucity of immunoglobulin localization in vessel walls distinguishes

专家们提出了具有自身免疫特征的间质性肺炎（IPAF）这一称谓，并定义了具体的分类标准，以更好地研究和描述这类患者。目前尚不明确 IPAF 患者的临床过程是更类似 CTD-ILD 还是更类似特发性间质性肺炎。

在已确诊的 CTD 患者中出现 ILD 时，一般不再建议肺活检，但如果进行了肺活检，则其组织病理学类型与特发性间质性肺炎（IIP）中的一些类型相似。非特异性间质性肺炎（NSIP）往往是 CTD-ILD 中最常见的组织病理学类型，而普通型间质性肺炎（UIP）和机化性肺炎（OP）也并不少见。某些 CTD-ILD 患者中，存在混合的组织病理学类型（如 NSIP-OP 重叠）。HRCT 的形态学类型一般与组织病理学类型一致。

CTD-ILD 的临床表现并无特异性，以劳力性呼吸困难和干咳常见。CTD-ILD 也可能并无明显的临床症状，在影像学检查时偶然发现 ILD，或在行 HRCT 筛查时才发现 ILD。CTD-ILD 患者的肺部查体可闻及双肺底爆裂音，肺功能检查常显示限制性通气功能障碍和弥散功能下降，若出现阻塞性通气功能障碍，则需要考虑结缔组织病相关性气道疾病，如类风湿关节炎患者的闭塞性细支气管炎。大多数 CTD-ILD 的临床表现呈现慢性病程、缓慢加重，特别是 SSc-ILD 和 RA-ILD 患者，这类患者常表现为 NSIP 型和（或）UIP 型的组织学和 HRCT 类型。更多的亚急性的临床表现可出现在 OP 样类型的 CTD-ILD 中（常见于 RA 或 PM/DM 中）。值得关注的是，某些 CTD-ILD 可呈现急性暴发性临床表现，常快速进展到呼吸衰竭 /ARDS。这种情况最常见于 PM/DM，其组织病理学和 HRCT 类型常表现为弥漫性肺泡损伤（DAD）或 DAD 和 OP 重叠型，或出现在 SLE 中，此时可看到 DAD 或毛细血管炎伴弥漫性肺泡出血（DAH）。

CTD 患者还可以出现 ILD 以外的其他类型的呼吸系统表现，而这些可为诊断潜在的 CTD 提供线索。非 ILD 相关性肺动脉高压可提示 SSc 或 MCTD，而胸腔积液提示 SLE 的可能。PM/DM 可因严重的呼吸肌无力出现呼吸困难、肺功能检测（PFT）异常和呼吸衰竭。最后，吞咽肌无力（PM/DM）和（或）食管功能障碍（SSc）可引起反复误吸。

治疗 CTD 常用的激素、免疫抑制剂也是用来治疗 CTD-ILD 的常用药物，不过，目前尚无大规模的随机对照临床试验来佐证。已有研究证实环磷酰胺和吗替麦考酚酯能延缓 SSc-ILD 的进展，另有小规模的研究也表明其他一些药物（如利妥昔单抗、硫唑嘌呤、钙调神经磷酸酶抑制剂等）对 SSc 和其他 CTD 可能有用。从某种程度上来说，对免疫抑制剂的疗效往往与 ILD 的类型相关（OP >细胞性 NSIP >纤维性 NSIP > UIP），这与 IIP 中的治疗反应类似。总体来说，CTD-ILD 患者对激素、免疫抑制剂的疗效优于 IPF 患者。然而，有不少 CTD-ILD 可主要呈现慢性和进展性的肺纤维化过程（如 UIP 型 SSc-ILD 和 RA-ILD），也可以尝试在这些 CTD-ILD 患者中应用治疗 IPF 的新型抗纤维化药物。近期也已有随机对照试验表明，抗纤维化药物尼

达尼布能够有效减缓 SSc-ILD 进展。

血管炎

血管炎是一组以血管壁炎症后引起的血管完整性丧失、出血和组织缺血为特征的疾病。包括 GPA、显微镜下多血管炎（MPA）、EGPA、寡免疫性肺毛细血管炎、抗肾小球基底膜（抗 GBM）病和与 CTD 相关性血管炎。许多影响肺部的血管炎与循环中针对中性粒细胞胞质抗原的自身抗体 [即抗中性粒细胞胞质抗体（ANCA）] 有关。在 ANCA 测试中有两种主要的免疫荧光类型：胞质型染色（cANCA）或核周型染色（pANCA）。ANCA 针对的特定抗原包括蛋白酶 3（PR3，对应 cANCA）和髓过氧化物酶（MPO，对应 pANCA）。

GPA 是一种系统性的坏死性肉芽肿性血管炎，常常累及上呼吸道、下呼吸道和肾脏的小型和中型血管。不过，并非所有的 GPA 患者首发症状中均包括上述三联征：在病初，仅 40% 的患者有肾病，但其实 80% ～ 90% 的 GPA 患者最终均会出现肾小球肾炎。肺部症状是 GPA 最常见的临床表现，以咳嗽、胸痛、咯血和呼吸困难多见。发热和体重减轻等全身症状，以及皮肤、眼睛、心脏、神经系统和肌肉骨骼系统受累时相应的症状在临床上也很常见。

胸部影像学检查可表现为双侧、逐渐加重的浸润影。肺部结节常见，部分可形成空洞。胸腔积液和淋巴结肿大不常见。鼻窦平片或 CT 可发现上呼吸道受累。GPA 的诊断依据包括相应的临床表现和外周血 ANCA 阳性（ANCA 阳性率为 90%）。剩余的 10% 患者 ANCA 阴性。在 ANCA 阳性患者中，cANCA 阳性多见，对应抗 PR3 抗体阳性；10% ～ 20% 的患者 pANCA 阳性，对应抗 MPO 抗体阳性。

确诊 GPA 往往需要活动性病变部位的组织活检。鉴于肾活检简单易行以及诊断阳性率高，建议首选肾活检。若无肾脏受累，则考虑肺活检。病理学上，GPA 特征性的病理表现为小至中等血管的坏死性血管炎和肉芽肿性炎。还应安排组织标本的特殊染色和培养以排除有相似病理表现的感染性疾病。

MPA 是一种系统性坏死性小血管炎，一般都会累及肾脏，10% ～ 30% 的患者会累及肺部。MPA 的发病率为（1 ～ 3）/100 000 人，它是致肺出血肾炎综合征的最常见病因。MPA 的前驱病程长，主要以全身症状为主；随后进展为快速进展的肾小球肾炎。毛细血管炎引起的弥漫性肺泡出血（DAH）是 MPA 最常见的肺部受累表现。还可以出现关节、皮肤、周围神经系统和胃肠道受累的症状。

70% 的 MPA 患者有 ANCA 阳性，大多数为抗 MPO 阳性的 pANCA。由于 MPA 和 GPA 患者中均可出现 pANCA/抗 MPO 和 cANCA/抗 PR3 抗体，因此无法仅凭 ANCA 类型来鉴别这两类疾病。但是，两者的病理表现有特异性，可用来鉴别诊断：MPA 特征性病理表现是局灶性、节段性坏死性血管炎，累及小静脉、毛细血管、微动脉和小动脉，但没有坏死性肉芽肿性炎症的临床或病理特征。无或寡血管壁免疫球蛋白沉积可以鉴别 MPA 与免疫复合物介

MPA from immune complex–mediated small vessel vasculitis such as Henoch-Schönlein purpura and cryoglobulinemic vasculitis.

Treatments for GPA and MPA are similar. Combination therapy with corticosteroids and cyclophosphamide is the standard of care to induce remission. Plasma exchange is added in cases of severe disease and provides better renal outcomes. Azathioprine or methotrexate can be substituted for cyclophosphamide if remission is achieved. Rituximab may be used for induction of remission in place of cyclophosphamide or for relapsing disease.

EGPA (formerly known as Churg-Strauss syndrome) is characterized by the triad of asthma, hypereosinophilia, and necrotizing vasculitis. Many other organ systems, including the nervous system, skin, heart, and gastrointestinal tract, may be involved. The vasculitis can be associated with skin nodules and purpura. Although DAH and glomerulonephritis may occur, they are much less common than in the other small vessel vasculitides. Morbidity and mortality often result from cardiac or gastrointestinal complications or status asthmaticus and respiratory failure.

ANCAs are less helpful in the diagnosis of EGPA because only 50% of patients are ANCA positive. Anti-MPO antibodies are more commonly seen in these patients. Pathologically, a necrotizing small vessel vasculitis and an eosinophil-rich inflammatory infiltrate with necrotizing granulomas are seen. Most patients respond well to corticosteroids, but other immunosuppressants such as cyclophosphamide may be required for patients with refractory disorders.

Other causes of pulmonary capillaritis include the connective tissue diseases (particularly SLE), pauci-immune pulmonary capillaritis, and anti–glomerular basement membrane (anti-GBM) disease (i.e., Goodpasture's syndrome). Pauci-immune pulmonary capillaritis is characterized by neutrophilic infiltration of the alveolar septae with negative ANCA testing and no other systemic manifestations of vasculitis. Goodpasture's syndrome causes DAH associated with glomerulonephritis due to anti-GBM antibodies to the α_3 chain of type IV collagen that is also found in the lung basement membrane. More than 90% of patients with Goodpasture's syndrome have anti-GBM antibodies detectable in the serum. For those without circulating antibodies, the diagnosis may be confirmed by lung biopsy, although the kidney is the preferred site. Up to 40% may also be ANCA positive, primarily with anti-MPO antibodies. Pathologically, linear deposition of antibody along the alveolar or glomerular basement membrane is visible by direct immunofluorescence. The treatment of Goodpasture's syndrome is plasmapheresis and immunosuppression. The disease is fatal if left untreated.

Sarcoidosis
Definition and Epidemiology
Sarcoidosis is a multisystem granulomatous disorder of unknown cause. The lungs and thoracic lymph nodes are frequent sites of involvement. Sarcoidosis is relatively common, with a prevalence of 1 to 40 cases per 100,000 people worldwide. A higher incidence of sarcoidosis is reported among Scandinavian, German, and Irish individuals residing in northern Europe. In the United States, the prevalence rates of sarcoidosis are 10.9 cases per 100,000 white individuals and 35.5 cases per 100,000 African Americans, with women in both groups being more frequently affected. Because sarcoidosis may be asymptomatic, the true prevalence may be higher. Sarcoidosis typically occurs in individuals between 10 and 40 years old.

Pathology and Pathophysiology
Sarcoidosis is characterized by the formation in tissues of noncaseating granulomas that organize in an inner core of epithelioid histiocytes, CD4+ T lymphocytes, and giant cells, which are surrounded by a rim of lymphocytes, fibroblasts, and connective tissue (Fig. 6.9).

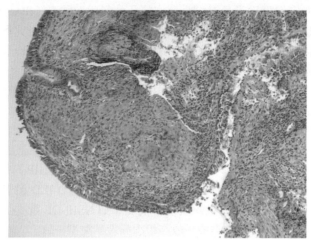

Fig. 6.9 Subepithelial noncaseating granuloma, which is characteristic of sarcoidosis, from an endobronchial biopsy.

Granulomas are found in the airways or lung parenchyma in more than 90% of patients with sarcoidosis. Granulomatous angiitis may also be found in the lungs. The upper respiratory system, lymph nodes, skin, and eyes are commonly involved. Virtually any other organ may be affected, including the liver, bone marrow, spleen, musculoskeletal system, heart, salivary glands, and nervous system.

The granulomas may be clinically silent or, if extensive, may disrupt normal organ structure and function. The cause of these lesions is unknown, but given the frequency of lung involvement, inhaled antigens ranging from bacteria (especially mycobacteria and *Propionibacterium*) to environmental substances have been hypothesized to trigger the onset of granulomatous inflammation. This inflammation may be self-limited or may be propagated, possibly by repeated exposure to the unknown antigen or because of defective immune regulation.

Familial susceptibility to sarcoidosis exists, and alleles of human leukocyte antigen (HLA) genes involved in antigen presentation and a mutation in the butyrophilin-like 2 gene *(BTNL2)*, a possible immunoregulatory gene, have been associated with susceptibility to sarcoidosis. A single causative antigen initiating granuloma formation may not exist, and sarcoidosis instead may represent a stereotypical inflammatory reaction to various antigens in a genetically susceptible host.

Sarcoidosis is associated with abnormal immune function as evidenced by cutaneous anergy and as exhibited in lung by an increased ratio of CD4+ to CD8+ T lymphocytes and increased concentrations of pro-inflammatory cytokines such as interferon-γ, interleukin-12, and tumor necrosis factor-α (TNF-α). These derangements can be detected in the bronchoalveolar lavage (BAL) fluid and are consistent with an imbalance in the production of type 1 (T_H1) and type 2 (T_H2) helper T-cell cytokines, favoring the production of the former and promoting persistent inflammation. Sarcoidosis may occur in the setting of immunomodulatory therapy, especially with interferon-α, or the immune reconstitution syndrome, occurring after initiation of antiretroviral therapy for human immunodeficiency virus (HIV) infection, highlighting the role of immune imbalances in the disorder.

Clinical Presentation
The clinical presentation of patients with sarcoidosis varies. The disease is frequently detected incidentally on routine chest radiographs of asymptomatic individuals. Others may have diverse acute or chronic symptoms. Patients may develop well-described acute syndromes such as Löfgren syndrome, which includes erythema nodosum, fever, arthritis, and hilar adenopathy, or uveoparotid fever (i.e., Heerfordt

导的小血管炎（如过敏性紫癜和冷球蛋白血症性血管炎）。

GPA 和 MPA 的治疗方法类似。糖皮质激素联合环磷酰胺治疗是诱导缓解的标准治疗方法。重症患者可加用血浆置换，以更好地改善肾病。在缓解期，可用硫唑嘌呤或甲氨蝶呤代替环磷酰胺。利妥昔单抗可代替环磷酰胺用于诱导缓解期或用于复发性病例。

哮喘、嗜酸性粒细胞增多和坏死性血管炎三联征是 EGPA（旧称 Churg-Strauss 综合征）的特征性表现。还可以累及其他多个器官/系统，包括神经系统、皮肤、心脏和胃肠道。血管炎还可出现皮肤结节和紫癜。虽然 EGPA 患者也会出现 DAH 和肾小球肾炎，但相较于其他类型小血管炎，上述表现在 EGPA 中要少见得多。心脏、胃肠道并发症或哮喘持续状态和呼吸衰竭是 EGPA 的常见发病形式和死亡原因。

鉴于仅有 50% 左右的 EGPA 患者 ANCA 阳性，ANCA 对 EGPA 的辅助诊断价值并不大，且以抗 MPO-ANCA 阳性多见。病理学上，可见坏死性小血管炎、嗜酸性粒细胞浸润性炎症伴坏死性肉芽肿。大多数患者对糖皮质激素反应好，环磷酰胺等免疫抑制剂可用于复发性 EGPA 患者。

其他可导致肺毛细血管炎的疾病包括结缔组织病（特别是 SLE）、寡免疫性肺毛细血管炎和抗肾小球基底膜（抗 GBM）病（即肺出血肾炎综合征）。寡免疫性肺毛细血管炎的特征是肺泡间隔内中性粒细胞浸润，ANCA 检测呈阴性，没有血管炎常见的其他系统受累的表现。肺出血肾炎综合征患者，由于体内的抗 GBM 抗体也能针对肺基底膜中的 IV 型胶原蛋白的 α3 链，从而同时引起肾小球肾炎和 DAH。90% 以上的肺出血肾炎综合征患者血清中可检测到抗 GBM 抗体。对于抗 GBM 抗体阴性的肺出血肾炎综合征患者，肾活检是首选措施，但其实也可通过肺活检来诊断。高达 40% 的肺出血肾炎综合征患者也可出现 ANCA 阳性，主要为抗 MPO 阳性的抗体。病理学上，直接免疫荧光可见沿肺泡或肾小球基底膜呈线性分布的抗 GBM 抗体沉积。肺出血肾炎综合征的治疗包括血浆置换和免疫抑制。若未及时治疗，肺出血肾炎综合征也是致命的。

结节病

定义和流行病学

结节病是一种原因未明的系统性肉芽肿性疾病。肺和胸部淋巴结是常见的受累部位。结节病相对常见，全球患病率在（1～40）/10 万人。据报道，居住在北欧的斯堪的纳维亚人、德国人和爱尔兰人中结节病发病率更高。在美国，结节病的患病率在白种人、非裔美国人中分别为 10.9/10 万人、35.3/10 万人，女性患病率均更高一些。由于结节病患者可能无症状，故而其实际患病率可能比上述报道率更高。结节病常发生在 10～40 岁的人群中（译者注：患者居住地、种族可能影响结节病患者的年龄分布）。

病理学和病理生理学

结节病的特征是受累组织中形成非干酪坏死性肉

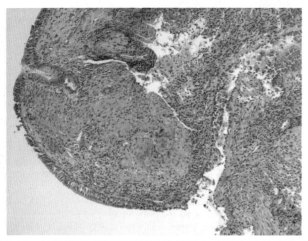

图 6.9 气管镜下支气管黏膜活检显示上皮下非干酪样肉芽肿，为结节病的特征性病理表现

芽肿，肉芽肿的内核由上皮样组织细胞、CD4+ T 淋巴细胞和巨噬细胞组成，周围环绕着淋巴细胞、成纤维细胞和结缔组织（图 6.9）。

90% 以上的结节病患者的气道或肺实质中存在肉芽肿。肺内也可出现肉芽肿性血管炎。结节病也常常会累及上呼吸道、淋巴结、皮肤和眼睛。其实，几乎所有器官都可能受累，包括肝脏、骨髓、脾脏、肌肉骨骼系统、心脏、唾液腺和神经系统。

肉芽肿形成后可无临床症状，但若肉芽肿病变广泛，会破坏器官的正常结构和功能。导致肉芽肿形成的原因尚不明确，不过因为肺部受累很常见，推测吸入的各种抗原，从细菌（尤其是分枝杆菌和丙酸杆菌）到环境中的物质，会触发肉芽肿性炎。这类炎症反应可呈自限性，但也可以因反复接触这些抗原物质或因免疫调节功能缺陷而在体内多处播散。

结节病也有家族易感性，参与抗原提呈的人类白细胞抗原（HLA）基因的等位基因、可能有免疫调节作用的基因——嗜乳杆菌样 2 基因（BTNL2）的突变等可能使得这些人群易患结节病。一般不认为是单一抗原刺激引起结节病肉芽肿，往往是具有结节病易感基因的人群接受多种抗原刺激后导致典型的肉芽肿形成的炎症反应而致病。

结节病患者存在免疫功能异常，表现为皮肤无反应，肺部表现为 CD4+/CD8+ T 淋巴细胞比值增加、促炎细胞因子［如干扰素-γ、白细胞介素-12 和肿瘤坏死因子-α（TNF-α）］浓度增加。这也可在支气管肺泡灌洗（BAL）液中出现，与 1 型（TH1）和 2 型（TH2）辅助 T 细胞的细胞因子失衡相关，其更促进持续性炎症反应。结节病可发生在免疫调节治疗，尤其是干扰素-α 治疗或免疫重建综合征中，以及人类免疫缺陷病毒（HIV）感染的抗逆转录病毒治疗后，凸显免疫失衡在结节病发病中的作用。

临床表现

结节病患者的临床表现多种多样、不尽相同。有些患者症状不明显，而是在常规胸部 X 线检查中偶然发现。有些患者则可出现多种急性或慢性症状。结节病患者可出现

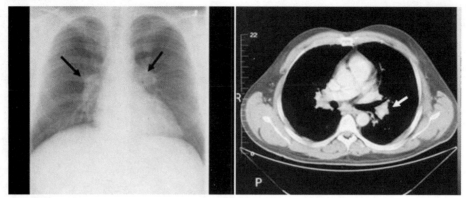

Fig. 6.10 Hilar adenopathy in a patient with sarcoidosis *(arrows)*. (A) Chest radiograph. (B) Chest computed tomography scan. (Courtesy Dr. Rafael L. Perez.)

syndrome), which exhibits the triad of uveitis, parotitis, and facial nerve palsy. Both syndromes are associated with better outcomes than for other clinical presentations of sarcoidosis.

In many cases, symptoms are vague and chronic, and they may include systemic symptoms such as low-grade fevers, fatigue, night sweats, or joint pains. Respiratory manifestations, including shortness of breath, wheezing, dry cough, and chest pain, occur in one third to one half of patients. Skin manifestations include erythema nodosum, plaques, nodules, and lupus pernio, a violaceous, often disfiguring, nodular lesion of the nose and cheeks. Ocular symptoms are also common, and the onset of uveitis may eventually lead to the diagnosis of sarcoidosis when granulomatous extraocular organ involvement is uncovered. Neurosarcoidosis may manifest with cranial nerve palsies or with headache in the setting of lymphocytic meningitis. Sarcoidosis can involve the heart, resulting in a cardiomyopathy. Arrhythmias and sudden cardiac death can occur as a result of the disruption of the conducting system by granulomatous infiltration. Pulmonary hypertension may result from pulmonary fibrosis or directly from granulomatous vasculitis.

In 90% of patients, the chest radiograph shows abnormalities that include bilateral hilar adenopathy (Fig. 6.10), parenchymal opacities, or both. The radiographic changes characteristic of sarcoidosis have been classified as stages 0 through IV (Table 6.6), but this staging system does not imply a typical chronologic progression. However, stage I patients have a better prognosis for resolution than those with more advanced stages of disease.

As in other ILDs, computed tomography (CT) is more sensitive for the detection of parenchymal abnormalities, and it more clearly demonstrates the extent of mediastinal adenopathy. Typical HRCT findings include bilateral, mid and upper lung zone predominant peribronchovascular opacities emanating from the hila, along with extensive micronodules that can be seen within the lung parenchyma and running along the interlobular septae, fissures, and pleural surfaces (Fig. 6.11). Positron emission tomography (PET) or gallium-67 scans may reveal other sites of organ involvement.

Pulmonary function tests show restriction, obstruction, or mixed deficits. Liver involvement may cause mild elevation of transaminase levels, and cirrhosis and liver failure have been reported, although they are rare. Hypercalcemia and hypercalciuria may be detected and are caused by increased intestinal absorption of calcium as a result of increased conversion of vitamin D to its active form in sarcoid granulomas. Kidney stones may result from the abnormal calcium metabolism. Elevated levels of angiotensin-converting enzyme (ACE) are common but are not specific. The use of ACE levels in the diagnosis or management of sarcoidosis is controversial.

TABLE 6.6   Radiographic Staging of Sarcoidosis

Stage	Radiographic Findings
0	Normal radiograph
I	Adenopathy without parenchymal abnormality
II	Adenopathy and parenchymal disease
III	Parenchymal disease without lymphadenopathy
IV	End-stage fibrosis

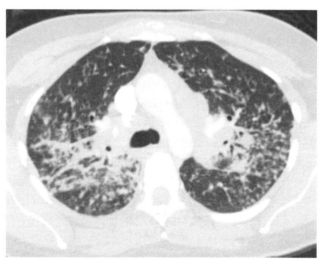

Fig. 6.11 CT image from a patient with sarcoidosis demonstrating bilateral, upper lung zone predominant peribronchovascular opacity and extensive micronodules.

Diagnosis

The diagnosis of sarcoidosis depends on a typical clinical, radiographic, and histologic picture and is a diagnosis of exclusion. Patients with classic syndromes such as the Löfgren syndrome or uveoparotid fever may not require biopsy; however, most patients require tissue biopsy of an affected organ. Tissue samples show noncaseating granulomas, but because this finding is nonspecific, careful attention should be given to ruling out other causes of granulomatous inflammation (e.g., mycobacterial infection) through stains and cultures.

Necrotizing granulomas have rarely been reported in sarcoidosis, but this finding should prompt an intense search for infection. In

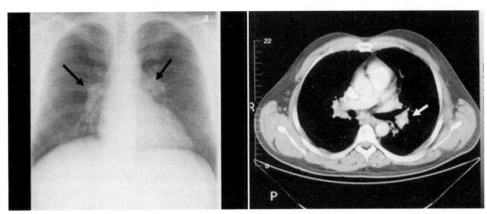

图 6.10　结节病患者肺门淋巴结肿大（箭头所示）。（**A**）胸部 X 线，（**B**）胸部 CT（经 Dr. Rafael L. Perez. 授权）

某些急性综合征，如 Löfgren 综合征，包括结节性红斑、发热、关节炎和肺门淋巴结肿大；或葡萄膜腮腺炎热（即 Heerfordt 综合征），表现为葡萄膜炎、腮腺炎和面神经麻痹三联征。这两类综合征的预后都优于其他结节病。

大多数结节病患者起病隐匿、呈慢性病程，临床症状不明显，可表现为全身症状，如低热、疲劳、盗汗或关节痛。约 1/3 至半数患者会出现呼吸系统症状，包括气短、喘息、干咳和胸痛。皮肤表现包括结节性红斑、斑块、结节和冻疮样狼疮（紫色的、分布在鼻和脸颊的结节，可明显影响患者容貌）。眼部症状也很常见，部分结节病患者可以眼葡萄膜炎起病，在之后出现眼外脏器受累后才被诊断为结节病。神经结节病可表现为脑神经麻痹或淋巴细胞性脑膜炎性头痛。结节病还会累及心脏引起心肌病。肉芽肿浸润破坏心脏传导系统后可致心律失常和心脏性猝死。肺纤维化或肉芽肿性血管炎可导致结节病患者的肺动脉高压。

90% 的结节病患者胸部 X 线片均可有异常表现，包括双侧肺门淋巴结肿大（图 6.10）、肺阴影或两者兼有。基于胸部 X 线片异常表现，结节病可以分为 0 至 Ⅳ 期（表 6.6），但胸部 X 线片分期并不与结节病的病程分期相关，即结节病并不从 0 期逐步进展到 Ⅳ 期。不过，Ⅰ 期患者的预后确实优于其他进展期结节病患者。

与其他 ILD 一样，计算机断层成像（CT）能更好地显示肺内病变和纵隔淋巴结的肿大程度。典型的胸部 HRCT 表现包括双中上肺野、肺门旁沿支气管血管束走行为主的肺部阴影，伴有肺内沿着小叶间隔、叶间裂及胸膜上的弥漫性微结节（图 6.11）。正电子发射断层成像（PET）或 ^{67}Ga 扫描可探测到肺外脏器受累的情况。

肺功能检查显示限制性、阻塞性或混合性通气功能障碍。肝脏受累时可引起转氨酶水平轻度升高，罕见有肝硬化和肝功能衰竭的报道。结节病肉芽肿中维生素 D 转化为活性形式增加会引起肠道对钙的吸收异常增加，从而导致结节病患者高钙血症和高钙尿症。钙代谢异常还会引起肾结石。血管紧张素转换酶（ACE）水平升高常见，但 ACE 并非结节病的特异性诊断指标。血清 ACE 水平作为结节病诊断或疗效评价指标还存在争议。

表 6.6　结节病影像学分期	
分期	胸部 X 线片表现
0	未见异常
Ⅰ	淋巴结增大，不伴肺内浸润影
Ⅱ	淋巴结增大，伴肺内浸润影
Ⅲ	肺实质浸润影，不伴淋巴结增大
Ⅳ	终末期肺纤维化

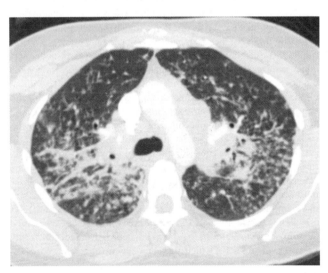

图 6.11　结节病患者 CT 表现为双上叶分布为主的、支气管血管束周边的斑片影和大量小结节影

诊断

结节病是一种排除性诊断，诊断结节病要基于典型的临床表现、影像学和组织病理学表现。Löfgren 综合征或葡萄膜腮腺炎热等典型综合征的患者可不需活检而诊断结节病，除此之外，都要基于受累器官的组织活检来确诊结节病。结节病的组织病理表现为非干酪坏死性肉芽肿，但这一病理表现并不具特异性，要全面结合特殊染色和微生物培养来排除可引起肉芽肿性炎的其他原因（如分枝杆菌感染）。

结节病患者出现坏死性肉芽肿罕见，故对于这样的患者需要强化感染性疾病的鉴别诊断。开胸肺活检是大多数 ILD 的活检方式，但结节病患者则可通过皮肤结节

contrast to most ILDs, in which tissue diagnosis requires open lung biopsy, the granulomas in sarcoidosis can be identified in skin nodules or in lymph nodes. Due to frequent lung and lymph node involvement, bronchoscopy is commonly used to diagnose sarcoidosis. Results of bronchoscopy with transbronchial lung biopsy are positive for 50% to 60% of patients, but the procedure poses the risks of hemorrhage and pneumothorax. Because airway involvement is common, endobronchial biopsies may also demonstrate granulomas. However, there is increasing evidence that transbronchial needle aspiration of mediastinal and hilar lymph nodes using endobronchial ultrasound guidance may have a higher diagnostic yield for granulomas than conventional bronchoscopic techniques.

As mentioned above, sarcoidosis is a multisystem disease, so careful attention must be paid to potential signs and symptoms of extra-pulmonary involvement. After the diagnosis is made, all patients should have an ophthalmologic evaluation to assess for ocular involvement and an ECG to look for conduction abnormalities. Further cardiac testing, including Holter monitoring, echocardiography, or cardiac magnetic resonance imaging (MRI) should also be done depending on the presence of symptoms (e.g., palpitations) or ECG abnormalities. PET scanning can also be helpful for detecting active cardiac involvement from sarcoidosis. Additional imaging studies and/or tissue biopsies may be needed when symptoms or basic lab testing suggests other organ involvement (e.g., headaches, abnormal liver function tests, etc.).

Treatment

Corticosteroids are the mainstay of therapy, although they are not required in all patients with sarcoidosis because many patients are minimally symptomatic and may undergo spontaneous remission. Whether corticosteroids alter the disease course is uncertain. However, corticosteroid therapy should be considered in patients with extra-pulmonary organ involvement, respiratory symptoms, or evidence of progressive pulmonary disease. In patients with pulmonary involvement, oral prednisone at a dosage of 20 to 40 mg per day is typically initiated and maintained for a 4- to 6-week course before being slowly tapered over a course of 3 to 6 months. Some patients may experience remission with this treatment approach and may be managed off therapy for an extended period of time. For patients with disease that is refractory to corticosteroids, or for those who experience disease worsening when steroids are tapered, additional treatments should be considered. Methotrexate is the most commonly used steroid-sparing agent in sarcoidosis, but leflunomide, azathioprine, and mycophenolate have also been used. Anti TNF-α inhibitors (e.g., infliximab) can also be used for refractory disease, and there are some small studies to support this approach in individuals with refractory sarcoidosis or with extra-pulmonary involvement.

Prognosis

The course of sarcoidosis varies. Spontaneous remission is common, and death and disability occur rarely, making decisions regarding treatment initiation difficult. The acute sarcoidosis syndromes tend to remit and not recur. However, about one third of patients with sarcoidosis have chronic, progressive disease, and some patients develop pulmonary fibrosis or other end-organ damage.

Lymphangioleiomyomatosis
Definition and Epidemiology
Lymphangioleiomyomatosis is a rare, slowly progressive, multisystem disorder resulting in cystic interstitial lung disease and kidney angiomyolipomas that occurs in either a sporadic form or in association with tuberous sclerosis complex (TSC-LAM). Sporadic LAM occurs almost exclusively in women of childbearing age.

Pathology

The disease is characterized by extensive infiltration of the lungs and lymphatics with growths of smooth muscle–like lymphangioleiomyomatosis cells. Mutations in the *TSC1* or *TSC2* gene, which encodes tumor suppressor proteins that normally act as inhibitors of protein synthesis and cell growth, may result in tuberous sclerosis or lymphangioleiomyomatosis. Mutations in *TSC2* are associated with greater disease severity.

Clinical Presentation

Dyspnea and spontaneous pneumothorax are the most common presentations, with chylous pleural effusions and hemoptysis also occurring. These clinical presentations result from lung parenchymal destruction, airway narrowing, and lymphatic obstruction caused by the abnormal proliferation of the smooth muscle–like cells.

Imaging studies show an interstitial pattern with middle and upper lung predominance; multiple, thin-walled cystic lesions; and characteristically preserved lung volumes. Pleural effusion or pneumothorax may be seen on imaging. CT of the abdomen may reveal fat-containing kidney lesions consistent with angiomyolipomas. Pulmonary function tests typically show a progressive obstructive pattern, although mixed obstruction and restriction may also be seen.

Diagnosis

Although the clinical features coupled with characteristic imaging are often diagnostic, lung biopsy may be necessary in some cases. It demonstrates interstitial nodules composed centrally of spindle-shaped cells that stain for smooth muscle cell actin and for HMB-45, an antibody to the melanocytic glycoprotein 100, with staining involving the alveolar walls, lobular septa, venules, small airways, and pleura.

Treatment

Treatment involves management of pleural complications, including the use of pleurodesis to prevent recurrent pneumothorax or effusion, bronchodilator and oxygen therapy, and avoidance of pharmacologic estrogens, which may exacerbate the disease. Progesterones have been used in an attempt to modulate disease progression, but efficacy data are limited.

Because the products of the *TSC1* and *TSC2* genes normally act as inhibitors of the mammalian target of rapamycin (mTOR), pharmacologic mTOR inhibitors such as sirolimus and everolimus have been studied in lymphangioleiomyomatosis. Sirolimus stabilized lung function in lymphangioleiomyomatosis, and sirolimus and everolimus treatment resulted in angiomyolipoma shrinkage. Lung transplantation can be performed in patients with severe pulmonary dysfunction.

Prognosis

Lymphangioleiomyomatosis is a slowly progressive disease that can result in potentially fatal complications, especially respiratory failure.

SUMMARY

The interstitial lung diseases (ILDs), or *diffuse parenchymal lung diseases* (DPLDs), are a heterogenous group of nonmalignant and noninfectious lung diseases characterized by varying amounts of inflammation and/or fibrosis (scarring) of the lung parenchyma. ILDs manifest with a wide range of overlapping clinical presentations, radiographic findings, and histologic abnormalities. Because of the similarities shared by many ILDs and the rarity of most of these conditions, establishing a definitive diagnosis can often be difficult and requires the incorporation of a detailed history, physical exam, imaging, and

或肿大的淋巴结活检等小标本活检来诊断。鉴于结节病患者经常有肺和胸内淋巴结受累，也常可通过支气管镜检查来诊断结节病。50% ～ 60% 的结节病患者可通过支气管镜透壁肺活检来诊断，但有出血和气胸的操作相关风险。结节病气道受累常见，因此，支气管内膜活检也常可取到肉芽肿病灶。不过，更多的研究证据表明，经支气管镜超声引导下对纵隔和肺门淋巴结针吸活检，获取肉芽肿病灶的阳性率高于上述传统的支气管镜下操作。

综上所述，结节病是系统性疾病，诊断结节病后还需要密切关注肺外脏器受累相关的体征和症状。诊断结节病后，建议所有患者均安排眼科检查以评价眼部受累情况，并接受心电图检查以排查心律失常。根据是否有临床症状（如心悸）或心电图异常，决定是否安排进一步的心脏检查，包括动态心电图（Holter）监测、超声心动图或心脏磁共振成像（MRI）。PET 扫描有助于发现结节病相关的活动性心脏病变。当出现其他器官受累相关的症状或实验室化验异常时（如头痛、肝功能指标异常等）时，需要额外安排针对性的影像学检查和（或）组织活检。

治疗

糖皮质激素是结节病的主要治疗药物，但并非所有结节病患者都需要使用糖皮质激素。对于许多症状轻微的结节病患者可以自愈。尚不明确，糖皮质激素的使用是否会改变结节病的疾病进程。不过，对于肺外器官受累、有呼吸道症状或肺部病变进行性进展时，要考虑给予糖皮质激素治疗。对于肺结节病患者，一般建议起始剂量为泼尼松 20 ～ 40 mg/d 口服，并维持4 ～ 6 周后开始缓慢减量，在 3 ～ 6 个月内减停。一些结节病患者通过上述治疗后可治愈并能停药。对于糖皮质激素抵抗或减停后复发的结节病患者，应考虑加用其他药物治疗。甲氨蝶呤是治疗结节病最常用的替代糖皮质激素的免疫抑制剂，此外，也可使用来氟米特、硫唑嘌呤和霉酚酸酯。TNF-α 抑制剂（如英夫利昔单抗）也可用于治疗难治性结节病，已有小宗报道表明这类药物可有效治疗难治性结节病或肺外结节病。

预后

结节病患者的病程多种多样：自愈常见，罕见会致死，因此很难决定每个结节病患者是否需要开启药物治疗。急性结节病综合征往往会缓解且不复发。然而，约1/3 的结节病患者会呈现慢性、进行性进展的病程，部分患者还会发展为肺纤维化或其他器官的终末期病变。

淋巴管平滑肌瘤病

定义和流行病学

淋巴管平滑肌瘤病（LAM）是一种罕见的、缓慢进展的多系统疾病，可引起囊性间质性肺疾病和肾血管平滑肌脂肪瘤，有散发性 LAM 和结节性硬化症 LAM（TSC-LAM）两型。散发性 LAM 几乎只出现于育龄女性。

病理学

LAM 的病理特征为肺和淋巴管广泛的平滑肌样淋巴管平滑肌瘤细胞的增生、浸润。*TSC1* 或 *TSC2* 基因突变可导致结节性硬化症或平滑肌瘤病，*TSC1* 或 *TSC2* 基因编码抑制蛋白质合成和细胞生长的肿瘤抑制蛋白。*TSC2* 基因突变时 LAM 病情更重。

临床症状

LAM 最常见的临床表现为呼吸困难和自发性气胸，也可出现乳糜性胸腔积液和咯血。这些临床表现是由于平滑肌样细胞异常增生引起的肺实质破坏、气道狭窄和淋巴管阻塞所致。

影像学检查显示中上肺野为主的肺内多发、薄壁囊腔，肺容积保留是 LAM 的特征。影像学检查还可见胸腔积液或气胸。腹部 CT 检查显示包含脂肪的肾脏病变，符合肾脏血管平滑肌脂肪瘤的表现。肺功能检查往往显示进行性加重的、阻塞性通气功能障碍，但也可能出现混合型通气功能障碍。

诊断

基于临床表现和特征性的胸部影像学表现可以诊断 LAM，但部分患者还需要借助于肺活检才能诊断。肺活检病理提示肺间质结节的中心由平滑肌细胞肌动蛋白和 HMB-45（黑色素细胞糖蛋白 100 的抗体）染色阳性的纺锤形细胞组成，这些细胞可以分布在肺泡壁、小叶间隔、小静脉、小气道和胸膜。

治疗

LAM 的治疗包括处理胸膜病变并发症（胸膜固定术预防复发性气胸或胸腔积液）、支气管扩张剂、氧疗和避免使用可能加重病情的雌激素类药物。已有研究尝试用孕酮来缓解 LAM 患者的病情进展，但疗效相关数据有限。

因为 *TSC1* 和 *TSC2* 基因产物可以抑制哺乳动物雷帕霉素靶蛋白（mTOR），已开展了雷帕霉素和依维莫司等mTOR 抑制剂治疗 LAM 的研究：雷帕霉素可稳定 LAM患者肺功能，雷帕霉素和依维莫司均可缩小血管平滑肌脂肪瘤。肺功能受损严重的 LAM 患者可安排肺移植。

预后

淋巴管平滑肌瘤病是一种缓慢进展的疾病，可导致致命性并发症，尤其是呼吸衰竭。

总结

间质性肺疾病（ILD）或弥漫性肺实质疾病（DPLD）是一组异质性的非恶性和非感染性肺病，其特征是肺实质出现不同程度的炎症和（或）纤维化（瘢痕形成）。不同的 ILD 可出现多种类似的临床表现、影像学表现和组织学异常。由于许多不同的 ILD 表现类似，且大多数

histologic data. Although there is no universally accepted classification system for ILDs, it can be useful to think of these entities as falling into the three broad categories of exposure-related ILDs, ILDs attributable to systemic diseases, and idiopathic ILDs.

The treatment approach for ILDs generally revolves around treating the underlying illness (if present) and removal of offending exposures (if identified), as well as suppressing inflammation in those settings where inflammation is thought to play a prominent role. However, pulmonary fibrosis is a characteristic feature of many ILDs, and fibrosis often progresses despite these approaches. Fortunately, we are now starting to see the emergence of treatments that target the aberrant wound-healing processes that are thought to contribute to the development of lung fibrosis. Antifibrotic treatments are now available for idiopathic pulmonary fibrosis (IPF) that slow the progression of this otherwise fatal disease process, and these treatments may also be effective for other types of fibrotic ILD. However, until therapies are developed that can completely arrest—and ideally even reverse—fibrogenesis, lung transplantation remains the only option for a chance at prolonged survival for many patients afflicted with IPF and other ILDs.

SUGGESTED READINGS

Caminati A, Cavazza A, Sverzellati N, Harari S: An integrated approach in the diagnosis of smoking-related interstitial lung diseases, *Eur Respir Rev* 21(125):207–217, 2012.

Distler O, Highland KB, Gahlemann M, et al: Nintedanib for systemic sclerosis-associated interstitial lung disease, N Engl J Med 380(26): 2518–2528, 2019.

Frankel SK, Schwarz MI: The pulmonary vasculitides, Am J Respir Crit Care Med 186(3):216–224, 2012.

Gupta N, Finlay GA, Kotloff RM, et al: Lymphangioleiomyomatosis diagnosis and management: high-resolution chest computed tomography, transbronchial lung biopsy, and pleural disease management. An official American Thoracic Society/Japanese Respiratory Society Clinical Practice Guideline, Am J Respir Crit Care Med 196(10):1337–1348, 2017.

King Jr TE, Bradford WZ, Castro-Bernardini S, et al: A phase 3 trial of pirfenidone in patients with idiopathic pulmonary fibrosis, N Engl J Med 370(22):2083–2092, 2014.

King Jr TE, Pardo A, Selman M: Idiopathic pulmonary fibrosis, Lancet 378(9807):1949–1961, 2011.

Lederer DJ, Martinez FJ: Idiopathic pulmonary fibrosis, N Engl J Med 378(19):1811–1823, 2018.

Mira-Avendano I, Abril A, Burger CD, et al: Interstitial lung disease and other pulmonary manifestations in connective tissue diseases, Mayo Clin Proc 94(2):309–325, 2019.

Raghu G, Remy-Jardin M, Myers JL, et al: Diagnosis of idiopathic pulmonary fibrosis. An official ATS/ERS/JRS/ALAT clinical practice guideline, Am J Respir Crit Care Med 198(5):e44–e68, 2018.

Richeldi L, du Bois RM, Raghu G, et al: Efficacy and safety of nintedanib in idiopathic pulmonary fibrosis, N Engl J Med 370(22):2071–2082, 2014.

Salisbury ML, Myers JL, Belloli EA, et al: Diagnosis and treatment of fibrotic hypersensitivity pneumonia. where we stand and where we need to go, Am J Respir Crit Care Med 196(6):690–699, 2017.

Spagnolo P, Rossi G, Trisolini R, et al: Pulmonary sarcoidosis, Lancet Respir Med 6(5):389–402, 2018.

Travis WD, Costabel U, Hansell DM, et al: An official American Thoracic Society/European Respiratory Society statement: update of the international multidisciplinary classification of the idiopathic interstitial pneumonias, Am J Respir Crit Care Med 188(6):733–748, 2013.

Vasakova M, Morell F, Walsh S, et al: Hypersensitivity pneumonitis: perspectives in diagnosis and management, Am J Respir Crit Care Med 196(6):680–689, 2017.

ILD 是罕见疾病，确诊某一特定的 ILD 有难度，往往需要整合患者详细的病史、体格检查、影像学和组织病理学表现才能做出诊断。目前尚无被普遍公认的 ILD 分类系统，但将其分为暴露相关 ILD、系统性疾病相关 ILD 和特发性 ILD 三大类有助于 ILD 的诊疗。

ILD 的治疗涉及治疗潜在的基础疾病（若存在）、消除有害暴露（若已确定），以及抗炎治疗（若以炎症反应为主）。然而，许多 ILD 患者会出现肺纤维化，即便采用了上述治疗措施仍未能阻断肺纤维化进程。所幸我们已开发了针对异常的损伤后修复过程的治疗措施。用于特发性肺纤维化（IPF）患者的抗纤维化治疗药物，可以减缓其疾病进展，也对其他类型的纤维化型 ILD 有效。不过，在开发出可完全阻止（理想情况下甚至逆转）纤维化进展的疗法之前，肺移植仍然是延长许多 IPF 和其他 ILD 患者生存期的唯一措施。

推荐阅读

Caminati A, Cavazza A, Sverzellati N, Harari S: An integrated approach in the diagnosis of smoking-related interstitial lung diseases, *Eur Respir Rev* 21(125):207–217, 2012.

Distler O, Highland KB, Gahlemann M, et al: Nintedanib for systemic sclerosis-associated interstitial lung disease, N Engl J Med 380(26): 2518–2528, 2019.

Frankel SK, Schwarz MI: The pulmonary vasculitides, Am J Respir Crit Care Med 186(3):216–224, 2012.

Gupta N, Finlay GA, Kotloff RM, et al: Lymphangioleiomyomatosis diagnosis and management: high-resolution chest computed tomography, transbronchial lung biopsy, and pleural disease management. An official American Thoracic Society/Japanese Respiratory Society Clinical Practice Guideline, Am J Respir Crit Care Med 196(10):1337–1348, 2017.

King Jr TE, Bradford WZ, Castro-Bernardini S, et al: A phase 3 trial of pirfenidone in patients with idiopathic pulmonary fibrosis, N Engl J Med 370(22):2083–2092, 2014.

King Jr TE, Pardo A, Selman M: Idiopathic pulmonary fibrosis, Lancet 378(9807):1949–1961, 2011.

Lederer DJ, Martinez FJ: Idiopathic pulmonary fibrosis, N Engl J Med 378(19):1811–1823, 2018.

Mira-Avendano I, Abril A, Burger CD, et al: Interstitial lung disease and other pulmonary manifestations in connective tissue diseases, Mayo Clin Proc 94(2):309–325, 2019.

Raghu G, Remy-Jardin M, Myers JL, et al: Diagnosis of idiopathic pulmonary fibrosis. An official ATS/ERS/JRS/ALAT clinical practice guideline, Am J Respir Crit Care Med 198(5):e44–e68, 2018.

Richeldi L, du Bois RM, Raghu G, et al: Efficacy and safety of nintedanib in idiopathic pulmonary fibrosis, N Engl J Med 370(22):2071–2082, 2014.

Salisbury ML, Myers JL, Belloli EA, et al: Diagnosis and treatment of fibrotic hypersensitivity pneumonia. where we stand and where we need to go, Am J Respir Crit Care Med 196(6):690–699, 2017.

Spagnolo P, Rossi G, Trisolini R, et al: Pulmonary sarcoidosis, Lancet Respir Med 6(5):389–402, 2018.

Travis WD, Costabel U, Hansell DM, et al: An official American Thoracic Society/European Respiratory Society statement: update of the international multidisciplinary classification of the idiopathic interstitial pneumonias, Am J Respir Crit Care Med 188(6):733–748, 2013.

Vasakova M, Morell F, Walsh S, et al: Hypersensitivity pneumonitis: perspectives in diagnosis and management, Am J Respir Crit Care Med 196(6):680–689, 2017.

Pulmonary Vascular Diseases

Christopher J. Mullin, James R. Klinger

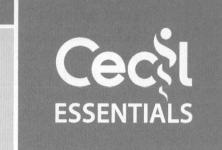

INTRODUCTION

Pulmonary vascular disease is a broad term for any disease that affects the blood vessels of the lungs. These diseases are a heterogeneous group of disorders with multiple causes, but most can be categorized as diseases of either pulmonary embolism or pulmonary hypertension. Some pulmonary vascular diseases, such as idiopathic pulmonary arterial hypertension (PAH), directly affect the pulmonary vessels, whereas other forms of pulmonary vascular disorders are compensatory responses to elevation of pulmonary venous pressure or recurrent hypoxia due to chronic heart and lung diseases. This chapter discusses pulmonary hypertension and pulmonary thromboembolism, with a focus on pulmonary arterial hypertension (PAH) and chronic thromboembolic pulmonary hypertension (CTEPH).

The normal pulmonary vasculature is a high-flow, low-resistance system with very high capacitance that can accept the entire output of the right ventricle with only slight increases in pressure. The right ventricle (RV) in health is well adapted to the pulmonary circulation and matches the cardiac output of the left ventricle with one fifth of the energy expenditure. However, the RV is unable to tolerate large increases in afterload, which occur acutely in the setting of pulmonary thromboembolism and more subacutely or chronically in pulmonary hypertension. As such, right ventricular function is important in the clinical manifestations, diagnosis, treatment, and prognosis of pulmonary vascular diseases.

❖ For a deeper discussion on this topic, please see Chapter 75, "Pulmonary Hypertension," in *Goldman-Cecil Medicine*, 26th Edition.

PULMONARY HYPERTENSION

Definition and Epidemiology

Normal pulmonary arterial pressure (PAP) in healthy adults at rest is about 25/10 mm Hg with a mean PAP (mPAP) of 14.3 mm Hg ± 3.0 mm Hg. Thus, mPAP above 20 mm Hg is two standard deviations above the mean and generally considered to be abnormal. However, mPAP increases slightly with age and is difficult to measure accurately due to limitations in normalizing intravascular pressure to atmospheric pressure. For these reasons, PH is usually defined as mPAP greater than or equal to 25 mm Hg. In 1998, the World Symposium on Pulmonary Hypertension proposed a classification of pulmonary hypertension that grouped diseases with similar pathologic and hemodynamic characteristics. In the most recent version of this classification (Table 7.1), PH is divided into five groups: (1) Pulmonary arterial hypertension (PAH), meant to infer disease of the pulmonary arteries, (2) pulmonary hypertension due to elevated pulmonary venous pressure caused by left-sided heart disease, (3) pulmonary hypertension due to chronic hypoxia or lung disease, (4) pulmonary hypertension

caused by chronic pulmonary emboli, and (5) pulmonary hypertension attributable to unclear or multifactorial mechanisms.

The most common types of pulmonary hypertension are WHO Groups 2 and 3. In one study, nearly 75% of adult cases of PH were due to left heart disease and 10% due to chronic lung disease. However, much of the attention on pulmonary vascular disease has focused on WHO Group 1 PAH. Despite representing a small minority of cases, PAH is the most severe form of pulmonary hypertension and often afflicts relatively young otherwise healthy individuals. Without treatment, median survival is about 3 years. In early registries, the peak incidence of PAH occurred in the fourth decade of life, but it can be seen at all ages and it affects women two to three times more frequently than men. The cause of PAH is unknown, but disease classification has been further subdivided into idiopathic PAH, heritable PAH, and associated PAH (APAH) in which PAH is associated with one of several diseases. Heritable PAH is caused primarily by mutations in the gene for bone morphogenetic protein receptor type 2 *(BMPR2)* representing nearly three quarters of the cases of familial PH and approximately 20% of patients with idiopathic PAH. Mutations in other related genes within the transforming growth factor-β family including (activin receptor-like kinase 1 [ALK1]) and endoglin (ENG) have also been described.

Idiopathic PAH is extremely rare with an incidence estimated at 1 to 10 in 1,000,000. However, APAH is not uncommon in patients with connective tissue disease, especially the limited cutaneous form of scleroderma and mixed connective tissue disease where it can be seen in up to 14% of patients. PAH also occurs in 2% to 3% of patients with portal hypertension and 0.5% of patients with HIV infection. It is also seen in patients exposed to methamphetamines, particularly the anorectic drug phentermine/fenfluramine, and is a common sequel of congenital heart diseases that result in significant left-to-right intracardiac shunt. Pulmonary veno-occlusive disease (PVOD) and pulmonary capillary hemangiomatosis (PCH) constitute a rare subgroup of PH that is characterized by vascular remodeling and occlusion of small pulmonary veins and venules, leading to severe hypoxia and in some cases interstitial edema.

Pulmonary Arterial Hypertension
Pathophysiology

Although the pathogenic mechanisms responsible for PAH are not well understood, the vascular remodeling associated with it has been well described. Prominent features include an obliterative vasculopathy characterized by medial vascular smooth muscle hypertrophy, adventitial thickening, and proliferation of pulmonary vascular endothelial cells. In situ thromboses of small pulmonary arteries and areas of perivascular inflammation are also frequently observed. Plexiform lesions consisting of abnormal proliferation of endothelial cells causing near complete obstruction of the vascular lumen of distal pre-acinar arterioles with areas of recanalization are considered pathognomonic of the

肺血管疾病

王诗尧 译 翟振国 侯刚 审校 代华平 王辰 通审

引言

肺血管疾病广义上是指影响肺部血管的所有疾病。这些疾病是由多种原因引起的一个异质性疾病群，但大多数疾病可以归类为肺栓塞或肺动脉高压（PH）。部分肺血管疾病，如特发性肺动脉高压，会直接影响肺部血管，而其他类型的肺血管疾病则可能是由于肺静脉压力升高，或由于慢性心肺疾病导致反复缺氧而出现的代偿性反应。本章讨论了肺动脉高压和肺血栓栓塞症，重点聚焦于动脉型肺动脉高压（PAH）和慢性血栓栓塞性肺动脉高压（CTEPH）。

正常的肺血管系统是一个高流量、低阻力系统，具有非常高的容纳能力，能够接受右心室的全部心输出量而仅产生轻微的压力增加。在健康人群中，右心室（RV）很好地适应了肺循环系统，并以左心室 1/5 的收缩力匹配其心输出量。然而，右心室无法耐受后负荷的大幅度增加，尤其是在急性肺血栓栓塞症和在亚急性或慢性肺动脉高压的情况下。因此，右心室功能在评价肺血管疾病的临床表现、诊断、治疗和预后中具有重要意义。

❖ 有关此专题的深入讨论，请参阅 *Goldman-Cecil Medicine* 第 26 版第 75 章 "肺动脉高压"。

肺动脉高压
定义和流行病学

在健康成人的静息状态下，肺动脉压（PAP）的正常值约为 25/10 mmHg，平均肺动脉压（mPAP）为 14.3 mmHg±3.0 mmHg。因此，mPAP 高于 20 mmHg，也就是比平均值高出两个标准差，通常被认为是异常的。然而，随年龄增长，mPAP 会略有增加，而且根据大气压力标化血管内的压力也存在很多局限，导致 mPAP 的准确测量较为困难。因此，PH 通常被定义为 mPAP 大于或等于 25 mmHg。1998 年，世界肺动脉高压研讨会上，基于相似的病理和血流动力学特征，提出了一种肺动脉高压的分类方法。在最新版本中（表 7.1），PH 被分为五大类：①动脉型肺动脉高压（PAH）：指肺动脉本身的病变；②左心疾病所致的肺静脉压力升高而引起的肺动脉高压；③慢性缺氧或肺病所致的肺动脉高

压；④由慢性肺栓塞导致的肺动脉高压；⑤机制未明或多因素机制引起的肺动脉高压。

最常见的肺动脉高压类型是 WHO 分组的第 2 大类和第 3 大类。在一项研究中，近 75% 的成人肺动脉高压是由左心疾病引起的，10% 是由慢性肺病引起的。然而，关于肺血管疾病的研究和关注大多集中在 WHO 第 1 大类，即 PAH。尽管 PAH 病例占比很小，但它是一种最严重的肺动脉高压形式，通常影响相对年轻且无基础病的个体。如不进行治疗，中位生存期约为 3 年。在早期的注册登记研究中，PAH 的发病高峰出现在 40 多岁，但在各个年龄段都可以见到，且女性患者的发病率是男性的 2～3 倍。PAH 的病因尚不明确，其疾病分类可进一步细分为特发性、遗传性和与其他疾病相关的 PAH（APAH）。遗传性 PAH 主要是由骨形成蛋白受体 2 型（*BMPR2*）基因突变引起，占家族性肺动脉高压病例的近 3/4，约 20% 的特发性 PAH 患者也存在这一基因突变。其他相关基因突变，包括转化生长因子 -β 家族内的基因，如激活素受体样激酶 1（ALK1）和内皮糖蛋白（ENG）基因突变，也有报道。

特发性 PAH 极为罕见，发病率估计为每 100 万人中 1～10 例。然而，APAH 在结缔组织病患者中并不少见，尤其是局限性硬皮病和混合性结缔组织病的患者中，其患病率可高达 14%。在门静脉高压的患者中，2%～3% 会发生 PAH；在 HIV 感染者中，这一比例为 0.5%。此外，PAH 也可见于使用甲基苯丙胺的患者、尤其是使用食欲抑制药苯丁胺 / 芬氟拉明的患者。PAH 同时也是存在显著左向右心内分流的先天性心脏病的常见后遗症。肺静脉闭塞病（PVOD）和肺毛细血管瘤病（PCH）构成了 PH 的一个罕见亚组，其特征是血管重塑和肺小静脉闭塞，导致严重缺氧，某些情况下还会引起间质性水肿。

动脉型肺动脉高压
病理生理学

尽管 PAH 的致病机制尚不完全清楚，但与其相关的血管重塑已有详细描述。肺血管重塑显著特征包括中层血管平滑肌肥大、外膜增厚以及肺血管内皮细胞的增生，这些特征构成了闭塞性血管病变。此外，也

TABLE 7.1   World Health Organization Classification of Pulmonary Hypertension

Group 1: Pulmonary Arterial Hypertension (PAH)
• Idiopathic PAH
• Heritable PAH
• Drug- and toxin-induced
• PAH associated with:
  • Connective tissue disease
  • Human immunodeficiency virus infection
  • Portal hypertension
  • Congenital heart disease
  • Schistosomiasis
Long-term responders to calcium-channel blockers
PAH with overt features of venous/capillary involvement (pulmonary veno-occlusive disease or pulmonary capillary hemangiomatosis)
Persistent pulmonary hypertension of the newborn

Group 2: Pulmonary Hypertension Due to Left Heart Disease • Heart failure with preserved left ventricular ejection fraction • Heart failure with reduced left ventricular ejection fraction • Valvular heart disease • Congenital/acquired cardiovascular conditions leading to post-capillary PH
Group 3: Pulmonary Hypertension Due to Lung Diseases and/or Hypoxia • Obstructive lung disease • Restrictive lung disease • Other lung diseases with mixed restrictive and obstructive pattern • Hypoxia without lung disease • Developmental lung diseases
Group 4: Pulmonary Hypertension Due to Pulmonary Arterial Obstructions • Chronic thromboembolic pulmonary hypertension • Other pulmonary artery obstruction: sarcoma, other malignant or nonmalignant tumors, arteritis without connective tissue disease, congenital pulmonary artery stenosis, parasites
Group 5: Pulmonary Hypertension With Unclear and/or Multifactorial Mechanisms • Hematologic disorders: chronic hemolytic anemia, myeloproliferative disorders • Systemic and metabolic disorders: sarcoidosis, pulmonary Langerhans cell histiocytosis, glycogen storage disease, Gaucher disease, neurofibromatosis • Others: chronic renal failure with or without hemodialysis, fibrosing mediastinitis • Complex congenital heart disease

Modified from Simonneau G, Montani D, Celermajer DS, et al. Haemodynamic definitions and updated clinical classification of pulmonary hypertension. Eur Respir J 2019; 53: 1801913.

disease. In some cases, vascular remodeling extends into pulmonary capillaries and proximal pulmonary veins. These varied changes result in narrowing of the vascular lumen and are thought to contribute to the increase in pulmonary vascular resistance and pressure. In addition, numerous changes in vascular cell function have been described. Pulmonary vascular endothelial cells show decreased expression of vasodilators such as prostacyclin and nitric oxide and increased expression of pulmonary vasoconstrictors such as thromboxane and endothelin. Pulmonary vascular smooth muscle becomes hypertrophic and proliferative leading to muscularization of distal normally nonmuscularized vessels. Adventitial fibroblasts display an inflammatory phenotype that may induce changes in smooth muscle cell growth. Finally, the loss of distal pulmonary vessels due to abnormal apoptosis of pulmonary vascular endothelial cells is also likely to contribute to the pathogenesis of PAH. It is unclear if the obliterative vascular remodeling characteristic of PAH is the primary cause of the disease or a compensatory response to the increase in blood flow through the remaining vessels. A leading hypothesis is that PAH is caused by a double hit mechanism, the first being vascular injury resulting in loss of distal pulmonary vessels and the second being the deregulation of vascular repair mechanisms that lead to abnormal pulmonary vascular remodeling.

Clinical Presentation

The initial presentation of PAH is often subtle. Initial symptoms include dyspnea on exertion, fatigue or exertional lightheadedness. As the disease progresses, right ventricular failure causes peripheral edema, decreased appetite, ascites, and occasionally exertional chest pain. Severity of PAH is often classified by the degree of exercise impairment using a WHO modification of the New York Heart Association functional class as follows: class I, asymptomatic; class II, symptoms with normal activity; class III, symptoms with less than normal activity; and class IV, symptoms with any physical activity or at rest.

Chest radiographs may reveal prominent pulmonary arteries or right ventricular enlargement. Pulmonary function testing usually shows normal spirometry, but diffusing capacity can be reduced reflecting the restricted circulation and decreased surface area available for gas exchange. Plasma brain natriuretic peptide levels rise as right ventricular pressure increases and a fall in oxygen saturation in response to exercise is often seen.

Diagnosis and Clinical Evaluation

The diagnosis of PAH depends on exclusion of other underlying heart or lung diseases that might cause pulmonary hypertension. Because PAH is

表 7.1　世界卫生组织肺动脉高压分类

第 1 类：动脉型肺动脉高压（PAH）
- 特发性肺动脉高压
- 遗传性肺动脉高压
- 药物和毒物相关肺动脉高压
- 疾病相关肺动脉高压
  - 结缔组织病
  - 人类免疫缺陷病毒感染
  - 门静脉高压
  - 先天性心脏病
  - 血吸虫病

对钙通道阻滞剂长期有反应的肺动脉高压

具有明显肺静脉 / 肺毛细血管受累征象的肺动脉高压（肺静脉闭塞病 / 肺毛细血管瘤病）

新生儿持续性肺动脉高压

第 2 类：左心疾病所致肺动脉高压
- 左心室射血分数保留的心力衰竭
- 左心室射血分数降低的心力衰竭
- 心脏瓣膜病
- 导致毛细血管后肺动脉高压的先天性 / 获得性心血管病

第 3 类：肺部疾病和（或）缺氧所致肺动脉高压
- 阻塞性肺疾病
- 限制性肺疾病
- 其他阻塞性和限制性并存的肺疾病
- 非肺部疾病导致的缺氧
- 肺发育障碍性疾病

第 4 类：肺动脉阻塞所致肺动脉高压
- 慢性血栓栓塞性肺动脉高压
- 其他肺动脉阻塞性疾病：肉瘤等恶性或良性肿瘤、肺血管炎（除外结缔组织病）、先天性肺动脉狭窄、寄生虫感染

第 5 类：未明和（或）多因素机制所致肺动脉高压
- 血液系统疾病：如慢性溶血性贫血、骨髓增殖性疾病
- 系统性和代谢性疾病：如结节病、肺朗格汉斯细胞组织细胞增生症、糖原贮积症、戈谢病、神经纤维瘤病
- 其他：伴或不伴血液透析的慢性肾衰竭，纤维素性纵隔炎
- 复杂性先天性心脏病

改编自 Simonneau G，Montani D，Celermajer DS，et al. Haemodynamic definitions and updated clinical classification of pulmonary hypertension. Eur Respir J 2019；53：1801913.

常观察到肺小动脉的原位血栓形成和血管周围炎症。病理学上，特征性病变包括内皮细胞异常增生形成的丛状病变，几乎完全阻塞了远端小动脉的血管腔，并伴有再通区域。在某些情况下，血管重塑延伸至肺毛细血管和近端肺静脉。这些不同的表现导致血管管腔变窄，并引起了肺血管阻力和压力增加。此外，血管细胞功能的多种变化也有报道。肺血管内皮细胞显示出血管扩张因子（如前列环素和一氧化氮水平）的表达减少，而血管收缩因子（如血栓素和内皮素）的表达增加。肺血管平滑肌肥大和增生，导致远端正常时无肌性血管发生肌化。外膜成纤维细胞呈现炎性表型，可能诱导平滑肌细胞过度生长。最后，由于肺血管内皮细胞异常凋亡导致的远端肺血管丧失，也可能在 PAH 的发病机制中发挥作用。目前尚不清楚 PAH 的闭塞性血管重塑是导致疾病发生的主要原因，还是对流经剩余血管的血流量增加的代偿性反应。一种主流的假说认为 PAH 是由双重打击机制引起的，首先是血管损伤导致远端肺血管丧失，其次是血管修复机制失调导致异常的肺血管重塑。

临床表现

PAH 的早期表现通常较为隐匿。早期症状包括活动后呼吸困难、疲劳或活动时头晕。随疾病进展，右心衰竭会引起外周性水肿、食欲减退、腹水，偶发劳力性胸痛。PAH 的严重程度通常根据活动能力受损的程度进行分级，目前采用的是 WHO 对纽约心脏协会（NYHA）功能分级的修改版本，具体如下：Ⅰ级：无症状；Ⅱ级：正常活动时出现症状；Ⅲ级：低于正常活动时出现症状；Ⅳ级：任何体力活动或静息时出现症状。

胸部 X 线片可显示肺动脉突出或右心室增大。肺功能检查通常显示肺通气功能正常，但弥散能力可能降低，反映了循环受阻和气体交换表面积减少。随着右心室压力的增加，血浆脑钠肽水平升高；活动后氧饱和度下降的现象也很常见。

诊断和临床评估

PAH 的诊断首先需要排除其他可能导致肺动脉高压的潜在心脏或肺部疾病。由于 PAH 在健康个体中

TABLE 7.2	Medications for Treatment of Pulmonary Arterial Hypertension		
Drug Class	**Drug Name**	**Route of Administration**	**Mechanism of Action**
Endothelin receptor antagonist	Ambrisentan	Oral	Inhibits vasoconstriction by blocking endothelin
	Bosentan	Oral	
	Macinentan	Oral	
Phosphodiesterase type 5 inhibitor	Sildenafil	Oral, intravenous	Promotes vasodilation by delaying metabolism of intracellular cGMP
	Tadalafil	Oral	
Prostacyclin derivative	Epoprostenol	Intravenous, inhaled[a]	Promotes vasodilation by increasing intracellular cAMP
	Iloprost	Inhaled, intravenous infusion[a]	
	Treprostinil	Oral, inhaled, subcutaneous infusion, intravenous infusion	
Prostacyclin receptor agonist	Selexipag	Oral	Activates prostacyclin receptor
Soluble guanylyl cyclase stimulator	Riociguat	Oral	Promotes vasodilation by increasing cGMP synthesis

[a]Currently no commercial preparation available for this route of administration in the United States.

extremely rare in healthy individuals, every effort should be made to look for connective tissue disease, portal hypertension, HIV infection, congenital heart disease, chronic pulmonary emboli, or history of exposure to a potentially causative drug or toxin. Most patients should have pulmonary function testing to exclude obstructive or restrictive defects and measure oxygen saturation. Nocturnal hypoxemia from sleep-disordered breathing should be considered. A lung ventilation/perfusion scan should be done to exclude chronic pulmonary embolism and blood tests for screening for autoimmune disease, HIV, or liver dysfunction should be obtained. Left heart disease is usually evaluated by echocardiography, but in some patients, additional studies to assess coronary artery disease or infiltrative cardiomyopathies may be needed. Although rare, PCH and PVOD should be considered, the latter characterized by severe hypoxemia, decreased D_{LCO}, and a triad of centrilobular nodules and ground-glass opacities and thickened interlobular septa on high-resolution chest CT.

Transthoracic echocardiography is often the first step in excluding left-sided heart disease and when used with Doppler ultrasound can provide an estimate of pulmonary artery systolic pressure. In addition, it provides important information on right atrial and ventricular size and function and the relative degree of right- versus left-sided filling pressure by examining the position of the interatrial and interventricular septa. Finally, the presence of significant intracardiac shunts can often be detected.

Definitive diagnosis of PAH requires right heart catheterization to confirm increased mPAP and assess left-sided filling pressure via measurement of pulmonary artery occlusion pressure. Hemoglobin oxygen saturation should be measured in the superior or inferior vena cava, right atrium, and pulmonary artery to exclude significant left-to-right shunt. In patients with PAH, pulmonary vasoreactivity should be tested by administration of a short-acting selective pulmonary vasodilator such as inhaled nitric oxide or intravenous epoprostenol. A decrease in mPAP of 10 mm Hg or greater to a mPAP less than 40 mm Hg without a decrease in cardiac output is considered a positive response and identifies a small group of PAH patients who can often be treated successfully with a calcium-channel blocker.

Treatment

In the last 25 years, five classes of drugs have been approved for the treatment of PAH (Table 7.2). These drugs act primarily as semiselective pulmonary vasodilators, although antimitogenic properties that may slow pulmonary vascular remodeling have also been described. There are insufficient data to compare the relative efficacy of the different drug classes, but in general most treatment guidelines agree on several points: (1) In the absence of severe right heart failure, patients with a positive response to pulmonary vasodilator testing should be given a trial of calcium-channel blocker, usually nifedipine. (2) Patients with the greatest risk of death,

including those in WHO functional class IV, should be treated with continuous intravenous infusion of a prostacyclin derivative. (3) Patients with less advanced PAH such as those in functional class II or III should be treated with a combination of a phosphodiesterase type 5 inhibitor (PDE5) inhibitor and an endothelin receptor antagonist (ERA). Patients who are unable to tolerate this combination or who do not improve while taking it should be considered for treatment with soluble guanylate cyclase (sGC) stimulators in place of a PDE5 inhibitor or use of an inhaled or oral prostacyclin derivative or a prostacyclin receptor agonist.

Response to treatment is assessed by (1) symptomatic improvement as measured by change in functional class, (2) objective improvement in exercise capacity as assessed by 6-minute walk distance or cardiopulmonary exercise testing, (3) enhanced right ventricular function as assessed by echocardiogram or cardiac MRI and brain natriuretic peptide levels, and when necessary, (4) pulmonary hemodynamics assessed by repeat right heart catheterization.

Other interventions include supplemental oxygen to keep resting oxygen saturation greater than 90%, judicious use of diuretics to reduce peripheral edema and right ventricular overload, and a supervised exercise program such as pulmonary rehabilitation. The role of anticoagulation to prevent thrombosis in situ remains controversial, but some guidelines recommend low-level anticoagulation unless patients are at increased risk of bleeding. Patients who remain in or progress to functional class IV despite maximum medical therapy should be considered for lung transplantation. Current treatment guidelines also recommend consideration of referral of PAH patients to regional centers with experience in managing this disease.

OTHER TYPES OF PULMONARY HYPERTENSION

Pulmonary hypertension is a normal complication of any left-sided heart disease that increases pulmonary venous pressure such as left ventricular systolic or diastolic dysfunction or valvular heart disease. Pulmonary hypertension is also a common development of chronic lung disease, especially those that are associated with hypoxemia. These conditions have been called *secondary pulmonary hypertension* but now are usually referred to as WHO Group 2 and 3 PH (see Table 7.1). Hypoxic pulmonary vasoconstriction contributes to increased pulmonary vascular resistance in chronic or recurrent hypoxia. Long-standing hypoxia causes vascular remodeling that is similar to plexogenic pulmonary arteriopathy but does not include in situ thrombosis or formation of plexiform lesions.

Due to the association of increased mortality when PH is present in patients with chronic heart and lung disease, there is considerable

表 7.2　动脉型肺动脉高压的治疗药物

药物类别	药物名称	给药途径	作用机制
内皮素受体拮抗剂	安立生坦 波生坦 马昔腾坦	口服 口服 口服	通过阻断内皮素，抑制血管收缩
磷酸二酯酶 5 型抑制剂	西地那非 他达拉非	口服，静脉 口服	通过延缓细胞内 cGMP 的代谢，促进血管扩张
前列环素类似物	依前列醇 伊洛前列素 曲前列尼尔	静脉，吸入 a 吸入，静脉 a 口服，吸入，皮下，静脉	通过增加细胞内 cAMP，促进血管扩张
前列环素受体激动剂	司来帕格	口服	激活前列环素受体
可溶性鸟苷酸环化酶激动剂	利奥西呱	口服	通过增加 cGMP 合成，促进血管扩张

a 目前在美国尚无这种给药途径的商业制剂。cGMP，环磷鸟苷；cAMP，环磷腺苷。

极为罕见，因此应尽力寻找结缔组织病、门静脉高压、HIV 感染、先天性心脏病、慢性肺栓塞或潜在致病药物或毒素暴露的病史。大多数患者应进行肺功能检查以排除肺阻塞性或限制性疾病，并监测血氧饱和度。如果出现夜间低氧血症需要考虑睡眠呼吸障碍的可能。进行肺通气/灌注扫描以排除慢性肺栓塞，并进行血液检查以筛查自身免疫性疾病、HIV 感染或肝功能不全。左心疾病通常通过超声心动图评估，但在某些患者中，可能需要额外的检查以评估冠状动脉疾病或浸润性心肌病。尽管罕见，PCH 和 PVOD 也需要警惕，PVOD 的特点是严重低氧血症、D_{LCO} 降低，以及高分辨率胸部 CT 上表现出的小叶中心性结节、磨玻璃影和小叶间隔增厚三联征。

经胸超声心动图通常是排除左心疾病的第一步，使用多普勒超声可以估算肺动脉收缩压。除此之外，多普勒超声还能提供有关右心房和右心室大小和功能的重要信息，并通过检查房间隔和室间隔的位置来评估右心与左心的充盈压。通常也能够检测到显著的心内分流。

PAH 的确诊需要通过右心导管检查，以确认 mPAP 的升高，并通过测量肺动脉楔压评估左心充盈压力。应在上腔静脉或下腔静脉、右心房和肺动脉水平测量血红蛋白氧饱和度，以排除显著的左向右分流。在 PAH 患者中，应通过给予短效选择性肺血管扩张剂，如吸入一氧化氮或静脉注射依前列醇，测试肺血管的反应性。如果 mPAP 下降 10 mmHg 或更多，且降至 40 mmHg 以下，同时心输出量不降，则被认为是血管反应试验阳性。阳性结果可以识别出能够使用钙通道阻滞剂成功治疗的一小部分 PAH 患者。

治疗

在过去的 25 年中，已有五类药物被批准用于治疗 PAH（表 7.2）。这些药物主要作为部分选择性肺血管扩张剂起作用，也有研究提示它们具有抗增殖特性，可能减缓肺血管重塑。虽然缺乏数据来比较不同药物类别的相对疗效，但大多数治疗指南通常在以下几个方面达成共识：①在没有严重右心衰竭的情况下，对于血管反应试验阳性的患者，应试用钙通道阻滞剂，通常为硝苯地平；②对于死亡风险较高（包括 WHO 心功

能分级Ⅳ级）的患者，应连续静脉输注前列环素衍生物进行治疗；③对于病情不太严重的 PAH 患者，如心功能分级为Ⅱ或Ⅲ级的患者，应使用磷酸二酯酶 5 型（PDE5）抑制剂和内皮素受体拮抗剂（ERA）联合治疗。对于无法耐受此联合治疗方案，或在使用期间病情未改善者，应考虑使用可溶性鸟苷酸环化酶（sGC）激动剂代替 PDE5 抑制剂，或使用吸入或口服前列环素衍生物或前列环素受体激动剂。

治疗反应的评估包括以下几个方面：①通过心功能分级的变化，衡量症状的改善；②通过 6 分钟步行距离或心肺运动试验，评估活动能力的改善；③通过超声心动图或心脏 MRI 以及脑钠肽（BNP）水平，评估右心室功能的改善；④在必要时，复查右心导管检查，评估肺循环血流动力学变化。

其他干预措施包括：①氧疗：保持静息时的氧饱和度大于 90%；②合理使用利尿剂：减轻外周水肿和右心室过负荷；③专业指导下的运动计划：如呼吸康复计划。抗凝治疗在预防原位血栓形成中的作用仍有争议，但一些指南建议在没有增加患者出血风险的情况下，进行低水平的抗凝治疗。对于接受最大药物治疗情况下，仍处于或进展到心功能分级Ⅳ级的患者，应考虑进行肺移植。当前的治疗指南还建议考虑将 PAH 患者转诊至有经验的区域中心，以便于更好地进行管理。

其他类型的肺动脉高压

肺动脉高压是任何导致肺静脉压力升高的左心疾病，如左心室收缩或舒张功能不全或心脏瓣膜病的常见并发症。肺动脉高压也是慢性肺病，尤其是与低氧血症相关的疾病的常见发展结局。这些情况既往被称为继发性肺动脉高压，但现在通常被称为 WHO 第 2 大类和第 3 大类肺动脉高压（见表 7.1）。在慢性或反复低氧的情况下，低氧性肺血管收缩会导致肺血管阻力增加。长期的低氧会导致类似于丛状肺动脉病变的血管重塑，但不包括原位血栓形成或丛状病变形成。

由于慢性心肺疾病患者在存在肺动脉高压时死亡率增加，因此人们对使用 PAH 药物治疗 WHO 第 2 大类和

interest in using PAH medications for the treatment of WHO Groups 2 and 3. There is currently insufficient evidence to suggest that any of the currently available medications are beneficial in these other types of pulmonary hypertension. Considering their high costs and ability to worsen gas exchange and pulmonary edema formation, their use in patients who do not have Group 1 PAH is not recommended, and treatment should be directed at the underlying heart or lung disease.

PULMONARY THROMBOEMBOLISM

Definition and Epidemiology

Pulmonary thromboembolism refers to the passage of a clot from the venous system or the right ventricle into a pulmonary artery. Several other materials can embolize to the pulmonary arterial bed, including air, fat, amniotic fluid, tumor, or injected foreign bodies (e.g., talc). These embolic phenomena have different risk factors and clinical manifestations but occur much less commonly than venous thrombosis with pulmonary thromboembolism.

Pulmonary thromboembolic disease is a relatively common entity, with an incidence ranging from 400,000 to 650,000 cases per year in the United States. The deep veins of the femoral and popliteal systems of the lower extremities are the most common sources of venous thrombosis, but upper extremity thrombosis and right heart thrombi can also embolize to the lung. Predisposing factors for pulmonary embolism are the same as those for venous thrombosis and include venous stasis, hypercoagulability, and endothelial injury, as well as congenital or acquired prothrombotic disorders (e.g., activated protein C deficiency, factor V Leiden).

❖　For a deeper discussion on this topic, please see Chapter 75, "Pulmonary Hypertension," in *Goldman-Cecil Medicine*, 26th Edition.

Pathophysiology

An acute pulmonary thromboembolism can obstruct a branch of the pulmonary artery, resulting in an increased $\dot{V}/\dot{Q}$ ratio. This increases overall dead space ventilation, which can lead to inefficient excretion of carbon dioxide, potentially raising the partial pressure of carbon dioxide in arterial blood ($Paco_2$). Blood flow is shifted from the obstructed site to other areas, leading to $\dot{V}/\dot{Q}$ mismatch, shunting, and hypoxemia.

Right ventricular dysfunction is commonly encountered in acute pulmonary thromboembolism, occurring when a substantial portion of the pulmonary vascular bed is occluded and there is an acute increase in PAP. Approximately 5% of patients present with cardiogenic shock from right ventricular failure, and somewhere between 30% and 70% of normotensive patients will have right ventricular dysfunction on transthoracic echocardiography, which is associated with a worse prognosis.

Clinical Presentation and Diagnosis

Common symptoms of pulmonary thromboembolism include shortness of breath, chest pain, hemoptysis, and syncope. When the diagnosis of acute pulmonary embolism is suspected, risk factors such as recent immobilization or surgery, malignancy, or a prior history of venous thrombosis should be clinically documented, and a validated clinical scoring system, such as the Wells or Geneva score, can be used to assess the pretest probability of pulmonary embolism. The most common physical examination findings are tachycardia and tachypnea, and chest examination may be normal or may reveal isolated crackles or even diffuse wheezing. Edema of the extremities, especially if the edema is asymmetrical, may indicate venous thrombosis. Signs of right ventricular strain, such as an increased pulmonary component

Approach to diagnosis

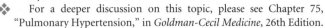

Fig. 7.1 A proposed diagnostic algorithm for the diagnosis of acute pulmonary embolism (PE). Clinical suspicion, often with the use of clinical decision rules, can determine if patients should proceed directly to an imaging study such as CT pulmonary angiography (CTPE) or ventilation-perfusion (V/Q) scan when the pretest probability is high. D-dimer testing is recommended in patients with a lower clinical suspicion for acute PE, where a negative D-dimer is a sensitive test and can exclude the diagnosis of venous thromboembolism (VTE).

of the second heart sound or a palpable right ventricular heave, can be observed in massive pulmonary embolus.

The electrocardiogram may show atrial tachyarrhythmias or evidence of right heart strain as shown by a new right bundle branch block or right ventricular strain pattern that mimics inferior myocardial infarction. The chest radiograph is often normal but may show atelectasis, isolated infiltrates, or a small pleural effusion, but in most cases, is not sufficiently sensitive to diagnose a pulmonary embolism.

Chest CT angiography is the main imaging modality used for the diagnosis of acute pulmonary embolism, although $\dot{V}/\dot{Q}$ scan and pulmonary angiography are used in certain clinical settings (Fig. 7.1). CT angiography provides a noninvasive, rapid, and sensitive way to detect pulmonary emboli, and most diagnostic algorithms combine CT pulmonary angiography with clinical suspicion, D-dimer determination, and assessment of the lower extremities for deep vein thrombosis by CT or ultrasound.

However, for individuals with absolute or relative contraindications to CT angiography, the $\dot{V}/\dot{Q}$ scan provides an alternative approach. A *high-probability* $\dot{V}/\dot{Q}$ scan, characterized by multiple perfusion defects in areas of normal ventilation, is more than 90% accurate in diagnosing pulmonary embolism. A *normal* $\dot{V}/\dot{Q}$ scan excludes pulmonary embolism in essentially all cases. The test is less reliable when interpreted as *low, intermediate,* or *indeterminate* probability. In these circumstances, pulmonary embolism is observed in 4% to 66% of patients, and in these situations the diagnostic certainty depends on the pretest probability of pulmonary embolism. With improvements in CT angiography, pulmonary angiography is now performed very infrequently but could be considered when other tests are inconclusive, a high likelihood of pulmonary embolism exists, and there is a need for diagnostic certainty.

Risk Stratification and Treatment

Once acute pulmonary thromboembolism is diagnosed, risk stratification is essential to guide treatment decisions. This typically incorporates

第 3 大类肺动脉高压有相当大的兴趣。然而，目前还没有足够的证据表明现有的任何药物对这些类型的肺动脉高压有益。考虑到这些药物的价格昂贵，以及可能导致气体交换恶化和肺水肿，不推荐在没有第 1 大类 PAH 的患者中使用这些药物，对于第 2 大类和第 3 大类肺动脉高压主要应针对基础心脏或肺部疾病进行治疗。

肺血栓栓塞症

定义和流行病学

肺血栓栓塞症是指血栓从静脉系统或右心室进入肺动脉的过程。其他几种物质也可以栓塞到肺动脉床，包括空气、脂肪、羊水、肿瘤或注射的异物（如滑石粉）。这些栓塞现象有不同的危险因素和临床表现，但发生率远低于伴静脉血栓形成的肺血栓栓塞症。

肺血栓栓塞性疾病是一种相对常见的临床情况，在美国每年的发病率约为 40 万至 65 万例。下肢股静脉和腘静脉是最常见的静脉血栓形成的来源，但上肢血栓和右心血栓也可栓塞到肺部。肺栓塞的诱发因素与静脉血栓形成相同，包括静脉血流淤滞、血液高凝状态和血管内皮损伤，以及先天性或获得性易栓症（如活化蛋白 C 缺乏症、V 因子 Leiden 突变）。

❖　有关此专题的深入讨论，请参阅 *Goldman-Cecil Medicine* 第 26 版第 75 章 "肺动脉高压"。

病理生理学

急性肺血栓栓塞症可以阻塞肺动脉的一个分支，导致 $\dot{V}/\dot{Q}$ 比率增加。这会增加整体的无效腔通气，导致二氧化碳排出效率降低，从而使动脉血中的二氧化碳分压（$PaCO_2$）升高。血流从阻塞部位转移到其他区域，导致 $\dot{V}/\dot{Q}$ 比例失调、分流增加和低氧血症。

在急性肺血栓栓塞症中，常出现右心室功能不全，见于肺血管床被阻塞的比例较高、肺动脉压（PAP）急剧增加时。大约 5% 的患者因右心室衰竭出现心源性休克，在正常血压的患者中，约有 30% ~ 70% 的患者在经胸超声心动图检查中会显示出右心室功能不全，而右心室功能不全与不良预后相关。

临床表现和诊断

肺血栓栓塞症的常见症状包括气短、胸痛、咯血和晕厥。当怀疑急性肺栓塞诊断时，应在临床中确证有无近期制动或手术、恶性肿瘤或静脉血栓形成病史等风险因素，并使用有效的临床评分体系，如 Wells 评分或 Geneva 评分来评估肺栓塞的验前概率。最常见的体征是心动过速和呼吸急促，胸部检查可能正常，也可能显示孤立的啰音甚至弥漫性喘鸣。四肢水肿，特别是非对称性水肿时，可能提示静脉血栓形成。右心室充盈的体征，如肺动脉瓣区第二心音亢进或触及右

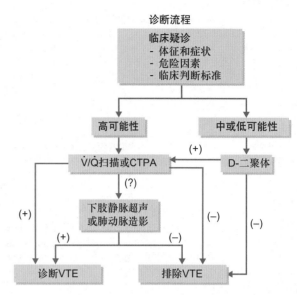

图 7.1　急性肺栓塞（PE）的诊断流程。临床疑诊（通常基于临床判断标准）可以确定患者是否应直接进行影像学检查，当验前概率较高时，应行 CT 肺动脉造影（CTPA）或通气/灌注（$\dot{V}/\dot{Q}$）扫描。对于临床疑诊急性 PE 可能性较低的患者，建议进行 D- 二聚体检测，因为 D- 二聚体阴性对排除静脉血栓栓塞症（VTE）的诊断颇具敏感性

心抬举样搏动，可在大面积肺栓塞中观察到。

心电图可显示房性心动过速或右心负荷增加的证据，如新发的右束支传导阻滞或类似于下壁心肌梗死的右心室劳损表现。胸部 X 线片通常正常，但可能出现肺不张、孤立性浸润影或少量胸腔积液等征象，在大多数情况下，其敏感性低，不足以诊断肺栓塞。

胸部 CT 血管成像（亦称 CT 血管造影，CTA）是诊断急性肺栓塞的主要影像学手段，某些临床场景下也会使用 $\dot{V}/\dot{Q}$ 扫描和肺动脉造影（图 7.1）。CT 血管成像是一种无创、快速且敏感的肺栓塞检测手段。大多数诊断流程将 CT 肺动脉造影（CTPA）与临床判断、D-二聚体检测以及通过 CT 或超声评估下肢深静脉血栓形成联合使用。

然而，对于存在绝对或相对禁忌证而不能进行 CT 血管成像的患者，$\dot{V}/\dot{Q}$ 扫描为一种替代方法。高概率诊断肺栓塞的 $\dot{V}/\dot{Q}$ 扫描特征是在正常通气区域存在多个灌注缺损，其诊断肺栓塞的准确率超过 90%。$\dot{V}/\dot{Q}$ 扫描正常几乎可排除肺栓塞。当结果解释为低概率、中等概率或不确定概率时，该检查的可靠性较低。在这些情况下，4% ~ 66% 的患者会出现肺栓塞，此时诊断的确定性取决于肺栓塞的验前概率。随着 CT 血管成像技术的改进，肺动脉造影现已很少进行，但在其他测试结果不明确、肺栓塞可能性高且需要确定诊断时可以考虑。

危险分层和治疗

一旦确诊急性肺血栓栓塞症，危险分层对于指导治疗决策至关重要。危险分层通常结合临床表现、生

clinical appearance, vital signs, validated PE risk scores, and RV function assessed by imaging modalities and cardiac biomarkers. Acute PE that causes hemodynamic instability is referred to as massive PE or high-risk PE and warrants immediate consideration of reperfusion therapies. In acute PE patients who present without shock or hemodynamic instability, multimodal risk stratification is used to identify patients at low and intermediate risk, the latter typically defined by signs of RV dysfunction on CT or echocardiography, or elevated levels of troponin or B-type natriuretic peptide (BNP).

Treatment of acute PE centers on supportive care, systemic anticoagulation, and consideration of reperfusion therapy. Unless there are contraindications, systemic anticoagulation should be started after the diagnosis of acute PE is established. Intravenous unfractionated heparin or subcutaneous low-molecular-weight heparin (LMWH) are typically the preferred agents. For patients with a contraindication to anticoagulation, an inferior vena cava filter should be placed. Reperfusion therapies include systemic thrombolysis and surgical thrombectomy and are indicated in massive PE. The use of systemic thrombolytics in intermediate risk PE remains controversial and is not practiced routinely. Catheter-directed thrombolysis and catheter embolectomy are other available reperfusion therapies that are less well studied and not recommended for routine use.

After stabilization and clinical improvement, patients are transitioned to their long-term anticoagulation therapy. Options for anticoagulation include vitamin K antagonists such as warfarin, non–vitamin K oral anticoagulants (NOACs), such as apixaban or rivaroxaban, or LMWH. NOACs have increasingly become the preferred oral anticoagulant due to their safety profile and ease of use, but risks and benefits of each agent should be discussed with patients to allow for individualized decision making. Duration of anticoagulation for an acute pulmonary embolism is at least 3 months, after which extended therapy can be considered based on clinical risk factors (e.g. provoked vs. unprovoked event) and bleeding risk.

Chronic Thromboembolic Pulmonary Hypertension

Chronic thromboembolic pulmonary hypertension (CTEPH) is a distinct type of pulmonary hypertension, classified as WHO group 4 PH. CTEPH is characterized by incomplete or abnormal resolution of acute pulmonary thromboembolism such that residual emboli become organized and fibrotic. This develops in approximately 4% of patients after acute pulmonary embolism. However, nearly half of CTEPH cases occur in patients without a prior history of venous thromboembolism. The diagnosis of CTEPH requires precapillary pulmonary hypertension on RHC in the presence of chronic/organized flow limiting thrombi/emboli in the elastic pulmonary arteries after at least 3 months of effective anticoagulation. Unlike other forms of pulmonary hypertension, the mainstay of treatment is surgical. Pulmonary endarterectomy (PEA) is performed via median sternotomy with cardiopulmonary bypass, after which deep hypothermic circulatory arrest allows for visualization, identification of the dissection plane, and complete endarterectomy. PEA is often curative, and is associated with improved symptoms, hemodynamics, and survival.

In patients for whom PEA is not feasible, medical therapy with pulmonary vasodilators, namely riociguat, has been shown to be effective in improving hemodynamics and functional capacity. Balloon pulmonary angioplasty is an emerging therapeutic option for CTEPH patients with inoperable disease or in whom the risk-to-benefit ratio of PEA is not favorable.

PROSPECTUS FOR THE FUTURE

Numerous advances in our understanding of pulmonary vascular biology over the last 35 years have markedly enhanced understanding of the pathogenesis of pulmonary hypertensive disorders and have led to the development of therapies that slow disease progression, increase functional capacity, and increase quality of life. However, most pulmonary vascular diseases are not curable and result in decreased survival. New therapies designed to prevent the loss of healthy vessels and reverse vascular remodeling are needed before substantial gains in disease reversal and cure can be achieved. Cellular mechanisms that regulate endothelial apoptosis, angiogenesis, and perivascular inflammation appear to have potential as future therapeutic targets. Modulation of sex hormones, cellular bioenergetics, and epigenetic factors may be other promising approaches. Little is understood about the adaptive changes of the right ventricle to chronically increased afterload. Furthermore, studies are needed in the area of genetic predisposition to thromboembolic disease and vascular dysfunction leading to thrombus formation as well as the determination of appropriate follow-up evaluation for patients after acute PE and who might benefit from screening for chronic thromboembolic disease. Finally, national studies currently underway that seek to provide deep phenotyping of pulmonary vascular disease and establish national biobanks and patient registries should provide important tools to help investigators find more effective therapies for these devastating diseases.

SUGGESTED READINGS

Girerd B, Weatherald J, Montani D, Humbert M: Heritable pulmonary hypertension: from bench to bedside, Eur Respir Rev 26(145), 2017.

Humbert M, Guignabert C, Bonnet S, et al: Pathology and pathobiology of pulmonary hypertension: state of the art and research perspectives, Eur Respir J 53(1), 2019.

Klinger JR, Elliott CG, Levine DJ, et al: Therapy for Pulmonary Arterial Hypertension in Adults: Update of the CHEST Guideline and Expert Panel Report, Chest 155(3):565-586, 2019.

Konstantinides SV, Meyer G, Becattini C, et al, ESC Scientific Document Group: 2019 ESC Guidelines for the diagnosis and management of acute pulmonary embolism developed in collaboration with the European Respiratory Society (ERS), Eur Heart J 41:543-603, 2020.

Mullin CJ, Klinger JR: Chronic thromboembolic pulmonary hypertension, Heart Fail Clin 14(3):339-351, 2018.

Simonneau G, Montani D, Celermajer DS, et al: Haemodynamic definitions and updated clinical classification of pulmonary hypertension, Eur Respir J 53(1), 2019.

Stacher E, Graham BB, Hunt JM, et al: Modern age pathology of pulmonary arterial hypertension, Am J Respir Crit Care Med 186:261-272, 2012.

命体征、验证过的 PE 风险评分，以及通过影像学和心脏生物标志物评估的右心室功能。导致血流动力学不稳定的急性 PE 称为大面积 PE 或高危 PE，需立即考虑再灌注治疗。对于没有出现休克或血流动力学不稳定情况的急性 PE 患者，采用多模式风险分层来识别低危和中危患者。中危通常定义为 CT 或超声心动图上显示的右心室功能障碍表现，或肌钙蛋白或脑钠肽（B 型钠尿肽，BNP）水平升高。

急性 PE 的治疗主要包括支持性治疗、全身抗凝和考虑再灌注治疗。除非有禁忌证，在确诊急性 PE 后，应立即开始全身抗凝治疗。常用的药物包括静脉普通肝素或皮下注射低分子量肝素（LMWH）。对于有抗凝禁忌证的患者，应放置下腔静脉滤器。再灌注治疗包括全身溶栓和外科取栓，适用于大面积 PE。中危 PE 患者中使用全身溶栓疗法仍有争议，尚未常规应用。导管引导的溶栓和导管取栓也是可选择的再灌注治疗方法，但研究较少，不推荐常规使用。

在病情稳定及临床表现改善后，患者会过渡到长期抗凝治疗。抗凝治疗的选择包括维生素 K 拮抗剂如华法林、非维生素 K 口服抗凝剂（NOAC）如阿哌沙班或利伐沙班，或 LMWH。由于 NOAC 的安全性和便捷性，逐渐成为首选口服抗凝剂，但应与患者讨论每种药物的风险和益处，以便进行个体化决策。急性肺栓塞的抗凝持续时间至少为 3 个月，之后可根据患者临床危险因素（如有诱因和无诱因）和出血风险考虑延展期治疗。

慢性血栓栓塞性肺动脉高压

慢性血栓栓塞性肺动脉高压（CTEPH）是一种特殊类型的肺动脉高压，被归类为 WHO 第 4 大类 PH。CTEPH 的特征是急性肺血栓栓塞症未完全恢复，残留的血栓逐渐机化并纤维化。约 4% 的急性肺栓塞患者会发展为 CTEPH。然而，近一半的 CTEPH 病例发生在没有静脉血栓形成病史的患者中。CTEPH 的诊断需要在至少 3 个月的有效抗凝治疗后、通过右心导管检查（RHC）证实存在毛细血管前肺动脉高压，且肺动脉中存在慢性 / 机化的限流性血栓 / 栓子。与其他形式的肺动脉高压不同，CTEPH 的主要治疗方法是手术。通过开胸和体外循环进行肺动脉内膜剥脱术（PEA），在深低温循环停滞下进行可视化、解剖平面识别和完全内膜剥除。PEA 通常可获得良好的疗效，并能改善症状、血流动力学和生存率。对于无法进行 PEA 的患者，可使用肺血管扩张剂进行药物治疗（如利奥西呱），已被证明可有效改善血流动力学和功能状态。肺动脉球囊成形术是一种新的治疗选择，适用于那些无法手术或 PEA 风险 / 收益比不佳的 CTEPH 患者。

未来展望

在过去的 35 年中，人们对肺血管生物学理解取得了许多进展，极大增强了对肺动脉高压疾病发病机制的认识，并研发出减缓疾病进展、改善功能状态和提高生活质量的治疗方法。然而，大多数肺血管疾病无法治愈，并导致生存率下降。在实现疾病逆转和治愈方面取得重大进展之前，需要开发预防健康血管丧失和逆转血管重塑的新疗法。调控内皮细胞凋亡、血管生成和血管周围炎症的细胞机制似乎是未来治疗的潜在靶点。性激素调节、细胞生物能量学和表观遗传因素可能是其他有前途的干预靶点。目前关于右心室对慢性血栓增加的后负荷适应性变化仍知之甚少。此外，还需在血栓栓塞性疾病的遗传易感性、血管功能障碍导致血栓形成的研究领域进行更多探索，以及确定急性 PE 后患者如何优化随访评估，并确定慢性血栓栓塞性疾病筛查的潜在受益者。最后，目前在全美正在进行的全国性研究，旨在提供肺血管疾病的深度表型分析，建立国家生物样本库和患者登记系统，这将为研究人员提供重要工具，帮助找到更有效的治疗这些难治性疾病的方法。

推荐阅读

Girerd B, Weatherald J, Montani D, Humbert M: Heritable pulmonary hypertension: from bench to bedside, Eur Respir Rev 26(145), 2017.

Humbert M, Guignabert C, Bonnet S, et al: Pathology and pathobiology of pulmonary hypertension: state of the art and research perspectives, Eur Respir J 53(1), 2019.

Klinger JR, Elliott CG, Levine DJ, et al: Therapy for Pulmonary Arterial Hypertension in Adults: Update of the CHEST Guideline and Expert Panel Report, Chest 155(3):565-586, 2019.

Konstantinides SV, Meyer G, Becattini C, et al, ESC Scientific Document Group: 2019 ESC Guidelines for the diagnosis and management of acute pulmonary embolism developed in collaboration with the European Respiratory Society (ERS), Eur Heart J 41:543-603, 2020.

Mullin CJ, Klinger JR: Chronic thromboembolic pulmonary hypertension, Heart Fail Clin 14(3):339-351, 2018.

Simonneau G, Montani D, Celermajer DS, et al: Haemodynamic definitions and updated clinical classification of pulmonary hypertension, Eur Respir J 53(1), 2019.

Stacher E, Graham BB, Hunt JM, et al: Modern age pathology of pulmonary arterial hypertension, Am J Respir Crit Care Med 186:261-272, 2012.

Disorders of the Pleura, Mediastinum, and Chest Wall

Eric J. Gartman, F. Dennis McCool

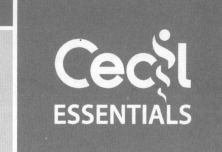

PLEURAL DISEASE

The pleura is a thin membrane that covers the entire surface of the lung, inner surface of the rib cage, diaphragm, and mediastinum. There are two pleural membranes: the visceral pleura, which covers the lung; and the parietal pleura, which lines the rib cage, diaphragm, and mediastinum. A layer of mesothelial cells lines both pleural surfaces. The closed space in between the surface of the lung and the chest cavity is called the *pleural space*. A small amount of fluid normally resides in this space and forms a thin layer between the pleural surfaces. Pleural fluid serves as a lubricant for the visceral and parietal pleurae as they move against each other during inspiration and expiration.

The blood vessels in the visceral pleura are supplied from the pulmonary circulation and have less hydrostatic pressure than the blood vessels in the parietal pleura, which are supplied by the systemic circulation. The pressure in the pleural space is subatmospheric during quiet breathing. Fluid is filtered from the higher-pressure vascular structures into the pleural space. The normal fluid turnover is about 10 to 20 mL per day, with 0.2 to 1 mL remaining in the pleural space. Pleural fluid usually contains a small amount of protein and a small number of cells that are mostly mononuclear cells. Although both parietal and visceral pleurae contribute to pleural fluid formation, most of the fluid results from filtration of the higher-pressure vessels supplying the parietal pleura.

After the fluid enters the pleural space, it is drained from the pleural space by a network of pleural lymphatics located beneath the mesothelial monolayer. The lymphatics originate in stomas on the parietal pleural surface. In abnormal circumstances of increased fluid production or impaired removal, fluid can accumulate in the pleural space. Factors that promote the entry of fluid into the pleural space include an increase in systemic venous pressure, an increase in pulmonary venous pressure, an increase in permeability of pleural vessels, and a reduction in pleural pressure. Conditions that increase hydrostatic pressure can be seen in congestive heart failure; changes in pleural membrane permeability can be seen in various inflammatory states or malignancy; and a reduction in pleural pressure can be seen with atelectasis. Occasionally, microvascular oncotic pressure may be sufficiently reduced to promote fluid entry into the pleural space in patients with hypoalbuminemia. Factors that block lymphatic drainage and interfere with the egress of fluid from the pleural space include central lymphatic obstruction and obstruction of lymphatic channels at the pleural surface by tumor.

Pleural Effusion

Pleural effusion is the accumulation of fluid in the pleural space. Pleural effusions usually are detected by chest radiography; however, the volume of fluid in the pleural space must exceed 250 mL to be visualized on a chest radiograph. When an effusion exists, there is blunting of the costophrenic angle on a posteroanterior chest film, which represents a fluid meniscus that can be detected posteriorly on the lateral chest radiograph, and fluid occasionally can be demonstrated in the minor or major fissures. Apparent elevation or changes in the contour of the diaphragm on a posteroanterior chest film may signify a subpulmonic effusion, so called because it retains the general shape of the diaphragm without blunting the costophrenic angle; however, it is evident on the lateral film.

A decubitus chest radiograph can be obtained to determine whether the fluid is free flowing or loculated. Computed tomography (CT) of the chest provides better definition of the pleural space than plain radiography. Chest CT is particularly useful in defining loculated effusions and in differentiating pulmonary parenchymal abnormalities from pleural abnormalities, atelectasis from effusion, and loculated effusion from lung abscess or other parenchymal processes. The edge of a parenchymal process usually touches the chest wall and forms an acute angle (0-90 degrees), whereas that of an empyema is usually an obtuse angle (90-180 degrees).

Thoracentesis is a procedure in which fluid is aspirated from the pleural space. To help minimize procedural complications and assist in needle placement, ultrasound or CT guidance should be used to direct the thoracentesis catheter into the pleural space.

Classifying pleural effusions as transudates or exudates greatly assists with the differential diagnosis. Further analysis of pleural fluid may provide a definitive diagnosis (e.g., malignancy); however, even without a definitive diagnosis, pleural fluid analysis can be useful in excluding possible causes of disease such as infection.

Transudates

Effusions that accumulate due to changes in oncotic and hydrostatic forces usually have a low protein content and are called *transudates* (Table 8.1). Congestive heart failure is the most common cause of a transudate, and the effusions are typically bilateral. If the effusion is unilateral, it involves the right hemithorax in most instances. Effusions due to heart failure almost universally are related to dysfunction of the left side of the heart, although they rarely can result from right heart failure (e.g., advanced pulmonary arterial hypertension).

Transudative effusions may be seen in cirrhosis, nephrotic syndrome, myxedema, pulmonary embolism, superior vena cava obstruction, and peritoneal dialysis. In patients with cirrhosis, the effusions are often right-sided, and the mechanism may be related to flow from the peritoneal space across diaphragmatic defects into the pleural space (i.e., hepatic hydrothorax). Transudative effusions are typically small to moderate sized and rarely require drainage to improve symptoms.

胸膜、纵隔与胸壁疾病

童润 译 侯刚 詹庆元 审校 代华平 王辰 通审

胸膜疾病

胸膜是一层覆盖在整个肺表面、胸廓内壁、横膈和纵隔的薄膜。胸膜分为两部分：覆盖肺脏的脏层胸膜，以及衬在胸廓、横膈和纵隔上的壁层胸膜。两部分胸膜表面都排列着一层间皮细胞。肺表面和胸腔之间的封闭空间称为胸膜腔。胸膜腔内通常存有少量的液体，并在脏层胸膜和壁层胸膜之间形成薄薄的一层浆液层。当脏层胸膜和壁层胸膜在吸气和呼气时相向运动，胸膜腔内的液体起到了润滑剂的作用。

脏层胸膜的血管来自肺循环，其静水压低于由体循环供应的壁层胸膜血管的静水压。在安静呼吸时，胸膜腔内的压力低于大气压。液体从高压血管结构过滤到胸膜腔。正常情况下，每天胸膜腔内液体交换量约为 $10 \sim 20$ ml，而胸膜腔内存留的液体约 $0.2 \sim 1$ ml。胸水通常含有少量蛋白质和少量细胞，这些细胞主要是单核细胞。尽管壁层胸膜和脏层胸膜都参与胸膜液的形成，但大部分胸水是由供应壁层胸膜的高压血管滤过引起的。

液体进入胸膜腔后，通过位于单层间皮下的胸膜淋巴管网络引流出胸膜腔。淋巴管起源于壁层胸膜表面的小孔。在异常情况下，液体生成增加或清除受阻，液体可积聚在胸膜腔内。促进液体进入胸膜腔的因素包括：体循环静脉压升高、肺静脉压升高、胸膜血管通透性增加以及胸膜腔压力降低。静水压升高可见于充血性心力衰竭；胸膜通透性改变见于各种炎症状态或恶性肿瘤；胸膜腔压力降低可见于肺不张。低白蛋白血症患者有时因微血管胶体渗透压显著降低，也可能促使液体进入胸膜腔。阻碍淋巴引流和妨碍胸膜腔内液体排出的因素包括中央淋巴回流受阻，以及肿瘤阻塞胸膜表面的淋巴管。

胸腔积液

胸腔积液是指胸膜腔内液体的积聚。胸腔积液通常通过胸部 X 线片（胸片）检查发现；但胸腔内的液体量必须超过 250 ml 才能在胸片上显示出来。当胸腔积液存在时，后前位胸片上肋膈角变钝，在侧位胸片上可以看到出现半月形的液体影，此外，积液有时可见于小叶间或者大叶间裂积聚。后前位胸片上膈肌轮廓的抬高或改变可能提示肺底积液，这种积液保留了膈肌的大体形状，不会使肋膈角变钝；但在侧位片上很明显。

侧位胸片可判断积液是否为游离性的或局限性的。胸部计算机断层成像（CT）比普通胸片能更好地显示胸膜腔。胸部 CT 特别有助于确定包裹性积液，以及鉴别肺实质与胸膜异常、肺不张与胸腔积液、包裹性积液与肺脓肿或其他引起肺实质轮廓突起的病变。肺实质突起接触胸壁时常形成锐角（ $0 \sim 90°$ ），而脓胸通常形成钝角（ $90° \sim 180°$ ）。

胸腔穿刺是一种将液体从胸膜腔中抽吸出来的操作。为了尽量减少操作相关并发症并辅助针刺定位，应使用超声或 CT 引导胸腔穿刺导管置入胸膜腔内。

将胸腔积液分为漏出液或渗出液有助于鉴别诊断。进一步分析胸腔积液可能提供明确的诊断（如恶性肿瘤）；即使没有明确诊断，胸腔积液分析也有助于排除可能的疾病原因，如感染。

漏出液

由于胶体渗透压或静水压改变产生的胸腔积液通常蛋白含量较低，称为漏出液（表 8.1）。充血性心力衰竭是漏出液最常见的原因，且通常为双侧胸腔积液。如果漏出液为单侧胸腔积液，多数累及右侧胸腔。心力衰竭所致的漏出液几乎普遍与左心功能障碍有关，罕见情况下也可由右心衰竭引起（如晚期肺动脉高压）。

漏出性胸腔积液还可见于肝硬化、肾病综合征、黏液性水肿、肺栓塞、上腔静脉阻塞及腹膜透析患者。肝硬化患者常出现右侧胸腔积液，其机制可能与积液自腹膜腔通过横膈缺损进入胸膜腔（即肝性胸腔积液）有关。漏出性胸腔积液通常量少到中等，极少需要引流来改善症状。

TABLE 8.1	Causes of Pleural Effusions

Conditions Associated With Transudates

Ascites
Cirrhosis
Congestive heart failure
Hypoalbuminemia
Intra-abdominal fluid
Malnutrition
Nephrotic syndrome
Peritoneal dialysis

Conditions Associated With Exudates

Asbestosis
Chylothorax
Collagen vascular disease
Complications of abdominal surgery
Dressler's syndrome (myocardial infarction, cardiotomy)
Drug-induced lupus
Empyema
Hemothorax
Infection
Intra-abdominal pathologic abnormalities (abscess)
Lymphedema
Malignancy (primary lung cancer, lymphoma, metastatic cancer)
Meigs' syndrome (benign ovarian tumor)
Myxedema
Pancreatitis
Parapneumonic causes (pneumonia, lung abscess, bronchiectasis)
Pulmonary embolism and infarction
Rheumatoid arthritis (pleurisy)
Ruptured esophagus
Subphrenic abscess
Systemic lupus erythematosus
Trauma
Uremia
Urinothorax
Miscellaneous sources

Modified from Light RW, Macgregor MI, Luchsinger PC, et al: Pleural effusions: the diagnostic separation of transudates and exudates, Ann Intern Med 77:507-513, 1972.

Exudates

Exudative effusions occur when there is an alteration in vascular permeability or pleural fluid resorption. They can be observed in inflammatory, infectious, or neoplastic conditions.

To distinguish an exudate from a transudate, one of three criteria must be fulfilled: (1) An exudate must have a pleural fluid–to-serum protein ratio greater than 0.5; (2) a pleural fluid–to-serum lactate dehydrogenase (LDH) ratio must be greater than 0.6; or (3) a pleural fluid LDH level must be greater than two thirds of the upper limit of normal (Table 8.2). When all three criteria are met, the sensitivity, specificity, and positive predictive value exceed 98% for defining an exudative effusion.

Measuring pleural fluid cholesterol may also help to distinguish an exudate from a transudate. Pleural fluid cholesterol is derived from degenerating cells within the pleural space and from vascular leakage due to increased permeability. A cholesterol level greater than 45 mg/dL is consistent with an exudative effusion.

Exudative effusions are commonly caused by infection. Parapneumonic effusion typically occurs in patients with bacterial pneumonia and can be further classified as an uncomplicated or complicated effusion.

TABLE 8.2	Differentiation of Exudative and Transudative Pleural Effusions	
Characteristic	Exudate	Transudate
Pleural fluid–to-serum protein ratio	>0.5	<0.5
Pleural fluid LDH level	>⅔ of the upper limit of normal	<⅔ of the upper limit of normal
Pleural fluid–to-serum LDH ratio	>0.6	<0.6

LDH, Lactate dehydrogenase.
Modified from Light RW, Macgregor MI, Luchsinger PC, et al: Pleural effusions: the diagnostic separation of transudates and exudates, Ann Intern Med 77:507-513, 1972.

Uncomplicated parapneumonic effusions do not require drainage and respond to antibiotic therapy alone used for treatment of the underlying pneumonia. In contrast, complicated parapneumonic effusions do not respond to antibiotic therapy alone and require drainage to prevent the formation of an empyema. The transition from uncomplicated to complicated can occur extremely rapidly, within a 24-hour period in some cases.

Typically, an uncomplicated parapneumonic effusion has a pH level greater than 7.3, a glucose level greater than 60 mg/dL, and an LDH level less than 1000 IU/L. A pH level of less than 7.2 usually identifies a complicated effusion. However, this finding is not specific for infection, and the cause may be malignancy, rheumatoid arthritis, or trauma with esophageal disruption causing an associated reduction in pH level.

Complicated exudative effusions require drainage to avoid development of loculation, cutaneous fistulas, bronchopleural fistulas, or fibrothorax. The findings of pus or bacteria by Gram stain or culture confirms the diagnosis of empyema and requires immediate drainage. The injection of fibrolytic agents and DNase into the pleural space can augment full drainage of infected pleural effusions; however, treatment of complicated pleural effusions occasionally requires surgical intervention and lung decortication.

Primary tuberculosis in endemic areas may be associated with pleural effusion in up to 30% of patients. The effusion is caused by increased vascular permeability of the pleural membrane because of a hypersensitivity reaction, not direct infection. Typically, the pleural fluid is lymphocyte predominant and acid-fast stain and culture negative. Adenosine deaminase levels greater than 50 U/L may be helpful in identifying tuberculous pleural effusions. Tuberculous empyema is distinct from a tuberculous pleural effusion and can occur when there is an extension of infection from the thoracic lymph nodes into the pleural space or hematogenous spread of tuberculosis to the pleural space.

Malignant effusions are the second most common cause of exudative pleural effusions and confer a poor prognosis. Seeding of the parietal or visceral pleura with malignant cells can change vascular permeability and impede resorption, resulting in effusion formation. However, the finding of a pleural effusion in an individual with malignancy does not necessarily imply that there is a malignant process in the pleural space. Effusions in these individuals may be caused by atelectasis, postobstructive pneumonia, hypoalbuminemia, pulmonary emboli, or complications from irradiation or chemotherapy.

The most common cause of malignant effusion is lung cancer, followed by breast cancer and lymphoma. An effusion that is bloody suggests a malignant process; however, other causes of bloody pleural effusions include trauma, asbestos exposure, tuberculosis, collagen vascular disease, and thromboembolic disease. To confirm the diagnosis of malignancy, cytologic examination of the fluid is needed. Malignant cells can be seen in 60% of malignant effusions on the first thoracentesis. Sensitivity rises to 80% if three separate samples are obtained. If needed, a biopsy

表 8.1 胸腔积液的原因
漏出性胸腔积液相关疾病
腹水
肝硬化
充血性心力衰竭
低白蛋白血症
腹腔积液
营养不良
肾病综合征
腹膜透析
渗出性胸腔积液相关疾病
石棉肺
乳糜胸
结缔组织病（胶原血管病）
腹部手术并发症
Dressler 综合征（心肌梗死，心脏切开术）
药物引起的红斑狼疮
脓胸
血胸
感染
腹腔内病理异常（脓肿）
淋巴水肿
恶性肿瘤（原发性肺癌、淋巴瘤、转移性癌）
Meigs 综合征（良性卵巢肿瘤）
黏液水肿
胰腺炎
肺炎旁原因（肺炎、肺脓肿、支气管扩张）
肺栓塞和梗死
类风湿关节炎（胸膜炎）
食管破裂
膈下脓肿
系统性红斑狼疮
创伤
尿毒症
尿胸
混杂性原因

改编自 Light RW，Macgregor MI，Luchsinger PC，et al：Pleural effusions：the diagnostic separation of transudates and exudates，Ann Intern Med 77：507-513，1972.

渗出液

渗出性胸腔积液可发生在血管通透性改变或胸水吸收异常时。它们可能出现在炎症、感染或肿瘤等情况下。

要将渗出液与漏出液区分开，必须满足以下三个条件中的任意一个：①胸水蛋白/血清蛋白比值大于 0.5；②胸水乳酸脱氢酶（LDH）/血清 LDH 比值大于 0.6；③胸水 LDH 水平大于实验室血清 LDH 正常值上限的 2/3（表 8.2）。如果同时满足这三个条件，诊断渗出性胸腔积液的敏感性、特异性和阳性预测值均超过 98%。

检测胸腔积液中胆固醇的含量也有助于区分渗出液和漏出液。胸腔积液中的胆固醇是由胸膜腔内细胞变性和血管通透性增加导致的血管渗漏引起的。胸腔积液中胆固醇含量超过 45 mg/dl 符合渗出液。

渗出性积液常由感染引起。肺炎旁胸腔积液通常见于细菌性肺炎的患者中，可进一步分为单纯性胸腔

表 8.2 渗出性与漏出性胸腔积液的鉴别		
特征	渗出液	漏出液
胸水蛋白/血清蛋白	> 0.5	< 0.5
胸水 LDH 水平	>血清 LDH 正常值上限的 2/3	<血清 LDH 正常值上限的 2/3
胸水 LDH/血清 LDH	> 0.6	< 0.6

LDH，乳酸脱氢酶。
改编自 Light RW，Macgregor MI，Luchsinger PC，et al：Pleural effusions：the diagnostic separation of transudates and exudates，Ann Intern Med 77：507-513，1972.

积液和复杂性胸腔积液。

单纯性肺炎旁胸腔积液无需引流，仅使用针对肺炎的抗生素治疗即可。相比之下，复杂性肺炎旁胸腔积液对单独抗生素治疗反应性差，需要进行引流以防止脓胸形成。从单纯性肺炎旁胸腔积液转变到复杂性肺炎旁胸腔积液可能非常迅速，有时在 24 h 内就会发生。

通常情况下，单纯性肺炎旁胸腔积液的 pH 值大于 7.3，葡萄糖水平大于 60 mg/dl，而 LDH 水平低于 1000 IU/L。pH 值低于 7.2 常提示复杂性胸腔积液。然而，这并不特异性地表明感染，其原因包括恶性肿瘤、类风湿关节炎或伴有食管破裂的创伤，以上情况都可能导致胸腔积液 pH 值降低。

复杂性渗出性胸腔积液需要引流以防止包裹、皮肤窦道形成、支气管胸膜瘘或纤维性胸膜炎。发现脓液或者通过革兰氏染色或培养确诊脓胸，则需要立即引流。向胸腔内注入纤溶剂和 DNA 酶有助于充分引流感染性胸腔积液；然而，复杂性胸腔积液的治疗有时需要手术干预和胸膜剥脱术。

在流行地区，原发性结核病患者中约有 30% 可能出现胸腔积液。胸腔积液的发生是由于胸膜的通透性增加，这是由超敏反应而非直接感染引起的。通常，胸腔积液以淋巴细胞为主，且抗酸染色和培养阴性。腺苷脱氨酶（ADA）水平大于 50 U/L 可能有助于鉴别结核性胸腔积液。结核性脓胸不同于结核性胸腔积液，当肺部淋巴结感染扩散至胸膜腔或结核经血行播散至胸膜时会出现这种情况。

恶性积液是渗出性胸腔积液的第二大常见原因，且预后不良。癌细胞侵犯壁层或脏层胸膜，改变血管通透性，妨碍了胸水的吸收，从而形成积液。然而，恶性肿瘤患者出现胸腔积液并不一定意味着胸膜腔内存在恶性病变。这些患者的积液可能由肺不张、阻塞性肺炎、低白蛋白血症、肺栓塞，或者放疗和化疗并发症所引起。

恶性积液最常见的原因是肺癌，其次是乳腺癌和淋巴瘤。血性胸腔积液提示恶性病变；然而，创伤、石棉暴露、结核病、结缔组织病和血栓栓塞等也可导致血性胸腔积液。为了确诊恶性肿瘤，需对积液进行细胞学检查。初次胸腔穿刺可见恶性细胞比例约为 60%，如果获取 3 次独立样本，细胞病理学的敏感度可

of the pleura may be useful in identifying a malignancy. Biopsies may be obtained via medical thoracoscopy, surgical video-assisted thoracoscopy or, less optimally, in a blinded fashion through a Cope or Abrams needle.

A low pleural fluid pH has prognostic and therapeutic implications for patients with malignant effusions. Patients with a low pleural fluid pH due to malignancy tend to have shorter survival times and poorer responses to chemical pleurodesis. Recurrent malignant pleural effusions may improve with chemical pleurodesis with talc or tetracycline derivatives, but effectiveness varies and a complete response is achieved in little more than 50% of patients. Alternatively, many patients with recurrent malignant effusions have tunneled indwelling pleural catheters placed, allowing intermittent drainage, relief of symptoms, and possibly mechanical pleurodesis over time.

Systemic inflammatory disorders such as rheumatoid arthritis and lupus erythematosus can be associated with exudative effusions. Rheumatoid pleural effusions are a common intrathoracic manifestation of rheumatoid disease and may be seen in as many as 5% of patients. Rheumatoid factor titers in pleural fluid are often greater than 1:320, and the pleural fluid glucose level is less than 60 mg/dL (or the pleural fluid–to-serum glucose ratio is less than 0.5). However, a low glucose level also may be found in complicated parapneumonic effusions or empyema, malignant effusion, tuberculosis pleurisy, lupus pleuritis, and esophageal rupture. In systemic lupus erythematosus, 15% to 50% of patients have pleural effusions, and the pleural fluid antinuclear antibody titer is greater than 1:160.

Measuring pleural fluid amylase concentrations may further refine the differential diagnosis for an exudative effusion. Finding a pleural amylase level greater than the upper limit of normal for serum amylase is consistent with acute pancreatitis, chronic pancreatic pleural effusion, esophageal rupture, or malignancy. Pancreatic disease is associated with pancreatic amylase isoenzymes, whereas malignancy and esophageal rupture are characterized by a predominance of salivary isoenzymes.

Pneumothorax

Pneumothorax is the accumulation of air in the pleural space. In this instance, pleural pressure becomes positive and there is compression of underlying lung. Patients with pneumothorax typically have acute onset of dyspnea. Findings include tachycardia, decreased breath sounds, decreased tactile fremitus, a pleural friction rub, subcutaneous emphysema, hyperresonance, and a tracheal shift to the opposite side.

The diagnosis can be made by obtaining an upright chest radiograph, and rapid assessment can be achieved with point-of-care ultrasound. Typically, the visceral pleura separates from the parietal pleura, and air can be seen between the visceral pleural lining and the rib cage. An end-expiratory radiograph increases the density of lung while reducing its volume, highlighting the difference between the lung parenchyma and the pleural gas.

Management of a significant pneumothorax usually requires insertion of a thoracostomy tube and suction followed by water-seal drainage. However, if the pneumothorax is small and the patient is not in distress, observation alone may be indicated. If there is not a continuing air leak, as from a bronchopleural fistula, the pleural air is reabsorbed into the blood with resolution of the pneumothorax.

A tension pneumothorax is a medical emergency that requires immediate decompression by placement of a chest catheter. A tension pneumothorax occurs when pleural pressure reaches levels sufficient to cause mediastinal shift, compression of the vena cava and heart, and hemodynamic compromise. This physiology implies an ongoing leak of air into the pleural space.

Pneumothorax is often associated with blunt or penetrating trauma. With penetrating trauma, air may leak into the pleural space through the chest wall or the lung. Mechanical ventilation has also been associated with pneumothorax. Patients with underlying lung disease receiving mechanical ventilation may acutely develop a pneumothorax. A sudden rise in peak airway pressures with a reduction in breath sounds can alert the clinician to this complication.

Pneumothorax may occur spontaneously or result secondarily from underlying lung disease. Typically, spontaneous pneumothorax occurs in tall, young, thin men, presumably a result of rupture of apical blebs. Underlying lung diseases that can be complicated by pneumothorax include emphysema, cystic fibrosis, granulomatous inflammation, necrotizing pneumonia, pulmonary fibrosis, and lung abscess. Catamenial pneumothorax occurs in women who have subpleural and diaphragmatic endometriosis, with rupture of the endometrial nodules at the time of menstruation causing pneumothorax.

Mesothelioma

Malignant mesotheliomas are neoplasms arising from the serosal membranes of the body cavities. Eighty percent of mesotheliomas originate in the pleura. Individuals usually are older than 55 years, and there is an association with asbestos exposure in the distant past. Symptoms include shortness of breath, chest pain, and weight loss.

The most common radiologic finding is a large, unilateral pleural effusion that may completely opacify the hemithorax. There may be circumferential pleural thickening, usually associated with various amounts of calcified pleural plaque and effusions. CT of the chest is the most accurate noninvasive method for assessing stage and progression of mesothelioma. Pleural fluid cytology frequently is insufficient for diagnosis, and the most efficient way of obtaining tissue is by CT-guided core biopsy or thoracoscopy.

The overall prognosis for patients with malignant mesothelioma is poor. No particular therapy has emerged as superior to supportive therapy alone in terms of survival.

MEDIASTINAL DISEASE

Lesion Location

The mediastinum is the central part of the thoracic cavity between the lungs that contains the heart and aorta, esophagus, trachea, lymph nodes, and thymus. The mediastinum is bordered by the two pleural cavities laterally, the diaphragm inferiorly, and the thoracic inlet superiorly. The mediastinal space can be divided into three compartments: anterior, middle, and posterior. The localization of mediastinal masses in one of these compartments assists in the differential diagnosis (Fig. 8.1).

The anterior mediastinal compartment is anterior to the pericardium and includes lymphatic tissue, the thymus, and the great veins. Lesions most commonly found in the anterior mediastinum are thymomas, germ cell tumors, lymphomas, intrathoracic thyroid tissue, and parathyroid lesions. Thymomas comprise 20% of mediastinal neoplasms in adults, and they are the most common anterior mediastinal primary neoplasm in adults. Symptoms due to myasthenia gravis may affect one third of patients with thymomas. Middle mediastinal lesions include tracheal masses, bronchogenic and pericardial cysts, enlarged lymph nodes, and proximal aortic disease (i.e., aneurysm or dissection). Posterior mediastinal masses include neurogenic tumors and cysts, meningocele, lymphoma, aneurysm of the descending aorta, and esophageal disorders such as diverticula and neoplasms.

Patients with systemic lymphoma often have mediastinal involvement, and 5% to 10% of patients with lymphoma have primary mediastinal lesions at clinical presentation. Mediastinal cysts can arise in the pericardium, bronchi, esophagus or stomach, thymus, and thoracic duct, and although benign, they can produce compressive symptoms. Lung cancer often presents with metastatic mediastinal adenopathy and is a sign of advanced stage.

提高至 80%。如有必要，胸膜活检有助于鉴别恶性肿瘤。胸膜活检可以经内科胸腔镜、手术视频辅助胸腔镜（VATS）来实现，次选活检方式是通过 Cope 针或 Abrams 针进行盲检。

恶性积液患者的胸水 pH 值降低具有预后和治疗意义。由恶性肿瘤导致的胸水 pH 值降低的患者往往生存时间更短，对化学胸膜固定术的反应较差。使用滑石粉或四环素衍生物进行化学胸膜固定术可以改善复发性恶性胸腔积液，但效果因人而异，只有不到 50% 的患者能完全缓解症状。许多复发性恶性胸腔积液患者也可以选择经皮植入胸腔引流管，进行间歇性引流、缓解症状、并可能随着时间推移实现机械性胸膜固定。

系统性炎症性疾病，如类风湿关节炎和系统性红斑狼疮，可伴有渗出性积液。类风湿性胸腔积液是类风湿病的一种常见胸内表现，可见于 5% 的患者。胸腔积液中的类风湿因子滴度常大于 1∶320，且积液中的葡萄糖水平低于 60 mg/dl（或积液 / 血清葡萄糖比值小于 0.5）。然而，复杂性肺炎旁胸腔积液或脓胸、恶性积液、结核性胸膜炎、狼疮性胸膜炎以及食管破裂等情况也可能导致胸水低葡萄糖水平。在系统性红斑狼疮患者中，15%～50% 会出现胸腔积液，胸腔积液中的抗核抗体滴度大于 1∶160。

检测胸水中的淀粉酶浓度有助于进一步区分渗出液的病因。胸水淀粉酶水平高于血清淀粉酶正常值上限，提示急性胰腺炎、慢性胰源性胸腔积液、食管破裂或恶性肿瘤。胰腺疾病与胰淀粉酶同工酶相关，而恶性肿瘤和食管破裂则以唾液淀粉酶同工酶为主。

气胸

气胸是指胸膜腔内气体积聚，此时胸膜腔内压力变为正压，导致肺组织受压。气胸患者通常会突然出现呼吸困难。临床表现为心动过速、呼吸音减弱、触觉震颤减低、胸膜摩擦音、皮下气肿、过清音以及气管向对侧移位。

通常通过直立位胸片来诊断气胸，床边超声可以提供快速评估。气胸的典型表现为脏层胸膜与壁层胸膜分离，脏层胸膜与胸廓之间可见气体。呼气末拍片可使肺密度增加而体积减小，从而凸显肺实质与胸腔气体之间的差异。

严重气胸通常需要插入胸腔闭式引流管并接水封瓶引流吸引。然而，如果气胸量较小且患者无明显不适，可考虑观察。如果不存在持续的气漏（如支气管-胸膜瘘），胸膜腔内的气体可被吸收，气胸也随之消失。

张力性气胸是一种需要立即通过放置胸管减压的医疗紧急情况。当胸腔内压力达到足以导致纵隔移位、腔静脉和心脏受压以及血流动力学障碍的程度时，就会发生张力性气胸。这种生理机制意味着胸膜腔内有持续的气体漏出。

气胸常与钝性或穿透伤有关。穿透伤时，空气可能经胸壁或肺部穿孔进入胸膜腔。气胸亦可与机械通气有关。有基础肺病的机械通气患者可能会突发气胸。当气道峰压突然升高和呼吸音减低时，临床医师需警惕这一并发症。

气胸可能是自发性的，也可能继发于基础肺病。通常，自发性气胸多见于高大、年轻、瘦削的男性，推测是由于肺尖的肺泡破裂所致。可并发气胸的基础肺病包括肺气肿、囊性纤维化、肉芽肿性炎症、干酪性肺炎、肺纤维化和肺脓肿。月经性气胸则发生在子宫内膜异位至胸膜下或横膈胸膜的女性中，月经期间子宫内膜结节破裂会导致气胸。

间皮瘤

恶性间皮瘤起源于体腔浆膜。80% 的间皮瘤源自胸膜。患者通常年龄超过 55 岁，并且与过去接触石棉有关。症状包括呼吸困难、胸痛和体重减轻。

最常见的影像学表现是大量单侧胸腔积液，可能完全填满一侧胸腔。胸膜增厚常常累及胸部周边，且常伴有不同程度钙化的胸膜斑块和积液。胸部 CT 是评估间皮瘤分期和进展情况最准确的无创方法。胸腔积液细胞学检查往往不足以做出诊断，而通过 CT 引导的活检或胸腔镜获取组织是最有效的手段。恶性间皮瘤患者的总体预后极差。就生存期而言，目前尚无任何特定的疗法能够优于单独的支持治疗。

纵隔疾病

病灶位置

纵隔位于两肺之间的胸腔中央，内含心脏、主动脉、食管、气管、淋巴结和胸腺。纵隔的边界是两侧的胸膜腔、下方的横膈、上方的胸腔入口。纵隔空间可以分为三个区域：前、中、后。纵隔肿物在纵隔的分区位置有助于疾病的鉴别诊断（图 8.1）。

前纵隔位于心包前方，包含淋巴组织、胸腺和大静脉。前纵隔中最常见的疾病有胸腺瘤、生殖细胞肿瘤、淋巴瘤、胸内甲状腺组织以及甲状旁腺病变。胸腺瘤占成年人纵隔肿瘤的 20%，是成人最常见的前纵隔原发性肿瘤。约 1/3 的胸腺瘤患者会出现重症肌无力相关症状。中纵隔病变包括气管肿块、支气管或心包囊肿、肿大的淋巴结以及主动脉近端疾病（如动脉瘤或夹层）。后纵隔肿块包括神经源性肿瘤和囊肿、脑（脊）膜膨出、淋巴瘤、降主动脉动脉瘤以及食管疾病（如憩室和肿瘤）。

系统性淋巴瘤常累及纵隔，约 5%～10% 的淋巴瘤患者在出现临床症状时即有原发性纵隔病变。纵隔囊肿可发生于心包、支气管、食管或胃、胸腺和胸导管，尽管通常为良性，但可产生压迫症状。肺癌晚期常常出现转移性纵隔淋巴结肿大。

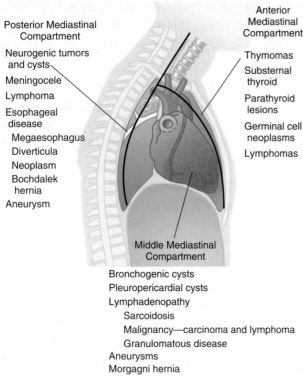

Fig. 8.1 Masses of the mediastinum and their anatomic locations.

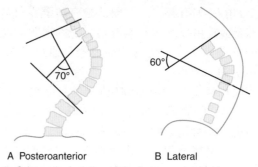

Fig. 8.2 Schematic depiction of the lines constructed to measure the Cobb angle of scoliosis (A) and kyphosis (B).

Treatment of a mediastinal mass depends on the underlying pathology. Many require surgical resection, irradiation, chemotherapy, or careful monitoring over time.

Mediastinitis

Inflammation of the mediastinal structures can be acute or chronic. Acute mediastinitis is a rapidly progressive condition due to infection, and it most commonly complicates cardiothoracic surgical procedures or occurs as a result of trauma. Chest imaging studies may show a widening of the mediastinum, pneumothorax, or hydrothorax. Treatment requires microbiological identification, antibiotics, pleural drainage, and mediastinal evacuation.

Chronic mediastinitis (i.e., fibrosing mediastinitis) is a progressive illness that results from fungal or granulomatous infections, neoplasms, radiotherapy, occasionally drugs (such as methysergide), or it may be idiopathic. Patients usually remain asymptomatic until vascular, respiratory, or neurologic structures are affected; tracheobronchial narrowing is the most common manifestation. Diagnosis and treatment often require surgical intervention, although no treatment is highly successful.

CHEST WALL DISEASE

The chest wall is composed of the bony structures of the rib cage, the articulations between the ribs and the vertebrae, the diaphragm, and other respiratory muscles. Normal function of this ventilatory pump is needed to bring oxygen from the atmosphere into the body. A wide variety of chest wall and neuromuscular disorders can result in dysfunction of the ventilatory pump. These disorders typically result in a restrictive dysfunction characterized by a reduction in total lung capacity and vital capacity with a normal residual volume. Hypoventilation may ensue, resulting in hypercapnia, atelectasis, and hypoxemia.

Skeletal Disease

Kyphoscoliosis and ankylosing spondylitis are disorders that involve the spine and its articulations. Pectus excavatum involves the sternum, flail chest affects the ribs, and obesity adds to the soft tissue mass of the chest wall. These disorders primarily affect the respiratory system by stiffening its tissues. Of these disorders, kyphoscoliosis produces the most severe restrictive impairment, and ankylosing spondylitis and pectus excavatum cause little respiratory compromise.

Kyphoscoliosis refers to a group of disorders characterized by excessive spinal curvature in the lateral plane (i.e., scoliosis) and sagittal plane (i.e., kyphosis). The degree of curvature can be assessed by measuring the Cobb angle (Fig. 8.2). Greater degrees of spinal curvature are associated with greater restriction and an increased risk of respiratory failure.

Kyphoscoliosis may be idiopathic, caused by neuromuscular disease, or associated with congenital vertebral malformations. Idiopathic kyphoscoliosis is the most common form, usually manifesting in late childhood or early adolescence and affecting females more than males (ratio of 4:1). It is thought to be a multigene condition with an autosomal or sex-linked inheritance pattern and variable phenotypic expression. A defect in the chromatin-remodeling gene (CHD7) has been associated with idiopathic kyphoscoliosis.

For a given degree of spinal deformity, individuals with kyphoscoliosis due to a neuromuscular disease have more respiratory impairment than those with idiopathic kyphoscoliosis. Factors that contribute to respiratory failure in patients with kyphoscoliosis include inspiratory muscle weakness, underlying neuromuscular disease, sleep-disordered breathing, and airway compression due to distortion of lung parenchyma and twisting of airways.

Treatment consists of general supportive measures such as immunizations against influenza and pneumococci, smoking cessation, maintenance of a normal body weight, supplemental oxygen, and treatment of respiratory infections. It is important to recognize nocturnal hypoventilation because it can be treated with noninvasive positive-pressure ventilation. This is typically delivered through a nasal or full face mask. Indications for instituting noninvasive ventilation include symptoms suggesting nocturnal hypoventilation, signs of cor pulmonale, nocturnal oxyhemoglobin desaturation, or an elevated daytime $Paco_2$.

Obesity

Obesity is a major health problem that affects children and adults throughout the world. Body fat usually constitutes 15% to 20% of body mass in healthy men and 25% to 30% of body mass in healthy women. In cases of obesity, the body fat content may increase by as much as 500% in women and 800% in men. The degree of obesity can be assessed by the body mass index, which is the ratio of body weight (BW) in kilograms to the square of the height (Ht) in meters (BW/Ht^2). Individuals with a BMI between 18.5 and 24.9 kg/m^2 are normal, and those with a BMI greater than 40 kg/m^2 are considered severely or morbidly obese.

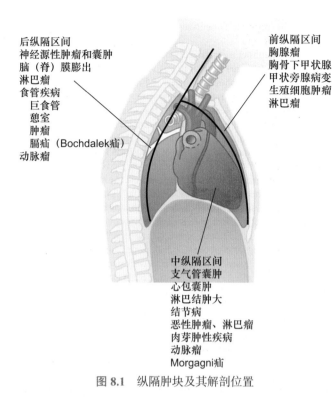

图 8.1　纵隔肿块及其解剖位置

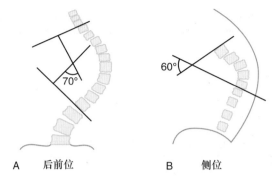

图 8.2　脊柱侧凸（**A**）和脊柱后弯（**B**）的 Cobb 角测量所需构建线条的示意图

中纵隔肿块的治疗取决于其潜在的病理。许多病例需要手术切除、放疗、化疗，或者长期观察随访。

纵隔炎

纵隔结构的炎症可以是急性或慢性的。急性纵隔炎是一种由感染引起的迅速进展的疾病，最常见并发于心胸外科手术，或由创伤引起。胸部影像学检查可能会显示纵隔增宽、气胸或胸腔积液。治疗需要微生物学鉴定、抗生素、胸腔引流以及纵隔引流。

慢性纵隔炎（如纤维性纵隔炎）是一种进展性疾病，由真菌或肉芽肿感染、肿瘤、放疗、偶尔药物（如甲基麦角胺）引起，也可能原因不明。患者通常在血管、呼吸或神经结构受累后才出现症状；气管-支气管狭窄是最常见的表现。诊断和治疗往往需要手术干预，但目前尚无非常有效的治疗方法。

胸壁疾病

胸壁由胸腔的骨性结构、肋骨与椎骨之间的关节、横膈膜和其他呼吸肌构成。正常的呼吸泵功能对于将氧气从大气带入体内至关重要。胸壁和神经肌肉系统的各种疾病可能导致呼吸泵功能障碍。这些疾病通常表现为限制性通气功能障碍，其特征是肺总量和肺活量下降，残气量正常。随后可能发生通气不足，导致高碳酸血症、肺不张和低氧血症。

骨骼疾病

脊柱侧后凸和强直性脊柱炎是累及脊柱及其关节的疾病。漏斗胸影响胸骨，连枷胸影响肋骨，而肥胖增加了胸壁软组织的量。这些疾病主要通过使呼吸系统的组织硬化来影响其功能。在这几种疾病中，脊柱侧后凸导致最严重的限制性通气功能障碍，而强直性脊柱炎和漏斗胸对呼吸的影响较小。

脊柱侧后凸是一组以侧面（即脊柱侧凸）和矢状面（即脊柱后弯）过度弯曲为特征的疾病。可以通过测量 Cobb 角来评估脊柱弯曲的严重程度（图 8.2）。脊柱弯曲度越大，呼吸受限的风险越高，可能导致呼吸衰竭。

脊柱侧后凸可能源于不明原因（特发性），也可由神经肌肉疾病引起，或与先天性脊柱畸形有关。特发性脊柱侧后凸最为常见，通常在儿童晚期或青少年早期出现，且女性受影响的比例高于男性（约为 4∶1）。它被认为是一种多基因疾病，具有常染色体或性连锁遗传模式，并表现出可变的表型表达。已发现染色质重塑基因（*CHD7*）缺陷与特发性脊柱侧后凸相关。

对于同一程度的脊柱畸形，由神经肌肉疾病导致的脊柱侧后凸患者相较于特发性脊柱侧后凸患者的呼吸功能障碍更严重。脊柱侧后凸患者出现呼吸衰竭的因素包括吸气肌无力、基础的神经肌肉疾病、睡眠呼吸障碍以及因肺实质变形和气道扭曲导致的气道压迫。

治疗包括一般支持措施（如流感和肺炎疫苗接种、戒烟、维持正常体重、补充氧气以及治疗呼吸道感染）。重要的是要识别并处理夜间低通气，因为其可以采用无创正压通气进行治疗，通常通过鼻罩或全脸面罩提供。开始无创通气的指征包括提示夜间低通气的症状、肺水肿体征、夜间血氧饱和度降低，或者日间动脉血 $PaCO_2$ 升高。

肥胖

肥胖是影响全球儿童和成人的重大健康问题。健康男性体脂约占体重的 15% ～ 20%，女性则占 25% ～ 30%。而在肥胖情况下，女性体脂含量可能增加高达 500%，男性则可能增加 800%。通过体重指数（BMI）可以评估肥胖程度，它是以千克为单位的体重（BW）除以以米为单位身高的平方（Ht^2）（BW/Ht^2）。个体 BMI 在 18.5 ～ 24.9 kg/m^2 属于正常范围，而 BMI 超过 40 kg/m^2 则被视为重度或病态肥胖。

Reductions in functional residual capacity and expiratory reserve volume are the most common pulmonary function abnormalities in obesity, whereas vital capacity and total lung capacity may be only minimally reduced. Obesity promotes breathing at low lung volumes, which reduces lung compliance and increases the work of breathing. A subgroup of individuals with obesity hypoventilate and become hypercapnic. When obesity is associated with hypoventilation, it is called the obesity-hypoventilation syndrome (i.e., Pickwickian syndrome). The mechanism underlying hypoventilation is unknown but may result from factors that reduce respiratory center chemosensitivity, such as hypoxia, sleep apnea, or adipokines such as leptin. The most important consequences of chronic hypoventilation are hypoxemia and pulmonary hypertension.

Nocturnal noninvasive positive-pressure ventilation can help to reverse these abnormalities. Weight loss is the optimal therapy, but it is not always attainable, and long-term weight loss maintenance is even more difficult. Pharmacotherapy or bariatric surgery should be considered for obese individuals who do not achieve weight control with conventional methods (i.e., diet, enhanced physical activity, and behavioral therapy).

Diaphragm Paralysis

The diaphragm separates the thorax from the abdomen and is the major muscle of inspiration. Diaphragm weakness or paralysis can involve one or both hemidiaphragms. Unilateral diaphragm paralysis is more common than bilateral diaphragm paralysis. The most frequent causes of unilateral paralysis include traumatic phrenic nerve injury, herpes zoster infection, cervical spinal disease, and compressive tumors. Patients may be asymptomatic, or the abnormality may be discovered as an incidental finding of an elevated hemidiaphragm on a chest radiograph (Fig. 8.3). The diagnosis is confirmed by seeing on fluoroscopy a paradoxical upward motion of the affected diaphragm during a vigorous sniff maneuver. There is no specific treatment for this disorder, but recovery after the initial injury occasionally occurs. When the patient has disabling symptoms and significant elevation of the diaphragm is seen on the chest radiograph, surgical plication of the diaphragm may provide some relief of symptoms.

Bilateral diaphragm paralysis is most often seen in the setting of a disease producing generalized muscle weakness or motor neuron disease such as amyotrophic lateral sclerosis. Pulmonary function test results are associated with severe restrictive impairments. When the patient assumes the supine position, there may be a further reduction ($\leq 50\%$) in vital capacity. It is not surprising that orthopnea is an especially prominent symptom, and patients often have difficulty sleeping

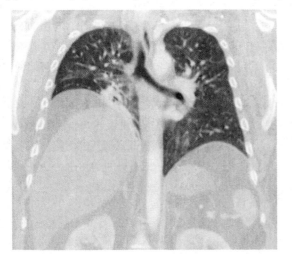

Fig. 8.3 Computed tomography of a patient with unilateral right hemidiaphragm paralysis and associated right lower lobe atelectasis.

in the supine position. Patients also complain of dyspnea when bending or lifting objects.

Bilateral diaphragm paralysis can be difficult to diagnose. Restriction evidenced by pulmonary function test results is nonspecific, as is the finding of low lung volumes on chest radiographs. Fluoroscopic sniff testing (i.e., diaphragm fluoroscopy) can yield false-negative and false-positive results. Measurement of transdiaphragmatic pressure is the gold standard, but it is somewhat invasive, requiring placement of catheters in the esophagus and stomach. Alternatively, B-mode ultrasound of the diaphragm in the zone of apposition is a very useful noninvasive means of diagnosing diaphragm paralysis, as it can directly assess the thickening of the diaphragm muscle (or lack thereof).

Treatment should address the underlying disease, which may or may not be reversible. If paralysis is idiopathic or caused by neuralgic amyotrophy (i.e., brachial plexus neuritis), more than 50% of individuals may recover. Phrenic nerve pacing may be used in patients with spinal cord injuries above C3, and noninvasive positive-pressure ventilation can be used to treat patients with nocturnal hypoventilation. Diaphragm plication is not indicated in patients with bilateral diaphragm paralysis.

PROSPECTUS FOR THE FUTURE

Numerous advances can be expected in treating individuals with pleural, mediastinal, and chest wall diseases. Progress in pleural fluid analysis using novel biomarkers and nucleic acid amplification tests may lead to more rapid and accurate diagnosis of tuberculous pleural effusions. Assays of pleural fluid tumor markers and chromosome analysis are promising developments for the differentiation of malignant from nonmalignant effusions. Mesothelioma remains resistant to traditional therapeutic approaches, but evolving technology centered on gene therapy may produce a new treatment modality.

Better visualization of mediastinal structures can be achieved as magnetic resonance imaging (MRI) evolves and becomes more routinely applied to examination of the chest. Molecular tracers targeting tumor receptors or proteins may be used with MRI and positron emission tomography imaging techniques to better differentiate malignant from benign mediastinal masses.

Noninvasive nocturnal ventilation remains a cornerstone of therapy for patents with chest wall and neuromuscular diseases, but compliance can be problematic. Continued evolution of techniques to deliver nocturnal noninvasive ventilation may improve compliance with treatment, and application of this technique to patients with obesity-hypoventilation syndrome may reduce morbidity and mortality for them.

Patients with diaphragm paralysis due to high cervical spinal cord lesions may benefit from advances in intramuscular diaphragm pacing. This technique may provide an alternative means of treating respiratory failure in these individuals and others with diaphragm paralysis.

For a deeper discussion on this topic, please see Chapter 92, ❖ "Diseases of the Diaphragm, Chest Wall, Pleura, and Mediastinum," in *Goldman-Cecil Medicine*, 26th Edition.

SUGGESTED READINGS

Brixey AG, Light RW: Pleural effusions occurring with right heart failure, Curr Opin Pulm Med 17:226-231, 2011.

Colice GE, Curtis A, Deslauriers J, et al: Medical and surgical treatment of parapneumonic effusions: an evidence-based guideline, Chest 18:1158-1171, 2000.

Davies HE, Davies RJ, Davies CW, BTS Pleural Disease Guideline Group: Management of pleural infection in adults: British Thoracic Society Pleural Disease Guideline 2010, Thorax 65: 2010.

功能残气量和补呼气容积减低是肥胖最常见的肺功能异常，而肺活量和肺总量可能仅轻度减低。肥胖会促进在肺容量较低时的呼吸，这降低了肺顺应性，增加了呼吸功。部分肥胖者通气不足并伴有二氧化碳潴留，称为肥胖-低通气综合征（即匹克威克综合征）。通气不足的确切机制不明，可能源于降低呼吸中枢化学感受性的因素，如低氧血症、睡眠呼吸暂停，或如瘦素之类的脂肪因子。慢性低通气的主要后果是低氧血症和肺动脉高压。

夜间无创正压通气有助于逆转这些异常。减重是首选的治疗方式，但并不总能实现，且长期维持减重更为困难。对于通过常规方法（即饮食、增强体力活动和行为治疗）未能控制体重的肥胖者，应当考虑药物治疗或进行减重手术。

膈肌麻痹

横膈膜将胸腔和腹腔分隔开，是吸气的主要肌肉。横膈肌无力或麻痹可能影响单侧或双侧横膈。单侧横膈麻痹比双侧横膈麻痹更为常见。单侧横膈麻痹的常见原因包括创伤性神经丛损伤、带状疱疹感染、颈椎病变及压迫性肿瘤。患者可能无症状，或者在胸部 X 线平片上偶然发现患侧横膈抬高（图 8.3）。可以通过 X 线透视观察患者在努力吸气时受影响的横膈出现反常的向上运动来确定诊断。该病无特定疗法，但初次损伤后偶尔会恢复。当患者有严重症状且胸部 X 线平片显示横膈显著抬高时，横膈折叠手术可能有助于缓解症状。

双侧膈肌麻痹最常出现在诸如肌萎缩侧索硬化症等导致全身肌肉无力或运动神经元疾病的患者中。肺功能检查结果通常表现为严重的限制性通气功能障碍。当患者采取仰卧位时，其肺活量可能会进一步减少（≤ 50%）。因此，端坐呼吸是一种特别突出的症状，仰卧位时患者往往难以入睡。当患者弯腰或提举重物

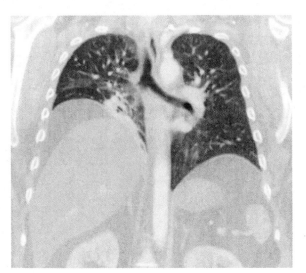

图 8.3　一名右侧半膈肌麻痹并伴有右下叶肺不张的患者的计算机断层成像图像

时也会主诉呼吸困难。

双侧膈肌麻痹的诊断颇具挑战性。肺功能检查结果和胸部 X 线片上显示的通气受限均缺乏特异性。透视下经鼻吸气试验（即膈肌 X 线透视）可能有假阴性和假阳性结果。跨膈压测定是金标准，但具有一定侵入性，需要在食管和胃中放置导管。作为一种非侵入性的替代方法，膈肌附着区 B 型超声检查能有效地诊断膈肌麻痹，还可以直接评估膈肌肌肉的增厚（或消失）。

治疗应当针对基础疾病，无论其是否可逆。如果膈肌麻痹是特发性的，或者由神经痛性肌萎缩（即臂丛神经炎）引起，超过 50% 的患者可能康复。对于 C3 及以上的脊髓损伤患者，可以使用膈神经起搏器；对于夜间通气不足的患者，可以采用无创正压通气。对于双侧膈肌麻痹的患者，不应进行横膈折叠术。

未来展望

在治疗胸膜、纵隔和胸壁疾病方面，预期将取得多项进展。利用新型生物标志物和核酸扩增试验检测胸腔积液可能会带来更快速、更准确的结核性胸腔积液诊断。检测胸腔积液肿瘤标志物和染色体分析是区分恶性与非恶性积液的有前景的发展领域。间皮瘤对传统治疗手段仍具抗药性，但基因疗法相关技术的进步可能开辟出新的治疗方式。

随着磁共振成像（MRI）技术的进步及其在胸部检查中的常规应用，可以更好地可视化纵隔结构。结合针对肿瘤受体或蛋白的分子探针，以及正电子发射断层成像（PET）技术，有助于区分恶性与良性纵隔肿物。

对于胸壁和神经肌肉疾病患者，夜间无创通气疗法仍然是治疗的基础，但依从性可能存在问题。夜间无创通气技术的不断改进可能会提高患者的依从性，而将这种技术应用于肥胖-低通气综合征患者可能有助于降低他们的发病率和死亡率。脊髓高位损伤导致膈肌麻痹的患者可能从膈肌起搏技术的进步中获益。这项技术为这类个体和其他膈肌麻痹患者的呼吸衰竭提供了一种治疗手段。

有关此专题的深入讨论，请参阅 *Goldman-Cecil* ❖ *Medicine* 第 26 版第 92 章 "膈、胸壁、胸膜与纵隔疾病"。

推荐阅读

Brixey AG, Light RW: Pleural effusions occurring with right heart failure, Curr Opin Pulm Med 17:226-231, 2011.

Colice GE, Curtis A, Deslauriers J, et al: Medical and surgical treatment of parapneumonic effusions: an evidence-based guideline, Chest 18:1158-1171, 2000.

Davies HE, Davies RJ, Davies CW, BTS Pleural Disease Guideline Group: Management of pleural infection in adults: British Thoracic Society Pleural Disease Guideline 2010, Thorax 65: 2010.

Duwe BV, Sterman DH, Musani AI: Tumors of the mediastinum, Chest 128:2893-2909, 2005.

Gottesman E, McCool FD: Ultrasound evaluation of the paralyzed diaphragm, Am J Respir Crit Care Med 155:1570-1574, 1997.

Heffner JE, Klein JS: Recent advances in the diagnosis and management of malignant pleural effusions, Mayo Clin Proc 83:235-250, 2008.

Jankowich MD, Gartman EJ, editors: Ultrasound in the intensive care unit, New York, 2015, Humana Press.

Light RW: The undiagnosed pleural effusion, Clin Chest Med 27:309-319, 2006.

McCool FD, Tzelepis GE: Current clinical aspects of diaphragm dysfunction, N Engl J Med 366:932-942, 2012.

Rahman NM, Maskell NA, West A, et al: Intrapleural use of tissue plasminogen activator and DNase in pleural infection, N Engl J Med 365:518-526, 2011.

Stafanidis K, Dimopolous S, Nanas S: Basic principles and current applications of lung ultrasonography in the intensive care unit, Respirology 16:249-256, 2011.

Tzelepis GE, McCool FD: Nonmuscular diseases of the chest wall. In Grippi MA, et al, editors: Fishman's Pulmonary Diseases and Disorders, 5th ed, McGraw-Hill, 2015.

Yusen RD: Medical and surgical treatment of parapneumonic effusions: an evidence-based guideline, Chest 118:1158-1171, 2000.

Duwe BV, Sterman DH, Musani AI: Tumors of the mediastinum, Chest 128:2893-2909, 2005.

Gottesman E, McCool FD: Ultrasound evaluation of the paralyzed diaphragm, Am J Respir Crit Care Med 155:1570-1574, 1997.

Heffner JE, Klein JS: Recent advances in the diagnosis and management of malignant pleural effusions, Mayo Clin Proc 83:235-250, 2008.

Jankowich MD, Gartman EJ, editors: Ultrasound in the intensive care unit, New York, 2015, Humana Press.

Light RW: The undiagnosed pleural effusion, Clin Chest Med 27:309-319, 2006.

McCool FD, Tzelepis GE: Current clinical aspects of diaphragm dysfunction, N Engl J Med 366:932-942, 2012.

Rahman NM, Maskell NA, West A, et al: Intrapleural use of tissue plasminogen activator and DNase in pleural infection, N Engl J Med 365:518-526, 2011.

Stafanidis K, Dimopolous S, Nanas S: Basic principles and current applications of lung ultrasonography in the intensive care unit, Respirology 16:249-256, 2011.

Tzelepis GE, McCool FD: Nonmuscular diseases of the chest wall. In Grippi MA, et al, editors: Fishman's Pulmonary Diseases and Disorders, 5th ed, McGraw-Hill, 2015.

Yusen RD: Medical and surgical treatment of parapneumonic effusions: an evidence-based guideline, Chest 118:1158-1171, 2000.

Respiratory Failure

Andrew E. Foderaro, Abhinav Kumar Misra

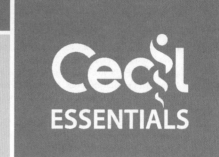

INTRODUCTION

The principle function of our lungs and respiratory system is gaseous exchange, absorption of oxygen and elimination of carbon dioxide produced by the body. Sudden inability to perform one or both of these functions leads to acute respiratory failure (ARF). Impairment of oxygen absorption will manifest as hypoxemia (arterial oxygen tension (Pao_2) <55-60 mm Hg) where impairment of carbon dioxide elimination (ventilation) is manifested by hypercapnia and respiratory acidosis (arterial carbon dioxide tension ($Paco_2$) >45 mm Hg). ARF is one of the most common causes for admission to an intensive care unit (ICU). The annual incidence of ARF in the United States is around 330,000 cases and carries significant short-term and long-term morbidity and mortality. Mortality rises with age, comorbidities, shock, or the presence of multiorgan failure. With an aging population in the United States the incidence of ARF is expected to rise.

PATHOPHYSIOLOGY

Respiratory failure can be classified as acute when derangements happen over hours to days or chronic when derangements occur more slowly over a longer period of time. Acute on chronic implies acute deterioration in someone with preexisting chronic respiratory failure. The respiratory system consists of two distinct parts: the lung (the gas exchanging organ) with the lung parenchyma and alveolar capillary interface, and the ventilatory pump comprising the lung and the chest wall (the respiratory muscles and airways that control ventilation).

Respiratory control is maintained by central neuronal respiratory centers in the medulla oblongata including the dorsal (DRG) and ventral respiratory groups (VRG). The DRG stimulates the diaphragm and intercostal muscles to contract causing inspiration and when activity ceases results in expiration. The VRG is involved in the forced inspiration and expiration through accessory muscles. The second respiratory center is located in the pons and consists of the pneumotaxic and apneustic center. These neurons are involved in control of rate and depth of breathing. Along with the central control there are peripheral chemoreceptors located in carotid bodies as well as aortic bodies constantly monitoring acidity and Pao_2 levels. Upon stimulation of respiratory muscles, the muscles contract generating a negative (subatmospheric) intrapleural pressure. This establishes a pressure gradient leading to flow of air towards alveoli where oxygen diffuses across the alveolar-capillary interface and forms oxyhemoglobin. The oxygen delivery to tissues is not only dependent on respiratory mechanics but also on hemoglobin and cardiac output.

Efficient gas exchange in our lungs is dependent on alveolar ventilation and pulmonary blood flow. This ratio is known as the ventilation-perfusion ($\dot{V}/\dot{Q}$) ratio. When there is alveolar ventilation without blood flow and thus without gas exchange this is referred to as dead space ventilation. Dead space consists of anatomic dead space (upper airway) as well as physiologic dead space (ventilation exceeding perfusion). In the case of physiologic dead space the $\dot{V}/\dot{Q}$ ratio is approaching infinity. Increased physiologic dead space ventilation can be seen when the alveolar-capillary interface is disrupted such as in emphysema, when pulmonary blood flow is reduced such as in low cardiac output, or when alveoli are overdistended due to positive-pressure ventilation. Alternatively, blood flow exceeding ventilation could lead to a portion of blood flow not partaking in gas exchange leading to intrapulmonary shunt. True shunt is when the $\dot{V}/\dot{Q}$ ratio is equal to 0. The fraction of cardiac output that does not partake in gas exchange is known as the shunt fraction, which is usually less than 10%. Increased shunt fraction can be seen when small airways are occluded (e.g., asthma), alveoli are collapsed (e.g., atelectasis), in alveolar filling diseases (e.g., pneumonia, pulmonary edema), or by bypassing the capillary bed (e.g., arteriovenous malformations).

Ideally, the oxygen that is present in the alveoli will equilibrate with the arterial blood. The difference between partial pressures of oxygen in alveolar space and arterial blood is known as the A-a gradient. This can be easily calculated with the help of the alveolar gas equation:

$$A\text{-}a \text{ gradient} = PAO_2 - PaO_2$$

$$PAO_2 = PIO_2 - (PACO_2 / RQ)$$

Here, PAO_2 represents partial pressure of oxygen in the alveolar space, Pao_2 represents partial pressure of oxygen in the arterial blood, PIO_2 is partial pressure of oxygen in inhaled gas, $PACO_2$ is partial pressure of carbon dioxide in alveolar space, and RQ is the respiratory quotient (the ration of CO_2 production to O_2 consumption). In a healthy subject eating a mixed diet, the respiratory quotient is 0.8. Furthermore, $PACO_2$ can be replaced by partial pressure of carbon dioxide in arterial blood ($Paco_2$) as CO_2 diffuses efficiently.

$$P_AO_2 = FiO_2 (P_A - P_{H2O}) - (Paco_2 / RQ)$$

FiO_2 is the fraction of oxygen, P_A is atmospheric pressure, and P_{H2O} is partial pressure of water vapor. Thus, for a normal healthy person breathing room air at sea level the A-a gradient equation would be as follows:

$$A\text{-}a \text{ gradient} = [FiO_2 (P_A - P_{H2O}) - (Paco_2 / RQ)] - PaO_2$$

$$A\text{-}a \text{ gradient} = [0.21 (760 - 47) - 40 / 0.8] - 90 = 10$$

Of note, the A-a gradient increases as a function of age. When patients are ventilated, their mean airway pressure needs to be added to atmospheric pressure to factor in the positive-pressure ventilation.

呼吸衰竭

吴小静 译 詹庆元 翟振国 审校 代华平 王辰 通审

引言

　　肺和呼吸系统的主要功能是气体交换，吸入氧气和排出身体产生的二氧化碳。当无法执行这两项功能之一时，就会发生急性呼吸衰竭（ARF）。氧气吸入功能受损表现为低氧血症［动脉血氧分压（PaO_2）< 55～60 mmHg］，二氧化碳排出功能受损则表现为高碳酸血症和呼吸性酸中毒［动脉血二氧化碳分压（$PaCO_2$）> 45 mmHg］。急性呼吸衰竭是入住重症监护病房（ICU）最常见的原因之一。美国每年ARF的年发病率约为33万例，具有显著的短期和长期病死率及发病率。病死率随着年龄、合并症、休克或出现多器官功能不全而升高。随着美国人口老龄化，ARF的发病率预计会继续升高。

病理生理学

　　呼吸衰竭可根据发病时间分为急性（发生在数小时至数天内）和慢性（在较长的时间段内缓慢发生）。慢性呼吸衰竭急性加重指那些已有慢性呼吸衰竭的患者出现急性恶化。呼吸系统由两部分组成：参与换气的肺组织（肺实质和肺泡毛细血管界面）和参与通气的肺和胸壁（呼吸肌和气道）。

　　呼吸控制由位于延髓的呼吸中枢神经元维持，包括背侧呼吸组（DRG）和腹侧呼吸组（VRG）。DRG刺激膈肌和肋间肌收缩，引起吸气，当刺激停止时就产生呼气。VRG通过控制辅助肌群参与吸气和呼气。第二个呼吸中枢位于脑桥，由呼吸调节中枢和呼吸暂停中枢组成。这些神经元参与控制呼吸的频率及深度。除了中央控制外，颈动脉体和主动脉体中还有外周化学感受器，持续监测酸碱度和PaO_2水平。刺激呼吸肌后，肌肉收缩，产生胸膜腔内负压（低于大气压）。这就建立了一个压力梯度，导致气体流向肺泡，在那里氧气弥散通过肺泡毛细血管界面，并形成氧合血红蛋白。氧气输送至组织不仅依赖于呼吸力学，还取决于血红蛋白数量和心输出量。

　　肺部的有效气体交换取决于肺泡通气量和肺血流量。这个比率称为通气-灌注（$\dot{V}/\dot{Q}$）比。当存在肺泡通气而无血流，导致没有气体交换时，称为无效腔（亦称死腔）通气。死腔通气包括解剖死腔（上呼吸道）和生理死腔（通气超过灌注）。在生理死腔情况下，$\dot{V}/\dot{Q}$比接近无穷大。当肺泡-毛细血管界面被破坏（如肺气肿），或肺血流量减少（如低心排血量），或正压通气导致肺泡过度扩张时，可以看到生理死腔增加。或者，当血流量远远超过通气量时，可能导致部分血流不参与气体交换，从而出现肺内分流。真性分流是指$\dot{V}/\dot{Q}$比等于0。心输出量不参与气体交换的部分就是分流部分，通常小于10%。当小气道闭塞（如哮喘）、肺泡塌陷（如肺不张）、肺泡充填性疾病（如肺炎、肺水肿），或毛细血管床旁路（如动静脉畸形）时，分流增加。

　　理想情况下，肺泡与动脉血中的氧气相平衡。肺泡腔和动脉血中的氧分压差被称为A-a梯度。可通过肺泡气体方程计算：

$$A\text{-}a \text{ 梯度} = PAO_2 - PaO_2;$$

$$PAO_2 = PIO_2 - (PACO_2/RQ)$$

　　这里的PAO_2表示肺泡腔内的氧分压，PaO_2表示动脉血中的氧分压，PIO_2表示吸入气体中的氧分压，$PACO_2$表示肺泡腔中的二氧化碳分压。RQ是呼吸熵（二氧化碳产生与消耗的比值）。在健康的混合饮食志愿者中，呼吸商为0.8。此外，由于二氧化碳的弥散效能高，$PACO_2$可使用动脉血二氧化碳分压（$PaCO_2$）代替。

$$PAO_2 = FiO_2 (P_A - P_{H2O}) - (PaCO_2/RQ)$$

　　FiO_2是吸氧浓度，P_A是大气压，P_{H2O}是水蒸气分压。因此，对于在海平面呼吸室内空气的健康年轻人来说，A-a梯度方程如下：

$$A\text{-}a \text{ 梯度} = [FiO_2 (P_A - P_{H2O}) - (PaCO_2/RQ)] - PaO_2$$

$$A\text{-}a \text{ 梯度} = [0.21 \times (760 - 47) - 40/0.8] - 90 = 10$$

　　值得注意的是，A-a梯度随着年龄的增长而增加。当患者进行机械通气时，他们的平均气道压需要加到大气压中，以叠加正压通气的因素。

TABLE 9.1   Classification of Respiratory Failure

Organ System	Disease Entity
Respiratory	Upper airway obstruction
	Airway obstructive disease
	COPD
	Asthma
	Pulmonary parenchyma
	Pneumonia
	ARDS
	ILD flare
	Pulmonary hemorrhage
	Alveolar proteinosis
Pulmonary Vascular	Pulmonary thromboembolism
	Pulmonary hypertension
	Right-to-left intrapulmonary shunts
Cardiac	Cardiogenic pulmonary edema
	Right-to-left intracardiac shunts
Neuromuscular	Myasthenia gravis
	ALS
	Guillain-Barré syndrome
Central Nervous System	Decrease respiratory drive
	Sedative medications
	Opioids
	Brain stem insult
	Space occupying lesion
	CVA
	Trauma

TABLE 9.2   Mechanisms That Cause Lower Partial Pressure in the Arterial Blood (Pao$_2$)

Etiologies of Hypoxia	Observed A-a Gradient
Low inspired oxygen	Normal
Hypoventilation	Normal
Ventilation-perfusion mismatch	Elevated
Shunt	Elevated
Diffusion Impairment	Elevated

CLASSIFICATION OF RESPIRATORY FAILURE

There are several ways to classify respiratory failure. A brief classification based on organ system can be found in Table 9.1.

Type I Hypoxemic Respiratory Failure

Mechanisms that cause lower Pao$_2$ are listed in Table 9.2. The first two mechanisms, low inspired oxygen and hypoventilation, lead to low Pao$_2$ through low Pao$_2$, thus the A-a gradient is normal. It is usually easy to eliminate the first two mechanisms in the clinical setting. Hypoventilation can be ruled out if hypercarbia is not present on arterial blood gas as the elevated Paco$_2$ leads to increased Paco$_2$ and lower Pao$_2$ (see the alveolar gas equation above).

The other three mechanisms result in an elevated A-a gradient. V̇/Q̇ mismatch and shunt are essentially a part of the same spectrum with shunt reflecting the extreme version of V̇/Q̇ mismatch. Administering supplemental oxygen will improve Pao$_2$. Supplemental oxygen cannot correct hypoxemia induced by pure shunt because the blood is completely bypassing the alveoli either physically or functionally. Impaired

diffusion is usually not clinically very important because oxygen transport across the alveolar-capillary interface is not diffusion limited even in individuals with preexisting interstitial disease.

Type II Hypercarbic Respiratory Failure

This represents incapability of the lungs to remove a sufficient amount of CO_2, due to either lower alveolar ventilation or, less commonly, higher production of carbon dioxide due to hyper-metabolic states such as sepsis, overfeeding, or fever. Minute ventilation is the product of respiratory rate and tidal volume. The dead space ventilation, both anatomic (in upper airways) and physiologic (areas where ventilation exceeds perfusion), does not take part in elimination of CO_2. Total alveolar ventilation is determined by the difference between total minute ventilation and dead space ventilation. As a result, both decreased tidal volume and increased dead space will lead to hypercarbia.

There are three major causes of ventilatory or hypercarbic failure: (1) Reduced central respiratory drive due to sedatives, drug overdoses or pathologic state of the medulla; (2) Mechanical defect in the chest wall (e.g., kyphoscoliosis, flail chest), disorders of the nerves or neuromuscular junctions such as myasthenia gravis, amyotrophic lateral sclerosis, or disorders of the respiratory muscles (e.g., myopathies); (3) Muscular fatigue usually seen when working against increased inspiratory load such as when hyperinflation is present or increased rate such that these muscles are no longer able to generate sufficient negative pleural pressure to maintain tidal volumes or required respiratory rate. Various etiologies of acute hypercarbic respiratory failure are summarized in Table 9.3.

TABLE 9.3   Causes of Hypercarbic Respiratory Failure

Etiology	Clinical Situation
Depressed CNS drive	Drugs: sedatives, opioids
	Brain stem/medulla lesions
	Sleep-disordered breathing
	Hypothyroidism
Neuromuscular transmission impairment	Spinal cord injury
	Phrenic nerve injury
	Demyelinating illness: ALS
	Neurotoxins: tetanus, botulism
	Neuromuscular junction disorders (e.g., myasthenia gravis, organophosphate poisoning)
	Muscle abnormalities: degenerative myopathies
Chest wall disease	Kyphoscoliosis
	Flail chest
	Obesity
	Pleural disruption: pneumothorax, pleural effusion
	Diaphragmatic rupture
Pulmonary disease	Upper airway obstruction
	Obstructive diseases
	Asthma
	COPD
	Alveolar filling process
	Pulmonary edema
	Atelectasis
	Pulmonary thromboembolism
	Bronchiectasis

表9.1　呼吸衰竭的分类	
器官系统	疾病
呼吸系统	上气道阻塞
	气道阻塞性疾病
	慢阻肺病
	哮喘
	肺实质病变
	肺炎
	ARDS
	间质性肺炎
	肺出血
	肺泡蛋白沉积症
肺血管疾病	肺血栓栓塞症
	肺动脉高压
	右向左肺内分流
心源性疾病	心源性肺水肿
	右向左心内分流
神经肌肉疾病	重症肌无力
	肌萎缩侧索硬化（ALS）
	吉兰-巴雷综合征
中枢神经系统疾病	降低呼吸驱动
	镇静药物
	阿片类药物
	脑干损伤
	占位性病变
	脑血管意外
	创伤

表9.2　导致动脉血氧分压（PaO_2）降低的机制	
低氧原因	A-a 梯度表现
吸入氧低	正常
低通气	正常
通气-灌注不匹配	升高
分流	升高
弥散受损	升高

呼吸衰竭分类

有几种方法可以对呼吸衰竭进行分类。基于器官系统的简要分类见表9.1。

Ⅰ型低氧血症型呼吸衰竭

表9.2 中列出了导致 PaO_2 降低的机制。前两种机制（吸入氧低和低通气），通过低 PAO_2 导致低 PaO_2，因此 A-a 梯度是正常的。在临床场景中通常很容易消除前两种机制。由于 $PACO_2$ 升高可导致 $PaCO_2$ 增加和 PAO_2 降低（见上文的肺泡气体方程），因此动脉血气中不存在高碳酸血症时可排除低通气的可能性。

其他三种机制都导致 A-a 梯度升高。$\dot{V}/\dot{Q}$ 不匹配和分流本质上是同一类问题，分流反映了 $\dot{V}/\dot{Q}$ 不匹配的极端情况。补充氧气可以改善 PaO_2。补充氧气不能纠正纯分流引起的低氧血症，因为血液在物理或功能

上均完全绕过肺泡。弥散受损通常在临床上不是很重要，因为即使在已经有间质性病变的个体中，通过肺泡-毛细血管界面的氧气输送也不受限制。

Ⅱ型高碳酸血症型呼吸衰竭

这表明肺无法清除足够量的 CO_2，这是由于肺泡通气量过低或因感染中毒症、过度喂养、发热等不常见的高代谢状态导致的二氧化碳产生过多。每分通气量是呼吸频率和潮气量的乘积。死腔通气，解剖死腔（上呼吸道）和生理死腔（通气超过灌注）都不参与 CO_2 的清除。肺泡总通气量由每分通气量和死腔通气量的差值决定。因此，潮气量的减少和死腔的增加都会导致高碳酸血症。

主要有三个原因导致通气或高碳酸血症型呼吸衰竭：①镇静剂、药物过量或脊髓病理状态导致的中枢性呼吸驱动降低；②胸壁机械性缺陷（如脊柱侧后凸、连枷胸）、神经或神经肌肉接头紊乱，如重症肌无力、肌萎缩侧索硬化或呼吸肌无力（如肌病）；③吸气负荷增高导致的呼吸肌疲劳，如当存在过度充气或呼吸频率增快时，这些肌肉不再能够产生足够的胸腔负压来维持潮气量或所需的呼吸频率。

表9.3 总结了急性高碳酸血症型呼吸衰竭的各种病因。

表9.3　高碳酸血症型呼吸衰竭的病因	
病因	临床情况
中枢性驱动降低	药物：镇静药、阿片类药物
	脑干/髓质病变
	睡眠呼吸障碍
	甲状腺功能减退
神经肌肉传递障碍	脊髓损伤
	膈神经损伤
	脱髓鞘疾病：肌萎缩侧索硬化（ALS）
	神经毒素：破伤风、肉毒素
	神经肌肉接头疾病：如重症肌无力、有机磷中毒
	肌肉异常：退行性肌病
胸壁疾病	脊柱侧后凸
	连枷胸
	肥胖
	胸膜疾病：气胸、胸腔积液
	膈肌破裂
肺部疾病	上气道阻塞
	阻塞性疾病
	哮喘
	慢阻肺病
	肺泡充填性疾病
	肺水肿
	肺不张
	肺血栓栓塞
	支气管扩张症

Clinical Manifestations

Common clinical manifestations of acute respiratory failure include tachycardia, tachypnea, anxiety, and cyanosis. For a patient to have cyanosis they must have 3 to 5 g/dL of deoxygenated hemoglobin, which usually corresponds to 80% peripheral capillary oxygen saturation (Spo_2). Patients may not be tachypneic if they are medicated with sedatives or opioids. Altered mental state is also a common finding. In the setting of acute hypercarbia, patients may experience increased somnolence, headaches, slurred speech, and eventually coma.

Chest radiography is an essential tool and shows one of three findings: (1) Normal or relatively normal, in which case etiologies such as airway disorders, right-to-left shunts, pulmonary embolism, and neuromuscular disorders come to the forefront; (2) Focal infiltrates as are seen with pneumonia or aspiration; (3) Diffuse infiltrates as can be seen in acute respiratory distress syndrome (ARDS) and interstitial lung disease flares. Initial evaluation for suspected respiratory failure should also include blood gas testing evaluating for presence of hypoxia. If hypoxia is present, calculating the A-a gradient can help point us in the direction of etiologic process. If a patient is hypercarbic, is that enough to cause hypoxemia? In this case, A-a gradient should remain normal. If A-a gradient is elevated it is likely $\dot{V}/\dot{Q}$ that mismatch or shunt is playing a role. These are usually the most common causes of respiratory failure.

Principles of Management

The differential diagnoses for acute respiratory failure are extensive; hence the specific management strategies depend on correcting the underlying cause. As part of the initial management it should be ensured that the airway is patent and the patient is breathing and has stable circulation. Strategies to supplement oxygen and improve oxygenation and ventilation remain cornerstones of supportive care until the etiology resolves.

Oxygen Delivery Systems

A large number of oxygen delivery systems exist. Each of these systems is characterized by the mechanism of delivery, some of which limit the concentration of oxygen (FiO_2) that can be delivered. Normal inspiratory flow rate at rest is 15 L/min, which is intermixed with the flow provided by the O_2 delivery device. Nasal cannula is one of the most commonly and widely accepted delivery systems. These provide 1 to 6 L/min of 100% FiO_2, which is mixed with room air. At rest these can provide an FiO_2 of 24% to 40% (nasal cannula oxygen intermixed with room air). Even though this modality is widely accepted by patients, its use has limitations in the acute setting due to inability to achieve high concentrations of FiO_2. Standard face masks are reservoir systems with 100 to 200 mL of reservoir around the patient's face. These use 5 to 10 L of flow to provide 35% to 50% FiO_2 to patients, which is variable depending upon the flow rate at which the patient is actually breathing. These need a minimum flow of around 5 L to clear exhaled gases. When an air entrainment device is attached, the FiO_2 can be regulated regardless of the flow. Air entrainment works by creating a high velocity stream of gas by narrowing the outlet of the oxygen, creating a pull that leads to room air getting mixed with oxygen. The greater the flow, the greater the force to pull room air, therefore keeping FiO_2 constant. This phenomenon was earlier thought to be due to the Venturi effect, lending these masks the name Venturi masks or Venti masks. These masks provide 24% to 50% FiO_2 in a constant fashion irrespective of the flow rates.

Non-rebreather masks are another form of reservoir system with attached reservoir bags of 600 to 1000 mL. As long as the bag is inflated, patients breathe air primarily contained in the bag. The masks are equipped with one-way expiratory ports to allow expired air to leave but don't allow room air to mix with oxygen in the reservoir bag. In ideal settings these masks can provide high FiO_2 up to 100%; however, due to leaks because of inadequate seal the true FiO_2 is often closer to 80%.

TABLE 9.4	Physiologic Benefits of HFNC
Improved oxygenation
Decreased anatomic dead space
Decreased carbon dioxide generation
Generation of positive nasopharyngeal and tracheal airway pressure
Increased lung volumes
Improved work of breathing
Preconditioning of inspired gas (heated and humidified)
Better secretion clearance
Superior comfort
Reduced room air entrainment

High-Flow Nasal Cannula

High-flow nasal cannula (HFNC) can provide up to 40 to 60 L/min of heated and humidified gas. An oxygen blender connected to the circuit enables precise titration of FiO_2 ranging from 21% to 100%. In order to actually match this to alveolar FiO_2, flow from the HFNC should be equal to the patient's flow. HFNC also creates a flow-dependent clearance of carbon dioxide from upper airways. In randomized trials HFNC has been shown to generate positive airway pressure between 0.35 (mouth open) and 0.69 (mouth closed) cm H_2O of pressure for every 10 L/min of flow. This pressure is higher in the expiratory phase of respiration, almost behaving like positive end-expiratory pressure (PEEP). It helps in recruitment of alveoli and may be more pronounced in people with higher BMI. HFNC has been shown to improve lung compliance, reduce respiratory rate, and increase tidal volume by as much as 10%. The heated and humidified nature of inhaled gas leads to increased mucociliary clearance as shown in patients with bronchiectasis. Physiologic effects of HFNC are summarized in Table 9.4.

The principles and mechanism of action make HFNC a very promising oxygen delivery device. In multiple prospective observational studies, it has been associated with reduction in respiratory rate, heart rate, use of accessory muscles, and dyspnea scores in ICU patients and is often better tolerated than bilevel positive airway pressure ventilation devices. Parke and colleagues conducted a prospective randomized trial in ICU patients with mild to moderate hypoxemic ARF and demonstrated fewer desaturations and less need of noninvasive ventilation (NIV) compared to face masks. However, until recently the effect of HFNC on intubation rates and mortality was not known. In the FLORALI trial, HFNC was shown to have lower mortality and higher ventilator-free days, albeit in secondary analyses. In contrast to the FLORALI trial, results of the HOT-ER trial concluded that HFNC was not superior to conventional oxygen therapy, although the intubation rate in the HFNC group was lower at 5.5% versus 11.6% in the conventional oxygen therapy group but did not reach statistical significance ($P = 0.053$). In a meta-analysis HFNC was associated with a much lower rate of intubation and as such HFNC should be considered first-line therapy in patients for acute hypoxemic respiratory failure.

In other population groups, retrospective studies found no difference in mortality between HFNC and NIV in immunosuppressed patients with ARF. In patients with cancer and patients who had a lung transplant HFNC was associated with lower mortality and lower intubation rates when compared to conventional oxygen therapy. HFNC was ineffective as a rescue therapy when NIV and conventional oxygen therapy had failed, suggesting benefit of early use. In 2014, Maggiore and colleagues showed that HFNC at 50 L/min for 48 hours when applied to a high-risk patient population who passed a spontaneous breathing trial but had a Pao_2/FiO_2 ratio of less than 300 had much lower reintubation rates at 3.8% versus 21% (Venturi mask).

临床表现

急性呼吸衰竭的常见临床表现包括心动过速、呼吸急促、焦虑和发绀。出现发绀的患者，至少有 3 ~ 5 g/dl 的脱氧血红蛋白，通常对应外周毛细血管血氧饱和度（SpO_2）80%。患者如果服用镇静剂或阿片类药物，可能不会出现呼吸急促。精神状态改变也是一个常见的表现。在高碳酸血症情况下，患者可能出现嗜睡、头痛、口齿不清，最终昏迷。

胸部 X 线片是急性呼吸衰竭评价中的重要检查，可表现如下 3 种类型中的一种：①正常或相对正常，在这种情况下，气道疾病、右向左分流、肺栓塞和神经肌肉病是最主要的病因；②局灶性浸润见于肺炎或吸入性病变；③弥漫性浸润见于急性呼吸窘迫综合征（ARDS）和间质性肺疾病。对疑似呼吸衰竭的初步评估还应包括血气分析以明确是否存在缺氧。如果存在缺氧，计算 A-a 梯度可以为病因诊断指明方向。如果患者是高碳酸血症，这是否足以引起低氧血症？如果引起低氧血症，A-a 梯度也应是正常的。如果 A-a 梯度升高，很可能是 $\dot{V}/\dot{Q}$ 失调或分流引起的。这些通常是呼吸衰竭最常见的原因。

管理原则

急性呼吸衰竭病因的鉴别诊断很广泛；因此，具体的管理策略取决于纠正其内在病因。作为初始管理的一部分，应保证患者气道通畅、呼吸和循环稳定。在病因解决前，补充氧气策略、改善氧合和通气是支持治疗的基石。

氧气输送系统

目前有众多氧气输送系统可供使用。每一个系统都以输送机制为特征，其中一些限制了可输送的氧气浓度（FiO_2）。静息时的正常吸气流速是 15 L/min，与氧气输送装置提供的流量混合。鼻导管是最常见和最广泛使用的输送系统之一。它们提供 1 ~ 6 L/min 的纯氧，与室内空气混合。静息状态下，可提供 24% ~ 40%（鼻导管吸氧与空气混合）的 FiO_2。尽管这种模式被患者广泛接受，但它在急性场景中的应用因其无法实现高浓度 FiO_2 而被限制。标准面罩是在患者面部周围储气 100 ~ 200 ml 的储存系统。其使用 5 ~ 10 L 的流量为患者提供 35% ~ 50% 的 FiO_2，这取决于患者的实际吸气流速。其大约需要最低 5 L 的流速来清除呼出的气体。当连接了空气卷吸装置时，FiO_2 的调节可以不考虑气流量。空气卷吸装置的作用是通过缩小氧气出口来产生高速气流，从而带动空气与氧气混合。流量越大，携带空气的力就越大，因此保持 FiO_2 稳定。这种现象被认为文丘里效应，因此这类面罩被称为文丘里面罩。无论流速如何，这些面罩都能提供 24% ~ 50% 切换范围的恒定 FiO_2。

非再呼吸式面罩是另一种储氧系统，附带 600 ~ 1000 ml 的储氧袋。只要袋子充满气，患者就可以主要吸入袋子中的气体。面罩设有单向呼气口，以呼出气体，但又不会让空气混入储氧袋。理想情况下，这类

表 9.4 HFNC 的生理获益
改善氧合
减少解剖死腔
减少二氧化碳产生
产生鼻咽和气道正压
增加肺容量
改善呼吸作功
吸入气体预处理（加温加湿）
分泌物清除更佳
极致的舒适性
减少空气卷吸

面罩可以提供 100% 的 FiO_2，但是由于密闭性不足导致的泄露，实际 FiO_2 通常接近 80%。

经鼻高流量吸氧

经鼻高流量吸氧（HFNC）可提供 40 ~ 60 L/min 的加温加湿气体。连接到电路的空氧混合器能精准滴定 21% ~ 100% 的 FiO_2。为了与肺泡 FiO_2 匹配，HFNC 的流量应等于患者的流量。HFNC 还可以形成流量依赖的上呼吸道二氧化碳清除。在随机试验中，HFNC 已被证实每 10 L/min 的流量可以产生 0.35（张嘴）~ 0.69（闭嘴）cmH_2O 的气道正压。这种压力在呼吸的呼气阶段更高，几乎表现为呼气末正压（PEEP）。它有助于肺泡复张，在 BMI 较高的人群中可能更显著。HFNC 已被证实可以改善肺顺应性，降低呼吸频率，并使潮气量增加 10%。如支气管扩张症患者中所示，吸入气体的加温加湿导致纤毛黏液清除率增加。HFNC 的生理效应总结于表 9.4。

HFNC 的原理和作用机制使其成为一种非常有前途的氧气输送装置。在多项前瞻性观察性研究中，它与降低 ICU 患者的呼吸频率、心率、辅助肌群的使用和呼吸困难评分相关，而且它通常比双水平正压通气设备的耐受性更好。Parke 及其同事在 ICU 轻至中度呼吸衰竭的患者中进行的一项前瞻性随机对照试验显示，与面罩相比，HFNC 患者氧饱和度下降率和无创通气（NIV）的需求都更低。然而，至今，HFNC 对气管插管率和死亡率的影响仍尚不清楚。在 FLORALI 研究的二次分析中，HFNC 组显示出更低的死亡率和更高的无机械通气天数。与 FLORALI 研究相比，HOTER 研究发现，HFNC 并不优于传统氧疗，尽管 HFNC 组的插管率低于传统氧疗组（5.5% *vs.* 11.6%），但是并没有达到统计学意义（$P = 0.053$）。在一项荟萃分析中，HFNC 与低得多的插管率相关，因此 HFNC 应该被作为急性低氧性呼吸衰竭患者的一线治疗。

对于其他人群，回顾性研究发现，免疫抑制 ARF 患者中，HFNC 和 NIV 的死亡率没有差异。在癌症和肺移植患者中，HFNC 相比传统氧疗，具有更低的死亡率和插管率。当 NIV 和传统氧疗治疗失败时，HFNC 作为挽救性治疗是无效的，这表明早期使用才能获益。2014 年，Maggiore 及其同事发现，在通过了自主呼吸试验但 PaO_2/FiO_2 < 300 mmHg 的高危人群中，使用 50 L/min 的 HFNC，再插管率显著低于使用文丘里面罩

Expanding on this trial, in 2016 Hernandez et al. showed this to be true even in a lower-risk population with reintubation rates being 4.9% in HFNC compared to 12.2% in conventional therapy group. Number needed to treat to prevent 1 reintubation was 14. HFNC has not been shown to be superior to conventional therapy or NIV in postcardiac surgical patients or postabdominal surgery patients. It can be used as a preoxygenation tool during intubation.

Patients who are failing HFNC need to be promptly intubated for invasive mechanical ventilation. Delaying intubation for greater than 48 hours has been shown to be associated with increased mortality. Poor prognostic signs include persistent tachypnea, hypoxia, asynchronous breathing, acidosis with pH less than 7.25, nonpulmonary organ failure or hypotension.

Mechanical Ventilation

Until the 1950s the "iron lung" and other forms of negative-pressure ventilation were the most common forms of mechanical ventilation, especially outside of the anesthesia suite. However, during the polio epidemic in Europe in 1955, the mortality benefit as well as safety outside of anesthesia suites of invasive positive-pressure ventilation was demonstrated, leading to increased use of positive-pressure ventilation. In the 1980s, noninvasive ventilation began to be used for patients with chronic respiratory failure and eventually moved from the outpatient to the inpatient setting. Since then it has become increasingly popular with as much as a 400% increase in use compared to 20 years ago.

Noninvasive Ventilation

NIV is the provision of ventilatory assistance to the lung without use of invasive interface such as endotracheal intubation. NIV uses a variety of noninvasive interfaces including oronasal masks, full face masks, and nasal prongs. Success of NIV depends on the tolerability of the interface as well as the seal provided by the interface. There are essentially two modes of ventilation: constant positive airway pressure (CPAP) and bilevel positive airway pressure (BiPAP).

CPAP provides a constant positive pressure while the patient breathes spontaneously. The degree of ventilatory support provided by this mode is limited. It does not lead to an increase in tidal volumes. It does provide benefit in patients without obstructive lung disease such as obesity hypoventilation and patients with cardiogenic pulmonary edema. BiPAP provides two different pressures during different phases of respiration. During inspiration it provides a higher pressure called inspiratory positive airway pressure (IPAP) and during expiration it maintains a lower airway pressure, which it maintains constantly, called expiratory positive airway pressure (EPAP). The EPAP essentially is the same as CPAP, with IPAP providing a pressure difference that assists during inspiration and provides ventilatory support. Because both of these modalities raise mean airway pressure they help with alveolar recruitment to a certain degree and have a role in providing hemodynamic support to patients with heart failure.

NIV has distinct advantages over invasive mechanical ventilation. Importantly, it eliminates intubation and it eliminates the risk of upper airway trauma by intubation. In addition, it reduces patient discomfort, lowers risk of ventilator-associated pneumonia (VAP), and preserves airway clearance. Patients can be provided breaks from ventilation to allow communication and normal eating and drinking. There are multiple specific etiologies where NIV has become first-line therapy, which are discussed below. There are specific clinical situations where NIV is contraindicated and clinicians should move to invasive mechanical ventilation (IMV). These are summarized in Table 9.5 .

TABLE 9.5	Contraindications for Noninvasive Ventilation (NIV)
Absolute Contraindications	**Relative Contraindications**
Cardiopulmonary arrest	Hemodynamically unstable
Facial surgery/trauma	Encephalopathy
Upper airway obstruction	Agitated or uncooperative
Vomiting	Unable to protect airway
Upper GI bleeding	Excessive secretions
	Multiple organ failure
	Swallowing impairment
	Inability to physically remove the mask

Hypercapnic respiratory failure. There are strong recommendations to use NIV in cases of acute COPD exacerbations with mild and moderate ARF with pH between 7.25 and 7.35 and $Paco_2$ of greater than 45 despite standard medical therapy. Early initiation of NIV has been shown to lower rates of intubation and the length of hospitalization as well as mortality. Though pH is the most important determinant, other clinical factors such as tachypnea, severity of dyspnea, and use of accessory muscles should also be considered. Although the mechanism of respiratory failure during asthma exacerbations resembles COPD exacerbation, the airway obstruction is less homogeneous and there is a higher risk of dynamic hyperinflation. Evidence to use NIV in this case is not as convincing. There is probably a narrow window to trial NIV and if respiratory failure does not improve to go ahead with invasive MV.

In patients with bronchiectasis such as cystic fibrosis patients, NIV has been shown to reduce the load on respiratory muscles as well as improve alveolar hypoventilation. NIV should be started if patients have hypercapnia either in the stable phase or during an exacerbation. It may be valuable supportive therapy as a bridge to lung transplantation. Similar to this patient population, in patients with neuromuscular disease respiratory pump impairment plays a pivotal role in alveolar hypoventilation. This usually presents initially as nocturnal hypoventilation, gradually getting worse as the disease progresses and leading to inspiratory muscle weakness, decreased chest wall compliance, and failure to clear secretions. Combining NIV with airway clearance therapies may delay intubation.

Hypoxemic respiratory failure. Several studies since the 1980s have looked at NIV in patients with cardiogenic pulmonary edema. Use of both forms of NIV (CPAP and BiPAP) have shown decreased mortality rate and decreased need for intubation in patients with ARF due to cardiogenic pulmonary edema and has been recommended as first-line therapy in the ATS 2017 guidelines. However, NIV should be used with caution in patients with acute coronary syndromes and cardiogenic shock because there is a slightly higher chance of myocardial infarction.

Guidelines recommend use of NIV in postsurgical patients who develop ARF. Use of both CPAP and BiPAP reduces intubation rates, nosocomial infections, as well as mortality once surgical complications have been ruled out.

Given the lower risk of VAP, NIV has been suggested in patients who are immune compromised with pooled analyses showing benefit and lower intubation risks. However, some studies have shown benefit of HFNC compared to NIV. In patients with ARF of unknown etiology NIV is not recommended. There are multiple disadvantages to consider, and the positive effects of NIV on alveolar recruitment are lost with any interruptions in therapy. NIV can mask clinical deterioration and delay intubations as well as cause lung injury if tidal volumes are too high. In patients with severe hypoxia with Pao_2/FiO_2 ratio of less than 150, use of NIV has been shown to have higher mortality.

（3.8% *vs.* 21%）。在这项研究的基础上，Hernandez 等人在 2016 年证实了，即使是在低风险人群中，HFNC 的再插管率为 4.9%，而传统氧疗组为 12.2%。针对 14 名患者进行 HFNC 治疗，可以成功预防其中 1 名患者再次插管（NNT = 14）。在接受心脏手术后或腹部手术后的患者中，HFNC 尚未被证明优于传统氧疗或 NIV。它可以作为插管过程中的预充氧工具。

HFNC 治疗失败的患者需要立即插管进行有创机械通气。延迟插管超过 48 h 已被证明与病死率增加相关。不良预后的征象包括持续呼吸窘迫、低氧、呼吸不协调、pH 值低于 7.25 的酸中毒、肺外脏器衰竭或低血压。

机械通气

直到 20 世纪 50 年代，"铁肺"和其他形式的负压通气都是最常见的机械通气模式，尤其是在麻醉室外。然而，在 1955 年欧洲脊髓灰质炎流行期间，有创正压通气的死亡率获益和麻醉室外安全性得到了证明，从而使正压通气的使用有所增加。在 20 世纪 80 年代，无创通气开始用于慢性呼吸衰竭患者，并最终从门诊转移到病房。从那时起，它变得越来越受欢迎，20 年来使用量增加了 400%。

无创通气

NIV 是在不使用气管插管等侵入性接口的情况下为肺部提供通气辅助。NIV 使用多种非侵入性接口，包括口鼻面罩、全脸面罩和鼻塞。NIV 的成功取决于接口的耐受性和密封性。有两种基本的通气模式：持续正压通气（CPAP）和双水平正压通气（BiPAP）。

CPAP 在患者自主呼吸时提供恒定的正压。该模式所提供的通气支持程度是受限的。它不会导致潮气量的增加，不会为非阻塞性肺病（如肥胖低通气和心源性肺水肿）患者带来获益。BiPAP 在呼吸的不同阶段提供两种不同的压力。在吸气阶段提供更高的压力，称为吸气正压（IPAP），在呼气阶段，保持持续较低的气道压力，称为呼气正压（EPAP）。EPAP 基本上与 CPAP 相同，IPAP 提供压差，以促进吸气并提供通气支持。由于这两种模式都能提高平均气道压，因此它们都可在一定程度上帮助肺泡复张，并为心力衰竭患者提供血流动力学支持。

NIV 与有创机械通气相比具有显著优势。重要的是，它消除了气管插管及其所带来的上呼吸道创伤风险。此外，它还能减少患者的不适、降低呼吸机相关肺炎（VAP）的风险，并保持气道廓清。患者可以在通气期间短时间中断，以便进行交流和正常饮食。NIV 已成为多种疾病的一线治疗，下文将对此进行讨论。在某些特定的临床情况下，NIV 是禁忌的，需要改为有创机械通气（IMV），这些情况总结于表 9.5。

表 9.5　无创通气（NIV）的禁忌证

绝对禁忌证	相对禁忌证
心肺骤停	血流动力学不稳定
面部手术 / 创伤	脑病
上气道阻塞	焦虑不安或不能配合
呕吐	丧失气道保护能力
上消化道出血	分泌物过多
	多器官衰竭
	吞咽障碍
	无法移除面罩

高碳酸血症型呼吸衰竭　强烈建议在慢阻肺病急性加重伴轻中度呼吸衰竭（pH 值 7.25 ～ 7.35 并 PaCO$_2$ > 45 mmHg）患者中，标准药物治疗同时使用 NIV。早期开始 NIV 已被证明与较低的插管率、住院时间和死亡率相关。尽管 pH 是最重要的因素，但呼吸窘迫、呼吸困难程度、使用辅助呼吸肌等其他临床指标也应被考虑。尽管哮喘急性发作期间呼吸衰竭的机制类似于慢阻肺病急性发作期，但气道阻塞更加不均一，动态过度充气的风险更高。这种情况下使用 NIV 的证据并不充分。NIV 的试验窗可能很窄，如果呼吸衰竭没有改善，就要进行有创通气。

在支气管扩张症（如囊性纤维化）患者中，NIV 已被证实可以减少呼吸肌负荷，并改善肺泡低通气。无论是在稳定期还是急性加重期，如果患者出现高碳酸血症，就应该开始 NIV。作为肺移植桥接，它可能是有价值的支持治疗。与此类患者相似，在神经肌肉疾病患者中，呼吸泵损伤在肺泡低通气中起着关键作用。最初表现为夜间通气不足，随着疾病的发展逐渐恶化，最终导致呼吸肌无力、胸壁顺应性下降和无法清除分泌物。结合 NIV 和气道廓清疗法可能会延迟插管。

低氧血症型呼吸衰竭　20 世纪 80 年代以来的几项研究关注于心源性肺水肿患者的 NIV。两种模式的 NIV（CPAP 和 BiPAP）都显示出降低心源性肺水肿导致呼吸衰竭患者的死亡率和插管率，并在美国胸科学会（ATS）2017 年指南中被推荐为一线治疗。然而，NIV 在急性冠脉综合征和心源性休克患者中应该谨慎使用，因为心肌梗死的概率略高。

指南建议术后 ARF 患者使用 NIV。使用 CPAP 和 BiPAP 都能降低气管插管率、院内感染，及除手术并发症外的死亡率。

鉴于 VAP 的风险较低，NIV 已被建议用于免疫抑制患者，联合分析显示出了获益和较低的气管插管率。然而，一些研究表明，HFNC 比 NIV 更能使患者获益。病因不明的 ARF 患者，不建议使用 NIV。有多种不利因素需要考虑，而且 NIV 对肺泡复张的积极作用会因为治疗过程中的任何中断而消失。NIV 可以掩盖临床恶化导致插管延迟，如果潮气量过高还会引起肺损伤。在 PaO$_2$/FiO$_2$ < 150 mmHg 的严重低氧患者中，使用 NIV 的死亡率更高。

TABLE 9.6	Risk Factors for Failure of NIV
Acute hypercarbic RF	Poor neurologic score: GCS <11
	Tachypnea: >35 breaths/min pH <7.25
	APACHE score >29
	Asynchronous breathing
	Excessive air leak
	Agitation
	Excessive secretions
	Poor tolerance
	Poor adherence to therapy
	No initial improvement within first 2 hrs of noninvasive ventilation
	No improvement in pH
	Persistent tachypnea, tachycardia
	Persistent hypercapnia
Acute hypoxic RF	Diagnosis of ARDS or pneumonia
	Age >40 yr
	Hypotension: systolic blood pressure <90 mm Hg metabolic acidosis: pH <7.25
	Low Pao_2/Fio_2 ratio <150
	Failure to improve oxygenation within first hour of noninvasive ventilation

Success of NIV is dependent on underlying disease. Disorders such as COPD exacerbation and cardiogenic edema are more responsive than hypoxemic respiratory failure of unknown etiology. Baseline severe acidosis (pH <7.25), severe hypoxia, respiratory distress with persistent high respiratory rate greater than 25, and nonpulmonary organ failure have been associated with NIV failure. Various risk factors for failure of NIV are summarized in Table 9.6.

Invasive mechanical ventilation. IMV is positive-pressure ventilatory assistance with the help of a tracheostomy or endotracheal tube connected to a ventilator. In the United States around 800,000 patients receive IMV annually. The fundamental operation of a ventilator involves four phases: (1) The trigger phase initiates the breath. This can be controlled by changing preset triggers such as flow or pressure in the circuit or by time (time-triggered) when the ventilation is completely controlled. (2) The target phase where the pressure or flow is maintained by the ventilator. (3) The cycling phase determines the end of the inspiratory phase. Once the variable—flow or pressure—reaches the preset value, the expiration phase starts. (4) The expiration phase is usually passive while maintaining a preset pressure (PEEP).

The simplest mode of ventilation is assist-control ventilation where the patient provides the initial trigger for a flow-targeted volume-cycled (volume assist-control ventilation, or VC) or pressure-targeted time-cycled (pressure assist control ventilation, or PC) ventilation. Both of these modes are usually on a simple feedback loop, so that if the patient's respiratory rate is too low then the ventilator will provide the set number of breaths per minute. When the patient's respiratory rate is higher, all breaths will be triggered by the patient and will get the set ventilatory assistance. Another simple mode is the pressure support mode (PS), where the patient triggers every breath. Apart from preset pressure assistance there is no cycling variable set and the patient controls the duration of the breath.

IMV is often lifesaving but it is fraught with complications. Many of these complications can be avoided and minimized. Initiation of IMV involves endotracheal intubation, which is a

critical procedure. Prior to intubation patients need to be evaluated for factors that could indicate presence of a difficult airway. Preoxygenation is essential and use of rapid-sequence intubation with sedative and neuromuscular blocking agents increases the rate of successful intubation. Following placement of an endotracheal tube IMV is not well tolerated in most fully awake patients, hence the need for sedation. Sedation agents are associated with their own complications; for example, long-term use of benzodiazepines, especially in the form of continuous infusions, has been linked with delirium and poor long-term outcomes.

In addition to sedation-related complications, ventilators can provide 100% FiO_2, which can cause oxygen toxicity when used inappropriately. Hyperoxemia has been linked to poor outcomes in patients suffering from strokes or cardiac illness.

Positive-pressure ventilation can cause direct pressure-related injuries from three mechanisms: barotrauma, volutrauma, and atelectrauma. Barotrauma is an increase in pressure in the airways that can lead to alveolar or distal airway rupture leading to air leaks and pneumothorax or pneumomediastinum. Volutrauma can lead to overdistension of alveoli, causing alveolar-capillary interface disruption leading to inflammation. In the 1980s, the first studies showed diffuse parenchymal infiltrates from high inflation volumes. Atelectrauma occurs during the expiratory phase when small airways can collapse, especially in cases where lung compliance is markedly reduced. Repetitive opening and closing of alveoli and small airways can lead to damage to airway epithelium and inflammation.

Weaning From Ventilation

As the underlying cause of respiratory failure improves, attempts need to be made to get the patient off of MV as soon as possible. Determining when a patient can be removed from ventilation is challenging. In the ICU, several studies have shown bedrest negatively affects musculoskeletal, cardiovascular, and respiratory systems. Profound weakness is common in ICU patients, persists beyond hospitalization, and is linked with reduced post-ICU survival. Recent guidelines recommend liberation from MV using protocols for sedation and weaning and mobilizing patients as early as possible. Daily use of spontaneous breathing trials (SBT) has not only been shown to be safe but also shown to reduce weaning times from ventilation when compared to gradual lowering of ventilator settings. For a SBT to be successful, a patient needs to be able to spontaneously breathe with no or minimal ventilator support for at least 30 mins, not be apneic, not be persistently tachypneic (>35 breaths/min), and remain hemodynamically stable without increased work of breathing. Minimizing sedation agents have been shown to reduce duration of ventilation. Daily interruption of sedation as well as stopping sedation prior to SBT increase the chances of successful SBT. Risk factors for unsuccessful extubation are listed in Table 9.7.

TABLE 9.7	Risk Factors for Failed Extubation
Failure of two or more SBTs
Chronic heart failure
Weak cough
Stridor postextubation
Hypercarbia during SBT or after extubation $Paco_2$ >45
Age >65
APACHE score >12 on day of extubation
Pneumonia as cause of ARF

表 9.6　NIV 失败的高危因素	
急性高碳酸血症型呼吸衰竭	神经功能评分差：GCS < 11
	呼吸急促：> 35 次 / 分，pH < 7.25
	APACHE 评分 > 29
	呼吸不同步
	漏气过多
	烦躁
	分泌物过多
	耐受性差
	治疗依从性差
	无创通气最初 2 h 内没有改善
	pH 值没有改善
	持续性呼吸急促、心动过速
	持续性高碳酸血症
急性低氧血症型呼吸衰竭	诊断为 ARDS 或肺炎
	年龄 > 40 岁
	低血压：收缩压 < 90 mmHg
	代谢性酸中毒：pH < 7.25
	PaO_2/FiO_2 < 150 mmHg
	无创通气第一小时内氧合无改善

GCS，格拉斯哥昏迷量表；APACHE，急性生理学和慢性健康状况评价。

NIV 的成功与否取决于潜在疾病。慢阻肺病急性加重和心源性肺水肿等疾病的反应性优于不明原因低氧性呼吸衰竭。基线严重酸中毒（pH < 7.25）、严重低氧、持续呼吸频率 > 25 次 / 分的呼吸窘迫和肺外脏器衰竭与 NIV 治疗失败相关。表 9.6 总结了 NIV 失败的各种风险因素。

　　有创机械通气（IMV）　IMV 是通过气管切开或气管插管连接呼吸机提供正压通气辅助。在美国，每年约有 80 万患者接受 IMV 治疗。机械通气的基本操作包括 4 个阶段：①触发阶段，启动呼吸。这可以通过改变预设触发器（如回路中的流量或压力）或完全控制通气时间（时间触发）来控制。②目标阶段，在此阶段呼吸机维持压力或流量。③循环阶段，决定吸气阶段的结束。一旦变量（流量或压力）达到预设值，呼气阶段开始。④呼气阶段，此阶段通常是被动的，同时保持预设压力（PEEP）。

　　最简单的通气模式是辅助控制通气，患者提供流量目标的容积曲线（容量辅助控制通气，VC），或压力目标的时间曲线（压力辅助控制通气，PC）通气的初始触发。这两种模式通常都是在一个简单的反馈回路上，因此，如果患者的呼吸频率过低，呼吸机将提供设置的每分钟呼吸次数。当患者的呼吸频率较高时，所有的呼吸都由患者触发，并获得设置的通气辅助。另一种简单模式是压力支持模式（PS），患者触发每一次呼吸。除了预设的压力辅助外，没有循环变量设置，由患者控制呼吸的持续时间。

　　IMV 通常是挽救生命的，但是并发症众多。许多并发症是可以避免和最小化的。IMV 的启动涉及气管

插管，这是一个关键的操作。插管前需评估患者是否存在困难气道的因素。预充氧至关重要，使用带镇静剂和神经肌肉阻滞剂的快速－顺序插管可提高插管成功率。放置气管插管后，大部分清醒患者都不能很好地耐受，因此需要镇静。镇静剂有其自身相关的并发症，如长期使用苯二氮䓬类药物，尤其是以连续输注的形式，与谵妄和不良的长期预后相关。

　　除了镇静相关并发症，呼吸机可以提供 100% FiO_2，如使用不当，会导致氧中毒。高氧血症与卒中或心脏疾病的不良预后相关。

　　正压通气可从三个机制引起直接的压力相关损伤：气压伤、容积伤和剪切伤。气压伤是指气道压升高，导致肺泡或远端气道破裂而出现漏气、气胸或纵隔气肿。容积伤可导致肺泡过度扩张，引起肺泡－毛细血管界面破坏，从而引发炎症反应。在 20 世纪 80 年代，首次研究发现高度膨胀的容积引起弥漫性实质浸润。剪切伤发生在呼气相，此时小气道可能塌陷，尤其是在肺顺应性显著降低的情况下。肺泡和小气道反复打开和关闭导致气道上皮损伤和炎症。

撤离机械通气

　　随着呼吸衰竭潜在病因得到改善，需要尽快尝试让患者脱离机械通气（MV）。决定患者何时脱机是具有挑战性的。在 ICU 内，几项研究显示卧床对肌肉骨骼、心血管和呼吸系统产生不利影响。严重虚弱在 ICU 患者中很常见，持续到出院后，并与 ICU 后存活率降低相关。最新的指南建议在镇静、脱机和早期活动方面使用标准化流程将患者尽早从 MV 中解放出来。与逐渐降低呼吸机参数相比，每日使用自主呼吸试验（SBT）不仅安全，而且能缩短脱机时间。要使 SBT 成功，患者需要在没有或少量呼吸机支持的情况下自主呼吸至少 30 min，没有呼吸暂停，没有持续呼吸急促（> 35 次 / 分），在不增加呼吸功耗的情况下保持血流动力学稳定。镇静剂最小剂量化已被证明可以缩短机械通气时间。每日镇静中断，同时在 SBT 前停止镇静，可以增加 SBT 成功的机会。表 9.7 列出了拔管失败的危险因素。

表 9.7　拔管失败的危险因素
SBT 失败 ≥ 2 次
慢性心力衰竭
咳嗽无力
拔管后喘鸣
SBT 期间出现高碳酸血症或拔管后 $PaCO_2$ > 45 mmHg
年龄 > 65 岁
拔管当天 APACHE 评分 > 12
肺炎是 ARF 的病因

APACHE，急性生理学和慢性健康状况评价。

SPECIFIC CLINICAL SITUATION: ACUTE RESPIRATORY DISTRESS SYNDROME

ARDS is one of the most severe forms of hypoxemic respiratory failure. Based on several observational studies, the incidence of ARDS has been estimated to be about 7 per 100,000. In 2012 a panel of experts established the Berlin definition of ARDS. ARDS is characterized by acute hypoxic respiratory failure from acute diffuse inflammatory lung injury. This leads to increased vascular permeability, increased lung weight, and loss of aerated lung tissue, resulting in decreased lung compliance. The lung injury can be direct (e.g., inhalational injury or multifocal pneumonia) or indirect (e.g., pancreatitis or severe sepsis).

For a patient to be defined as having ARDS the onset must be within 1 week of a known clinical insult or new or worsening respiratory symptoms. Based on the degree of hypoxia, severity of ARDS was quantified as mild when Pao_2/FiO_2 ratio was between 200 to 300 mm Hg on PEEP of 5 or higher via invasive or noninvasive MV, moderate ARDS with a Pao_2/FiO_2 ratio less than 200 mm Hg, and severe with a Pao_2/FiO_2 ratio less than 100 mm Hg.

The majority of the cases of ARDS occur in the setting of predisposing clinical risk factors such as bacterial pneumonia, severe sepsis, severe trauma, drug or alcohol overdose, systemic inflammation (e.g., acute pancreatitis), and massive aspiration. These risk factors can be divided into those that cause direct lung injury and those that cause indirect lung injury likely via inflammatory cytokines. It is estimated that 30% to 40% of patients with severe sepsis will go on to develop ARDS. Direct inhalational injury, acute exacerbation of interstitial lung disease, burns, head trauma, and near-drowning are less common causes of ARDS.

ARDS is a complex and heterogeneous disorder with a pathophysiology that is only partially understood. During the initial phase, described as the exudative phase, after exposure to a risk factor, there is injury to the type I pneumocytes and disruption of the alveolar capillary interface. This leads to leakage of protein-rich plasma into the alveolar spaces, release of proinflammatory cytokines (e.g., IL1, IL8, TNF-α) and lipid mediators such as leukotriene B, and neutrophilic accumulation, resulting in predominantly dependent alveolar edema. Unlike cardiogenic edema, which is mostly due to hydrostatic forces, the alveolar fluid is rich in proteins leading to dysfunction of the surfactant activity and a proteolytic process. The process leads to diminished aeration, atelectasis, decreased lung compliance, intrapulmonary shunting, increased physiologic dead space, and significant hypoxemia. The chest radiograph at this stage shows diffuse bilateral alveolar and interstitial opacities that are nonspecific and difficult to distinguish from cardiogenic pulmonary edema, multifocal pneumonia or diffuse alveolar hemorrhage. As ARDS improves there is organization of alveolar exudates and a shift from neutrophilic to lymphocyte predominant pulmonary infiltrate. Type II pneumocytes proliferate and repair the alveolar basement membrane, differentiate into type I pneumocytes, and synthesize surfactant.

In most patients ARDS will resolve after the acute phase. Rarely, some patients enter a fibrotic phase. In these patients there is extensive interstitial fibrosis and disruption of normal pulmonary architecture as well as pulmonary vascular intimal changes predisposing them to pulmonary hypertension and right ventricular failure. This leads to a prolonged phase of decreased lung compliance and oxygenation and prolonged need for continued MV. This phase can last for weeks and is complicated by nonpulmonary organ dysfunction, deconditioning, and hospital-acquired infections.

General principles of management of ARDS patients include recognition and treatment of underlying causes and secondary illnesses. Patients with ARDS frequently require mechanical ventilation for support. Historically, these patients were ventilated with tidal volumes set at 12 to 15 mL/kg. However, in 2000 the ARDS Network published the results of their first study comparing tidal volumes of 6 mL/kg versus 12 mL/kg and revealed a 9% absolute reduction in mortality in the lower tidal volume group. Along with the mortality benefit, both ventilator-free days and organ failure–free days were also increased in the low tidal volume group. Currently the American Thoracic Society in conjunction with the European Respiratory Society recommends using lower tidal volumes of 4 to 8 mL/kg of predicted ideal body weight and lower inspiratory pressures (P_{plat} <30 mm Hg).

Further, although higher PEEP may improve alveolar recruitment, oxygenation, and prevent atelectrauma, there are risks of alveolar overdistension, increased intrapulmonary shunt, and hemodynamic effects. There have been multiple studies comparing high PEEP with lower PEEP, including studies from ARDS Network comparing average PEEP of 13 versus 8 with similar clinical outcomes. None of these studies showed evidence of barotrauma related to higher PEEP. In an individual patient meta-analysis from three randomized controlled trials, patients with moderate or severe ARDS (Pao_2/FiO_2 <200 mm Hg) had significant mortality benefit from higher PEEP while patients with mild ARDS did not have statistically significant benefit.

There have been multiple studies addressing fluid management in ARDS. The ARDS Network conducted a large multicenter randomized controlled trial looking at a liberal fluid strategy versus a conservative fluid strategy targeting lower intravascular pressures. Patients in the conservative group had a higher number of ventilator-free days, better oxygenation, and did not have a higher incidence of shock or need for dialysis. The 2010 ACURASYS trial looking at neuromuscular blockade for patients in moderate to severe ARDS showed a lower incidence of barotrauma and higher adjusted overall survival. However, the 2019 ROSE trial did not show a similar benefit between the two groups. From a physiological perspective, neuromuscular blockade needs to be administered when patient-ventilator desynchronies exist. However, some patients' ventilatory pattern predisposes them to ventilator-induced lung injury despite use of sedation strategies.

Rescue therapies need to be applied to patients in the setting of refractory hypoxia. Prone positioning was initially shown to improve oxygenation but not affect mortality in several small studies; however, in prespecified subgroup analyses of these studies, prone position for greater than 12 hours a day in patients with moderate to severe ARDS showed mortality benefit. This was subsequently confirmed in the PROSEVA trial, in which proning led to a mortality benefit in patients with severe ARDS. Hence, proning is recommended by ATS in patients with severe ARDS. Other rescue therapies such as inhaled nitric oxide can improve oxygenation in some patients. This therapy can also lead to loss of hypoxia-induced vasoconstriction in poorly ventilated portions of the lung, leading to worsening oxygenation. Extracorporeal membrane oxygenation (ECMO) refers to circulation of blood externally over a gas exchanger to oxygenate blood and eliminate carbon dioxide. This was first studied in the 1970s and did not show any benefit; however, mortality from ARDS at that time was close to 90% in both arms of the study. In 2009 the CESAR trial was published, which showed a mortality benefit in the treatment arm; however, 25% of the patients in the treatment arm ended up getting conservative management. There were no fixed ventilation protocols for patients in the control arm, therefore it was difficult to predict how much benefit was attributable to ECMO. Another randomized trial in 2018 did not show mortality benefit using ECMO versus reserving it as a rescue therapy with conventional lung-protective ventilation.

特定临床情况：急性呼吸窘迫综合征

ARDS 是低氧血症型呼吸衰竭最严重的形式之一。基于几项观察性研究，ARDS 的发病率约为十万分之七。2012 年一个专家小组确定了 ARDS 的柏林定义。ARDS 的特点是急性弥漫性炎症性肺损伤引起的急性低氧血症型呼吸衰竭。这导致血管通透性增加，肺重量增加，充气肺组织减少，肺顺应性下降。肺损伤可以是直接的（如吸入性损伤或多灶性肺炎），也可以是间接的（如胰腺炎或严重感染中毒症）。

对于被定义为 ARDS 的患者，其发病必须是有已知诱因，1 周以内出现新发或恶化的呼吸道症状。基于低氧的程度，ARDS 的严重程度被定义为：轻度——无创或有创通气 PEEP ≥ 5cmH$_2$O 时，200 mmHg ＜ PaO$_2$/FiO$_2$ ＜ 300 mmHg；中度——100 mmHg ＜ PaO$_2$/FiO$_2$ ＜ 200 mmHg；重度——PaO$_2$/FiO$_2$ ＜ 100 mmHg。

大多数 ARDS 病例发生在易感临床风险的环境中，如细菌性肺炎、严重脓毒症、严重创伤、药物或酒精过量、全身炎症（如急性胰腺炎）和大量误吸。这些风险因素可以分为直接导致肺损伤的因素或通过炎症因子间接导致肺损伤的因素。大约 30% ～ 40% 严重脓毒症患者将继发 ARDS。直接吸入性损伤、间质性肺疾病急性加重、烧伤、头部创伤和淹溺是 ARDS 的不常见病因。

ARDS 是一种复杂的异质性疾病，其病理生理学仅被部分了解。在最初阶段，即渗出阶段，暴露于危险因素后，Ⅰ 型肺泡细胞受到损伤，肺泡-毛细血管界面破坏。这导致富含蛋白质的血浆泄露到肺泡腔，释放促炎因子（如 IL1、IL8、TNF-α）和脂质介质（如白三烯 B），中性粒细胞聚集，导致肺泡水肿。不同于主要由静水压引起的心源性水肿，肺泡液富含蛋白，导致表面活性物质和蛋白水解功能障碍。这一过程导致通气减少、肺不张、肺顺应性下降、肺内分流、生理死腔增加和严重低氧血症。这一阶段的胸部 X 线片显示双侧弥漫性肺泡和间质渗出，这是非特异性的，很难与心源性肺水肿、多灶性肺炎或弥漫性肺泡出血相鉴别。随着 ARDS 的改善，肺泡渗出物机化，肺浸润从中性粒细胞为主变为淋巴细胞为主。Ⅱ 型肺泡细胞增殖并修复肺泡基底膜，分化为 Ⅰ 型肺泡细胞，并合成表面活性剂。

大多数患者的 ARDS 会在急性期后消退。很少一部分患者进入纤维化阶段。在这些患者中存在广泛的肺间质纤维化、正常肺结构破坏和肺血管内膜改变，使他们容易出现肺动脉高压和右心功能不全。这导致低肺顺应性和低氧阶段延长，进而 MV 需求期延长。这一阶段可持续数周，并因肺外器官功能障碍、院内感染而使病情复杂化。

ARDS 患者管理的一般原则包括识别和治疗潜在病因和继发疾病。ARDS 患者常常需要机械通气支持。从历史上看，这些患者的潮气量通常设定为 12 ～ 15 ml/kg。

然而，在 2000 年，ARDS Network 团队发表了他们的第一项研究结果，比较 6 ml/kg 和 12 ml/kg 潮气量，并显示小潮气量组的死亡率降低了 9%。除了死亡率获益，小潮气量组的无机械通气时间和无脏器衰竭时间也有所增加。目前美国胸科学会（ATS）和欧洲呼吸病学会建议使用 4 ～ 8 ml/kg（预测理想体重）的小潮气量和低吸气平台压（P$_{plat}$ ＜ 30 mmHg）。

此外，尽管较高的 PEEP 可能改善肺复张、氧合，并预防剪切伤，但也存在肺泡过度扩张、肺内分流增加和血流动力学受影响的风险。有多项研究比较了高 PEEP 和低 PEEP，包括来自于 ARDS Network 的研究，比较了平均 PEEP 为 13 cmH$_2$O 和 8 cmH$_2$O，临床结局相似。这些研究均没有显示气压伤与高 PEEP 有关的证据。在一项来自 3 项随机对照研究的个体化荟萃分析中，中重度 ARDS（PaO$_2$/FiO$_2$ ＜ 200 mmHg）患者从高 PEEP 治疗中得到显著的死亡获益，而轻度 ARDS 患者则没有统计学意义的获益。

已有多项研究涉及 ARDS 的液体管理。ARDS Network 进行了一项大型多中心随机对照研究，着眼于宽松液体策略和维持较低血管内压的保守液体策略。保守液体策略组患者无机械通气时间更长，氧合更好，休克或透析发生率也没有更高。2010 年 ACURASYS 研究着眼于中重度 ARDS 患者使用神经肌肉阻滞剂的结果，显示更低的气压伤发生率和更高的调整后生存率。然而，2019 年的 ROSE 研究并没有显示出两组之间相似的获益。从生理学角度来看，当存在人机对抗时，需要进行神经肌肉阻滞。然而，尽管使用了镇静策略，一些患者的通气模式使他们更易发生呼吸机相关肺损伤。

挽救疗法需要应用于难治性低氧患者。在几项小型研究中，俯卧位最初被证明可以改善氧合，但不会影响死亡率，然而，在这些研究预先设定的亚组分析中，中至重度 ARDS 患者每天俯卧位超过 12 h 显示出了死亡率下降。这在随后的 PROSEVA 研究中得到了证实，在这项研究中，重度 ARDS 患者从俯卧位中实现死亡率下降。因此，俯卧位被 ATS 推荐用于重度 ARDS 患者。其他挽救疗法，如一氧化氮吸入，可以改善一些患者的氧合。这种治疗也会导致肺内通气不良区域低氧诱导的血管收缩消失，从而引起氧合恶化。体外膜肺氧合（ECMO）是指血液在气血交换器上进行外部循环，以给血液充氧并清除二氧化碳。从 20 世纪 70 年代首次开始对其进行研究，但没有显示出任何获益，然而，那个时候两组 ARDS 的死亡率都接近 90%。2009 年，CESAR 研究发表，显示治疗组有死亡率下降，然而 25% 治疗组患者最终接受了保守治疗。对照组患者没有固定的通气策略，因此很难预测 ECMO 的益处有多大。2018 年的另一项随机试验对使用 ECMO 与将其作为传统肺保护通气的挽救疗法进行比较，并未显示死亡率降低。

SUGGESTED READINGS

Acute Respiratory Distress Syndrome Network, et al: Ventilation with lower tidal volumes as compared with traditional tidal volumes for acute lung injury and the acute respiratory distress syndrome, N Engl J Med 342:1301-1308, 2000.

Brodie D, Bacchetta M: Extracorporeal membrane oxygenation for ARDS in adults, N Engl J Med 365:1905-1914, 2011.

Combes A, Hajage D, Capellier G, et al: Extracorporeal membrane oxygenation for severe acute respiratory distress syndrome, N Engl J Med 378:1965-1975, 2018.

Drake, MG: High-flow nasal cannula oxygen in adults: an evidence-based assessment, Ann Am Thorac Soc 15:145-155, 2018.

Fan E, Del Sorbo L, Goligher EC, et al: An official American Thoracic Society/European Society of Intensive Care Medicine/Society of Critical Care Medicine clinical practice guideline: mechanical ventilation in adult patients with acute respiratory distress syndrome, Am J Respir Crit Care Med 195:1253-1263, 2017.

Frat J-P, Ricard J-D, Coudroy R, et al: Preoxygenation with non-invasive ventilation versus high-flow nasal cannula oxygen therapy for intubation of patients with acute hypoxaemic respiratory failure in ICU: the prospective randomised controlled FLORALI-2 study protocol, BMJ Open 7:e018611, 2017.

Guérin C, Reignier J, Richard JC, et al: Prone positioning in severe acute respiratory distress syndrome, N Engl J Med 368:2159-2168, 2013.

Hernández G, Vaquero C, González P, et al. Effect of Postextubation High-Flow Nasal Cannula vs Conventional Oxygen Therapy on Reintubation in Low-Risk Patients: A Randomized Clinical Trial. JAMA 315(13):1354-1361, 2016.

Ischaki E, Pantazopoulos I, Zakynthinos S: Nasal high flow therapy: a novel treatment rather than a more expensive oxygen device, Eur Respir Rev 26:170028, 2017.

Maggiore SM, Idone FA, Vaschetto R, et al. Nasal high-flow versus Venturi mask oxygen therapy after extubation. Effects on oxygenation, comfort, and clinical outcome. Am J Respir Crit Care Med 190(3):282-288, 2014.

Mas A, Masip J: Noninvasive ventilation in acute respiratory failure, Int J Chron Obstruct Pulmon Dis 9:837-852, 2014.

Ouellette DR, Patel S, Girard TD, et al: Liberation from mechanical ventilation in critically ill adults: an official American College of Chest Physicians/American Thoracic Society clinical practice guideline: inspiratory pressure augmentation during spontaneous breathing trials, protocols minimizing sedation, and noninvasive ventilation immediately after extubation, Chest 151:166-180, 2017.

Parke RL, McGuinness SP, Eccleston ML. A preliminary randomized controlled trial to assess effectiveness of nasal high-flow oxygen in intensive care patients. Respir Care 56(3):265-270, 2011.

Pham T, Brochard LJ, Slutsky AS: Mechanical ventilation: state of the art, Mayo Clinic 92:1382-1400, 2017.

Rochwerg B, Brochard L, Elliott MW, et al: Official ERS/ATS clinical practice guidelines: noninvasive ventilation for acute respiratory failure, Eur Respir J 50:1602426, 2017.

Roussos C, Koutsoukou A: Respiratory failure, Eur Respir J Suppl 47:3s-14s, 2003.

Scala R, Pisani L: Noninvasive ventilation in acute respiratory failure: which recipe for success? Eur Respir Rev 27:180029, 2018.

Thompson BT, Matthay MA: The Berlin definition of ARDS versus pathological evidence of diffuse alveolar damage, Am J Respir Crit Care Med 187:675-677, 2013.

推荐阅读

Acute Respiratory Distress Syndrome Network, et al: Ventilation with lower tidal volumes as compared with traditional tidal volumes for acute lung injury and the acute respiratory distress syndrome, N Engl J Med 342:1301-1308, 2000.

Brodie D, Bacchetta M: Extracorporeal membrane oxygenation for ARDS in adults, N Engl J Med 365:1905-1914, 2011.

Combes A, Hajage D, Capellier G, et al: Extracorporeal membrane oxygenation for severe acute respiratory distress syndrome, N Engl J Med 378:1965-1975, 2018.

Drake, MG: High-flow nasal cannula oxygen in adults: an evidence-based assessment, Ann Am Thorac Soc 15:145-155, 2018.

Fan E, Del Sorbo L, Goligher EC, et al: An official American Thoracic Society/ European Society of Intensive Care Medicine/Society of Critical Care Medicine clinical practice guideline: mechanical ventilation in adult patients with acute respiratory distress syndrome, Am J Respir Crit Care Med 195:1253-1263, 2017.

Frat J-P, Ricard J-D, Coudroy R, et al: Preoxygenation with non-invasive ventilation versus high-flow nasal cannula oxygen therapy for intubation of patients with acute hypoxaemic respiratory failure in ICU: the prospective randomised controlled FLORALI-2 study protocol, BMJ Open 7:e018611, 2017.

Guérin C, Reignier J, Richard JC, et al: Prone positioning in severe acute respiratory distress syndrome, N Engl J Med 368:2159-2168, 2013.

Hernández G, Vaquero C, González P, et al. Effect of Postextubation High-Flow Nasal Cannula vs Conventional Oxygen Therapy on Reintubation in Low-Risk Patients: A Randomized Clinical Trial. JAMA 315(13):1354-1361, 2016.

Ischaki E, Pantazopoulos I, Zakynthinos S: Nasal high flow therapy: a novel treatment rather than a more expensive oxygen device, Eur Respir Rev 26:170028, 2017.

Maggiore SM, Idone FA, Vaschetto R, et al. Nasal high-flow versus Venturi mask oxygen therapy after extubation. Effects on oxygenation, comfort, and clinical outcome. Am J Respir Crit Care Med 190(3):282-288, 2014.

Mas A, Masip J: Noninvasive ventilation in acute respiratory failure, Int J Chron Obstruct Pulmon Dis 9:837-852, 2014.

Ouellette DR, Patel S, Girard TD, et al: Liberation from mechanical ventilation in critically ill adults: an official American College of Chest Physicians/ American Thoracic Society clinical practice guideline: inspiratory pressure augmentation during spontaneous breathing trials, protocols minimizing sedation, and noninvasive ventilation immediately after extubation, Chest 151:166-180, 2017.

Parke RL, McGuinness SP, Eccleston ML. A preliminary randomized controlled trial to assess effectiveness of nasal high-flow oxygen in intensive care patients. Respir Care 56(3):265-270, 2011.

Pham T, Brochard LJ, Slutsky AS: Mechanical ventilation: state of the art, Mayo Clinic 92:1382-1400, 2017.

Rochwerg B, Brochard L, Elliott MW, et al: Official ERS/ATS clinical practice guidelines: noninvasive ventilation for acute respiratory failure, Eur Respir J 50:1602426, 2017.

Roussos C, Koutsoukou A: Respiratory failure, Eur Respir J Suppl 47:3s-14s, 2003.

Scala R, Pisani L: Noninvasive ventilation in acute respiratory failure: which recipe for success? Eur Respir Rev 27:180029, 2018.

Thompson BT, Matthay MA: The Berlin definition of ARDS versus pathological evidence of diffuse alveolar damage, Am J Respir Crit Care Med 187:675-677, 2013.

Transitions in Care From Pediatric to Adult Providers for Individuals With Pulmonary Disease

Kate E. Powers, Debasree Banerjee, Robin L. McKinney

INTRODUCTION

With advances in technology and pharmaceuticals, more than 90% of children born with life-shortening diseases will survive to adulthood. The transition of care from pediatric to adult providers is high risk, with the potential for poor clinical outcomes. There are few resources and limited formal education for pediatric and adult providers on transition of care for individuals with underlying pulmonary disease. This gap in knowledge among health care providers has significant effects on patient outcome, including accelerated progression of disease and increased health care cost.

The Society for Adolescent Health and Medicine defines transition in care as "the purposeful, planned movement from adolescents and young adults with chronic physical and medical conditions from child-centered to adult-oriented health care systems." Despite the recognized need for detailed and active measures to ensure the transfer of patient care, there are no standardized approaches for transition of care for individuals with underlying pulmonary disease. Many individuals experience gaps of care during the transfer phase of transition before definitively establishing care with an adult provider. These gaps in care are multifactorial including individual, cultural, geographic, logistic, and financial etiologies. Adolescents and young adults may lack the skill or neurocognitive development to fully assume management of their own care. This is further compounded by moving away from home, loss of insurance as a dependent, and lack of engagement of family or caretakers in adult practices. If not adequately planned for, parents' lack of legal right of their child at the age of majority significantly impacts care and consent in neurocognitively impaired individuals. Fragmented care may lead to poor health maintenance, decreased adherence to medical therapies, and avoidance of medical intervention in earlier stages of illness. An organized transition process establishes individual trust in new adult providers, especially for young adults with chronic disease. A smooth transition of health care allows for developmentally appropriate care in a system that can support the individual patient throughout life.

Our goal for this chapter is to illustrate successful methods to transition adolescents and young adults with underlying pulmonary disease and those chronically critically ill individuals into adult clinics utilizing specific pulmonary disease examples.

CYSTIC FIBROSIS AND OTHER MUCOCILIARY DISEASES

Cystic fibrosis (CF) is an autosomal recessive genetic multisystem disease with primary involvement occurring in the respiratory and gastrointestinal tracts. Mucus plugging, inflammation, and bacterial infections lead to lung damage with progressive small airway obstruction and lung scarring known as bronchiectasis that eventually contributes to worsening lung function and respiratory failure. In the gastrointestinal and hepatobiliary tracts as well as the exocrine pancreas, inspissation of viscous secretions leads to intestinal obstruction, cholestasis, and fat and protein malabsorption. CF affects approximately 30,000 individuals in the United States and 70,000 worldwide. It is the most common life-shortening inherited disease in Caucasians but impacts all races and ethnicities. CF is caused by mutations in a gene on chromosome 7 that encodes the CF transmembrane conductance regulator (CFTR) protein. The CFTR protein primarily functions as a chloride and bicarbonate receptor responsible for the movement of fluid into and out of epithelial cells lining the respiratory tract, biliary tree, intestines, vas deferens, sweat ducts, and pancreatic ducts. As of 2017, the median predicted survival is about 50 years. Improvement in survival has resulted from specialized care centers, early diagnosis, timely screening, therapies to optimize pulmonary function and nutrition as well as clinical care guidelines to standardize symptom-based treatments. Newly developed CFTR modulator therapies target the basic defect in CF and are now clinically available for more than 60% of the US CF population. Although modulator therapies cannot reverse existing disease, they have already further altered the CF-disease trajectory improving overall health, quality of life, and survival.

With improved survival into adulthood, successful transition and transfer of individuals from pediatric to adult CF programs is essential. A timeline for recommended CF-related milestones has been developed to support an individual with CF and his or her parent or support person through transition. CF R.I.S.E. (Responsibility. Independence. Self-care. Education.) is a transition resource that includes patient assessments and checklists, care team progress reports, and educational resource guides to optimize the transition process over time.

Specific educational goals are established by age: early school age (6-9 years old), late elementary and middle school (10-12 years old), early high school (13-15 years old), late high school (16-18 years old) and young adults (18-25 years old). Modules assist individuals with CF and their families to better understand the disease, CF-related care including medications and therapies, as well as planning for the future (Table 10.1).

Primary ciliary dyskinesia (PCD) is an autosomal recessive disease with more than 30 different genetic variants, characterized by congenital impairment of mucociliary clearance. These defects lead to ciliary immotility, ciliary dyskinesia or ciliary aplasia. Considerable variation exists in the clinical presentation of PCD, but most present in childhood with recurrent upper and lower respiratory infections. It is characterized by chronic cough, bronchiectasis, chronic rhinosinusitis, and recurrent otitis media. Individuals with PCD generally live an active

肺病患者从儿童到成年的医疗衔接

石穿 译 徐燕 王孟昭 审校 黄慧 王辰 通审

引言

伴随着技术与药物治疗的进步，出生时患有减寿疾病的儿童中超过 90% 已能够存活至成年。儿科与成人医学团队间的医疗衔接具有高度风险，可能引起不良临床结局。然而，针对患有肺病的患者如何进行医疗衔接的学习与教育资源十分有限。医务工作者在该领域的知识缺陷可能加速患者疾病进展、增加医疗费用，对患者结局产生显著影响。

美国"青少年健康和医学协会"（Society for Adolescent Health and Medicine）将医疗衔接（transition in care）定义为"有目的、有计划地将伴有慢性身体和医疗状况的青少年从以儿童为中心的医疗保健系统转移到服务于成人的医疗保健系统"。尽管医学界已广泛认同应当采取积极、细致的措施确保医疗系统间衔接的顺利进行，现阶段对于肺病患者具体应当如何进行衔接尚无标准方案。许多患者在与成人医疗团队建立稳定联系前，都经历过医疗服务的临时中断。这种医疗服务中断与个体、文化、地理、组织、经济等多方面因素有关。青少年因为自身社会经验或认知功能发育的不足，可能难以担负起管理自身健康的重任。背井离乡、脱离原有保险、成人医疗实践中亲属参与不足等因素让局面变得更为复杂。此外，由于子女在成年时父母不再拥有法律层面的监护权，对于神经认知功能受损的患者，如果事先未进行充分规划，医疗衔接期间的医疗照护和知情同意将面临严重困难。割裂的医疗照护可能导致患者健康水平下降、治疗依从性不佳、丧失疾病早期干预机会。有序的医疗衔接则有利于患者建立对成人医疗团队的信任，尤其是对本身患有慢性疾病的年轻人。应当认为，医疗照护的平稳过渡是建立终生性、不断发展的适宜性医疗保健系统的重要环节。

本章旨在以具体疾病为例，展示如何成功地将患有肺病或慢性危重症的青少年转诊至成人医疗机构。

囊性纤维化和其他黏液纤毛疾病

囊性纤维化（CF）是一种遗传性多系统疾病，呈常染色体隐性遗传，主要累及呼吸道和胃肠道。黏液栓、炎症和反复细菌感染造成以进行性小气道阻塞、瘢痕形成为特征的肺部病变，即支气管扩张，最终引起肺功能恶化和呼吸衰竭。黏性分泌物在胃肠道、胆道及胰腺外分泌部中凝结，则可引起肠梗阻，胆汁淤积及蛋白质、脂质吸收不良等一系列临床表现。美国约有 3 万人患有该病，世界范围内患病人数达 7 万人。本病是高加索人种中最常见的缩短寿命的遗传性疾病，在其他种族与民族中亦有一定发病率。CF 系由 7 号染色体上编码囊性纤维化跨膜传导调节因子（CFTR）的基因突变引起。CFTR 作为氯离子和碳酸氢根通道蛋白，参与调节呼吸道、肠道、胆管、胰管、输精管、汗腺管上皮细胞的细胞内外液体转运。截至 2017 年，CF 患者的中位生存期约为 50 年。专业化的医疗团队、早期诊断、及时筛查、旨在改善肺功能与营养状态的治疗方案，以及依照指南的标准化对症治疗有利于改善疾病生存。近年来研发的 CFTR 调节剂（CFTR modulators）可直接作用于缺陷蛋白，现已覆盖美国 60% 以上的 CF 患者。该疗法虽然难以逆转已经发生的病理生理改变，但足以改变疾病后续发展轨迹，从而改善患者一般情况、生活质量及生存时间。

随着更多的 CF 患儿生命延续至成年，顺利实现儿科与成人医学团队间的衔接显得至关重要。目前已有成熟的 CF 里程碑时间表供患者及其父母或其他照护人员参考，以帮助他们渡过这一时期。CF R.I.S.E.（Responsibility. Independence. Self-care. Education.）是一个专门提供 CF 医疗衔接相关资源的项目，其内容覆盖患者评估清单、医疗团队进度报告及相应教育资源。

在 CF 里程碑时间轴上，根据患者年龄段（学龄早期，6 ～ 9 岁；小学后期与初中，10 ～ 12 岁；高中早期，13 ～ 15 岁；高中后期，16 ～ 18 岁；成年早期，18 ～ 25 岁）划分相应的患者教育目标。（译者注：原文根据美国中小学学制划分，与我国存在差异。）相应的模块有助于 CF 患者及其家人更好地了解疾病本身、药物与其他疗法，并对未来进行规划（表 10.1）。

原发性纤毛运动障碍（PCD）是一种以先天性纤毛清除功能障碍为特征的常染色体隐性遗传病。目前报道的遗

TABLE 10.1 Specific Educational Goals by Age

Milestones	6-9 Years Old	10-12 Years Old	13-15 Years Old	16-18 Years Old	18-25 Years Old
Understanding CF	Basics of CF	Many aspects of CF care	Most aspects of CF	All aspects of CF	Understands and learns about all adult-related CF care issues
Managing CF care					
Clinic visits	Able to answer some questions about general health status and symptoms with support person's input	Able to independently answer more questions	Independently answers most questions	Independently takes the lead including answering questions	Plans for and takes the lead
Health status	Begins to identify and report changes in symptoms or health to a parent/support person	Proactively identifies and reports changes in health and symptoms to parent/support person	Reports health/symptom changes to parents and care team	Implements recommended nutrition/ treatment changes after clinic and hospital visits	Implements recommended nutrition/ treatment changes after clinic and hospital visits
Coordination of care		Can report to care team all of the health care providers seen outside CF center	Can report to care team all of the health care providers seen outside CF center, reasons for and outcomes from those appointments	Works with parent to coordinate care with health care providers outside CF Center	Coordinates all care with health care providers outside CF center
Insurance and financial			Begins to watch parent/ support person order medication and supplies and starts to call for their own refills when needed	Monitors medications and supplies and calls in refills	Monitors medications and supplies, calls in refills, owns all medication and insurance-related management and reaches out to parent/ support person if questions arise
Transfer to adult care				Participates in key meetings and fills out paperwork associated with transfer	Participates in key meetings and fills out paperwork associated with transfer
Taking CF treatments and therapies					
Taking treatments	Begins taking steps towards remembering to take and carry pills and enzymes; Helps to set up nebulizer and airway clearance equipment; Takes and participates in all treatments with close oversight	Responsible for remembering to take and carry enzymes; Independently performs airway clearance with some oversight; Knows and sticks to treatment plan expectations	Independently administers enzymes and airway clearance; Responsible for following treatment plan in school and while on vacation with some supervision	Primarily responsible for taking all treatments with little parental supervision	Completely responsible for taking all treatments with little parental/support person supervision
Medication management		Begins tracking and sorting all medicines and proper storage plan for medicines	Tracks and sorts all medicines and tells parent when medicine is running low	Tracks and sorts all medications; demonstrates and calls for refills when medicine is running low	Responsible for tracking and sorting all medicines and identifying need for refills
Living with CF					
Planning for future	Pictures a future as an adult	Pictures a future and is able to talk about hopes and dreams	Begins to plan for future (big picture) and plan for how CF may impact future life plan and adulthood	Actively plans for future including college life, work, and/or living independently	Actively plans for future
Anxiety and depression	Aware of anxious or sad feelings and alerts a parent/support person	Can identify feelings of sadness and anxiety and bring to the attention of a parent/support person	Can identify warning signs of anxiety and depression and alert parent/support	Can identify warning signs of anxiety and depression and alert parent/support person	Can identify warning signs of anxiety and depression and alert parent/support person

里程碑	6～9岁	10～12岁	13～15岁	16～18岁	18～25岁
表 10.1　囊性纤维化按年龄划分的患者教育目标					
理解 CF	CF 基本知识	CF 照护的主要方面	CF 照护的大多数方面	CF 照护的各个方面	理解和学习成人 CF 照护事项
管理 CF					
门诊就诊	能在家长帮助下回答关于一般情况和症状的部分提问	能独立回答更多提问	独立回答大多数提问	主导就诊过程，包括主动回答提问	规划并主导就诊过程
健康监测	开始识别症状与健康状态变化并向家长汇报	主动识别症状与健康状态变化并向家长汇报	向家长与医疗团队报告症状与健康状态变化	就诊后执行饮食与治疗调整	就诊后执行饮食与治疗调整
医疗团队协调		能向医疗团队报告 CF 中心以外其他就诊	能向医疗团队报告 CF 中心以外其他就诊的原因及处理	能与家长一同协调 CF 中心以外其他医疗团队	自我协调所有 CF 中心外其他医疗团队
医疗保险与财务管理			学习家长如何取药并开始独立预约取药	监管药品与其他需求品消耗，常规取药	监管药品与其他需求品消耗，常规取药，自我管理医疗保险，必要时求助
转诊至成人医疗系统				参与转诊相关的重要会面并填写相应文书	参与转诊相关的重要会面并填写相应文书
接受 CF 治疗					
接受治疗	开始学习携带、服用胰酶；参与安装雾化器及其他气道廓清设施；在密切监督下进行所有治疗	自我携带、服用胰酶；能在监督下独立进行气道廓清；了解并遵从治疗计划	独立管理胰酶和气道廓清；在家长监督下负责在校和假期中遵从治疗方案	基本接管所有治疗，仅家长少许监督	负责实施所有治疗，仅需家长少许监督
药物管理		开始参与药品分类、追踪，制订适当的药品储存计划	分类并追踪所有药品，提醒家长余量偏低	分类并追踪所有药品；余量不足时安排取药	自我管理所有药物分类和追踪，及时取药
与 CF 共存					
规划未来	构想成年后的生活	构想未来的同时能描述愿望和梦想	开始规划人生方向，思考 CF 对人生规划可能产生的影响	积极规划未来的大学生活、工作和（或）独立生活	积极规划未来
焦虑与抑郁	对焦虑或伤感情绪有意识，提醒家长注意	能识别伤感与焦虑感受，提醒家长注意	能识别焦虑与抑郁的警兆，提醒家长注意	能识别焦虑与抑郁的警兆，提醒家长注意	能识别焦虑与抑郁的警兆，提醒家长注意

TABLE 10.1	Specific Educational Goals by Age—cont'd				
Milestones	6-9 Years Old	10-12 Years Old	13-15 Years Old	16-18 Years Old	18-25 Years Old
Exercise	Participates in sports, exercise, or other health activities	Maintains an exercise routine/participates in sports of other healthy activities	Maintains an exercise routine/participates in sports or other healthy activities	Works with care team to develop an exercise routine	
Self-advocacy	Can answer very basic questions about CF from family, friends, and teachers	Has a short statement to answer basic questions about CF	More comfortable independently answering common questions from peers/others about CF	Able to answer questions from peers/others about CF	Able to answer questions from peers/others about CF
Support system	Understands the importance of a support system of peers with CF	Understands the importance of a support system and starts to develop a group of peers with CF	Understands the importance of and starts to develop a support system of peers with CF	Understands the importance of and utilizes a support system of peers with CF	Understands the importance of and utilizes a support system of peers with CF

life and have a normal lifespan. The rate of lung function decline is much slower than that with CF. Similar to CF, individuals with PCD benefit from implementation of a preventative airway clearance regimen to mobilize retained pulmonary secretions. Retained pulmonary secretions can be corrosive leading to chronic inflammation, recurrent infections, and bronchiectasis.

Bronchiectasis is a structural abnormality characterized by abnormal dilatation and distortion of the bronchial tree with resultant chronic obstructive lung disease. A range of pathophysiologic and disease processes other than CF contribute to bronchiectasis, and most include some combination of bronchial obstruction and infection. Bronchiectasis is frequently associated with atelectasis, emphysema, pulmonary fibrosis, and bronchial vasculature hypertrophy. Improving airway clearance and preventing further airway damage are the cornerstones of therapy. Prognosis and outcome in non-CF related bronchiectasis depends primarily on the underlying etiology. Prediction of outcomes is limited, but with early diagnosis and appropriate therapies, including a preventative airway clearance regimen, lung function in children can stabilize or improve over time. Non-CF related bronchiectasis typically progresses much more slowly than CF-related bronchiectasis and often improves if an airway clearance regimen is implemented to minimize retained pulmonary secretions.

Consensus guidelines for transitioning individuals with PCD or non-CF related bronchiectasis from pediatric to adult providers have not been established to date. Both benefit from continued implementation of a preventative airway clearance regimen to mobilize pulmonary secretions.

ASTHMA AND BRONCHOPULMONARY DYSPLASIA

Asthma and bronchopulmonary dysplasia (BPD) are two of the most common chronic lung diseases in pediatrics. While adult health care providers will likely have experience and be comfortable managing asthma, BPD is a disease that few will be familiar with. BPD results from premature birth with an incidence of 10,000 to 15,000 new cases annually in the United States.

In premature infants, the type II pneumocytes of the lung are underdeveloped and produce insufficient quantities of surfactant, a surface-active substance produced by specific alveolar epithelial cells that helps to decrease surface tension and prevent alveolar collapse. This disorder is called respiratory distress syndrome (RDS). The treatment of RDS is administration of exogenous surfactant and corticosteroids to enhance lung maturation. To sustain life while allowing maturation, mechanical ventilation and oxygen supplementation are required but contribute to the development of BPD.

BPD is defined as the need for 30% or greater oxygen and/or positive pressure at 36 weeks postgestational age (PGA) or discharge, in infants born before 32 weeks gestational age. The neonatal and pediatric provider is likely to be more familiar with the immediate sequela and morbidity associated with BPD than adult health care providers who may inherit an individual years after symptoms have become silent. Birth history is often overlooked by both pediatric and adult health care providers but may provide health information relevant well into adulthood. BPD is often clinically silent by age four, but there is increasing evidence that abnormal spirometry can be detected in early childhood and significantly contributes to adult diseases including chronic obstructive pulmonary disease (COPD) and asthma.

Recent studies challenge the traditional teaching that lung function continuously improves from birth until the third decade of life. Evidence suggests childhood illnesses such as BPD and asthma can contribute to lower-than-expected lung function. Given this lower-than-expected lung function, pathology such as COPD is more likely to occur earlier in life and potentially have a more severe course.

It is essential for pediatric providers to begin early with age-appropriate conversations on the management of asthma in preparation for transfer and transition of health care in adolescence and young adulthood. A minority of patients with moderate to severe childhood asthma will experience remission as they enter adulthood. The majority of individuals will have persistent symptoms. There is an association between severe asthma in childhood with decreased peak lung function and a more rapid decline of lung function compared to children without asthma that ultimately leads to COPD later in life. Pediatric and adult providers should be aware of these long-term outcomes, appropriately monitor lung function, and manage symptoms accordingly to try and prevent long-term lung remodeling leading to persistent disease.

DIFFUSE LUNG DISEASE (INTERSTITIAL LUNG DISEASE)

Diffuse lung disease (DLD) consists of a diverse group of disorders that impact the pulmonary parenchyma and interfere with gas exchange reflecting a spectrum of underlying pathology. These disorders are associated with extensive alteration of alveolar and airway architecture in addition to interstitial changes, therefore the term DLD is now preferred to ILD. Childhood interstitial lung disease (chILD) is still a term utilized when DLD is suspected based on clinical and radiologic features without an established etiology. Some conditions that cause DLD are similar in children and adults, they occur in different proportions, and certain diseases are unique to infants. All diseases are rare in childhood.

表 10.1　囊性纤维化按年龄划分的患者教育目标（续表）				
里程碑	6～9 岁	10～12 岁	13～15 岁	16～18 岁	18～25 岁
锻炼	参加锻炼、体育运动或其他健康活动	坚持一种锻炼方式，或参与体育运动或其他健康活动	坚持一种锻炼方式，或参与体育运动或其他健康活动	与医疗团队一道制订日常锻炼计划	
自我倡权	能够回答来自亲属、朋友、老师的有关 CF 的非常基本的问题	形成一份简短声明，回答有关 CF 的基本问题	更加独立、从容地回答来自同辈或他人的有关 CF 的常见问题	能够回答来自同辈或他人的有关 CF 的问题	能够回答来自同辈或他人的有关 CF 的问题
互助组织	了解病友互助的重要性	了解病友互助的重要性、开始组建 CF 病友小组	了解病友互助的重要性、开始组建 CF 病友互助组织	了解病友互助的重要性、使用来自互助组织的帮助	了解病友互助的重要性、使用来自互助组织的帮助

传变异形式已超过 30 种。这些遗传缺陷可引起包括纤毛不动、纤毛运动不良、纤毛发育不全在内的一系列表型。PCD 临床表现多样，常以儿童时期反复发作的上、下呼吸道感染起病，其特征为慢性咳嗽、支气管扩张、慢性鼻窦炎和复发性中耳炎。PCD 通常不影响日常活动与寿命。相较于 CF，PCD 患者肺功能恶化的速度较慢。与 CF 相似的是，PCD 患者也可通过预防性气道廓清排出滞留的气道分泌物得到临床获益，因为纤毛运动障碍而滞留的气道分泌物可能引起慢性炎症、反复感染和支气管扩张。

支气管扩张症指以支气管异常扩张、变形为特征的结构改变及由此引起的慢性气道阻塞性疾病。除 CF 外，许多以气道阻塞和感染为核心的疾病和病理生理过程均可能引起支气管扩张症。支气管扩张症常伴随肺不张、肺气肿、肺纤维化和支气管血管增生。改善气道清除功能、防止进一步结构破坏是治疗支气管扩张症的基石。非 CF 相关支气管扩张症的预后和结局根据潜在病因的不同差异较大、预测困难。不过，儿童期早期诊断和及时启动预防性气道廓清等治疗，有利于维持和改善患者肺功能。相较于 CF，非 CF 相关的支气管扩张症进展相对缓慢。在充分气道廓清，尽可能减少残留气道分泌物的治疗下，患者症状一般能够得到改善。

迄今为止，尚未颁布涉及 PCD 或其他非 CF 相关支气管扩张症患者成年时医疗衔接的指南共识。不过，现有证据表明，PCD 和其他非 CF 相关支气管扩张症患者均能通过持续的气道廓清治疗获益。

哮喘和支气管肺发育不良

哮喘和支气管肺发育不良（BPD）是儿科最常见的两种慢性肺病。以成人为服务对象的医疗团队在哮喘的管理上往往具备经验与把握，但对于 BPD 则相对陌生。BPD 与早产相关。据统计，美国每年有（1～1.5）万新发 BPD 病例。

早产儿中，因 II 型肺泡上皮细胞发育不全，分泌的用以降低表面张力、防止肺泡塌陷的肺表面活性物质不足，可引起新生儿呼吸窘迫综合征（RDS）。RDS 的治疗方法包括外源性补充肺表面活性物质和给予糖皮质激素促进肺成熟。为维持患儿生命和等待肺成熟，往往需要机械通气和氧疗支持，但上述支持治疗增加 BPD 风险。

BPD 的定义是：胎龄 32 周前分娩的婴儿，在 36 周或出院时，仍需要 30% 以上的氧浓度或正压通气支持。新生儿与儿童医疗团队对于 BPD 的发病和直接后遗症往往较为敏感，而成人医疗团队在接手患者时症状可能已沉寂多年。儿科与成人医师在接诊时容易忽略患者出生史，实际出生史对患者健康的影响可能延续至成年。当患儿成长至 4 岁以上时，BPD 通常已没有临床症状。不过，越来越多的证据表明，BPD 患者在儿童早期仍能检测到通气功能异常，发生慢阻肺病、哮喘等疾病的概率也显著增加。

近期的研究结果对人体肺功能从出生到 20 余岁不断增长的传统观点发起了挑战。有证据显示，儿童期疾病，如 BPD、哮喘，可能导致肺功能低于预期。这一后果使得 BPD 患者更可能在生命早期出现慢阻肺病等疾病，且其病情可能更为严重。

儿科医师应当尽早与患儿及其亲属讨论如何在不同年龄阶段管理哮喘病情，并帮助患儿提前准备未来青春期的医疗衔接。少数在儿童期患有中-重度哮喘的患者，在进入成年后病情将得到自然缓解，大多数个体的哮喘症状则将持续存在。与健康对照相比，儿童期患有严重哮喘的患儿肺功能峰值水平更低，肺功能下降速度更快，日后慢阻肺病患病率更高。儿童与成人医疗团队应当认识到上述远期结局，定期监测肺功能，管理症状，预防长时间肺结构重塑最终导致持续性疾病。

弥漫性肺疾病（间质性肺疾病）

弥漫性肺疾病（DLD）是一组由不同病因引起的，累及肺实质，干扰气体交换的异质性疾病。除间质病变外，该类疾病中也可观察到广泛的肺泡和气道结构改变。因此，近来倾向于用 DLD 取代过去间质性肺疾病（ILD）的概念。不过，在儿科语境下，对于临床和影像学怀疑 DLD 而病因不明的病例，仍保留儿童间质性肺疾病（chILD）这一术语。部分引起 DLD 的病因在儿童与成人中均可存在，仅占比不同；也有特定的疾病仅在婴幼儿阶段发病。应当指出的是，在儿童期 DLD 整体相对少见。

For many forms of DLD, treatment options are limited and often include medications with unproven efficacy and substantial side effects. Lung transplantation is an option for children with severe and progressive disease without a response to therapy. Consensus guidelines for transitioning individuals with DLD from pediatric to adult providers have not been established to date. Given the spectrum of underlying pathology and possible post–lung transplant status, individuals with DLD benefit from a focused transition of care.

INDIVIDUALS WITH TECHNOLOGY DEPENDENCE OR OTHER SPECIAL HEALTH CARE NEEDS

Children and youth with special health care needs (CYSHN) is defined as those who have one or more chronic physical, developmental, behavioral, or emotional condition requiring additional health and related services beyond that of children generally. Approximately 750,000 CYSHN transition into adulthood annually. While these individuals make up a small fraction of the pediatric patient population, they utilize the largest fraction of health care resources. Individuals with technology dependence include those who have tracheostomy dependence requiring part- or full-time mechanical ventilatory support.

Home oxygen therapy is often required in children with chronic respiratory conditions including CF, BPD, sleep-disordered breathing, sickle cell disease, pulmonary hypertension with and without congenital heart disease, and DLD. Despite a lack of empirical evidence regarding implementation, monitoring, and discontinuation of supplemental oxygen therapy, an expert panel through the American Thoracic Society published clinical practice guidelines in 2018. Optimal implementation includes age-appropriate oxygen equipment to maintain acceptable oxygen saturations according to age and respiratory condition and pulse oximetry.

Important steps to optimal transfer and transition include updating insurance status to reflect the coordination of special services with durable medical equipment companies and qualifying patients for certain state or national services. Adult providers frequently have a more patient-centered than family-centered approach to care than pediatric counterparts. Adolescence and young adulthood is often a time of educational transition with variation in access and medical support provided for children and youth with special health care needs. Lack of disease-specific education and few evidence-based guidelines may contribute to adult pulmonologists' limited expertise caring for an individual with technology dependence. General pediatric recommendations for improving transition include the preparation of a transition plan written in early adolescence starting at age 14. This plan includes individual patient and family perspectives, anticipated health care services the individual will need, and a financial plan. It should include preventative as well as disease-specific therapies and insurance coverage strategies for the transition period to decrease gaps of care.

IMPORTANCE OF A SUCCESSFUL TRANSITION

Data from 10 years ago suggested that more than 500,000 adolescents with special health care needs in the United States reach adulthood annually. As life expectancy for individuals with chronic lung disease, technology dependence or other special health care needs has increased, so has the need for a guided, structured transfer and transition of care and transition from pediatric to adult-focused care. The transition of individuals from pediatric to adult care should begin years before the actual transfer. The transition process should include individual- and family-specific education, patient understanding of disease including

TABLE 10.2	Multilevel Suggestions for Transition of Health Care
Patient level	Begin discussions of transition early in life
	Develop a road map in preparation for transition readiness, disease knowledge, and skills assessment to share with patients and families
	Create a personalized medical summary to ensure seamless continuity of care, especially where an electronic medical record is not shared by pediatric and adult programs
CF team level	Create an open and transparent dialogue between the pediatric and adult CF programs
	Develop a working transitional care policy at all levels of the multidisciplinary team (include input from patients and parents)
	Create a registry of eligible patients and a plan to discuss them periodically
	Identify outcome measures to monitor progress and success, including establishment of best practices and communication among pediatric and adult care teams
Institutional level	Seek institutional leadership buy-in
	Collaborate with other hospital programs focused on transition
	Invest in EMR systems with patient access to personal health records and built-in transition tools

rationale for therapies and overall prognosis, as well as a patient readiness assessment indicating if the patient can independently manage therapies and navigate the health care system.

The goals of a planned transition are to improve quality of life, maximize independence, and minimize interruption in care as a patient transfers from pediatric to adult primary and subspecialty care. A designated transition coordinator or champion allows for streamlined communication between health care providers and helps to ensure individual access to medications, interventions, and medical devices through to establishment of care with the adult provider. Although no single process for transition will work in all health care systems, it is essential that an approach that best meets the needs of patient populations and fits within the health care system constraints be established (Table 10.2).

Transition of health care is a complex process involving multiple factors for which a multidisciplinary care team will provide the best chance for success for the individual patient and family (Table 10.3).

Effective transition of care can prevent the deterioration of chronic health conditions while engaging the adolescent to become involved and take over their own care. Poor transition of care has been associated with missed health care visits, loss to follow-up, poor compliance with medications, and increased morbidities. All of these lead to increased emergency care utilization and worse outcomes. Research has identified obstacles that can make transition challenging, including the limited number of capable providers for adults, lack of individual readiness, cognitive disability, instability of mental health (anxiety/depression), and communication issues between pediatric and adult providers.

CF is an example of a chronic pulmonary disease in which much effort has been placed into implementing models to optimize the process of transition. The CF Foundation supported the training of additional providers and developed Adult Care Consensus Guidelines to provide goals and help standardize care. Research and

对于许多类型的 DLD，治疗选择十分有限，且可能包含疗效未经证实、副作用明显的药物。肺移植是针对病情严重或进行性恶化、其他治疗无效的患儿的挽救性选项。迄今为止，尚未有涉及 DLD 患者成年时医疗衔接的指南或共识发布。考虑到潜在疾病谱的异质性，以及可能的移植后状态，在医疗衔接期对该类患者进行重点关注有利于他们的远期健康。

存在技术依赖或其他特殊医疗保健需求的个体

存在特殊医疗保健需求的儿童与青年（CYSHN）指的是患有一种或多种慢性躯体、发育、行为或情绪障碍，需要额外医疗保健及相关服务的青少年群体。每年，美国约有 75 万 CYSHN 步入成年。这部分群体人数有限，但所消耗的医疗卫生资源占比很高。技术依赖个体主要包括接受了气管切开术，需要全天或部分时间机械通气的人群。

患有慢性呼吸疾病（如 CF、BPD、睡眠呼吸障碍、镰状细胞病、伴或不伴先天性心脏病的肺动脉高压、DLD）的儿童通常需要家庭氧疗。尽管关于实施、监测和停止氧疗的经验性证据尚不够充分，美国胸科学会组织的专家小组已于 2018 年发布了针对儿童家庭氧疗的临床实践指南。指南推荐，最佳的氧疗实施方案应选择与年龄相适配的供氧设备，将脉氧饱和度维持于根据年龄和具体疾病确定的可接受范围内。

对于上述人群，实现顺利医疗衔接的重要步骤包括：更新保险状态以协调特殊医疗服务与医疗设备公司；申请进入国家或州层次的特殊医疗保健项目。成人医师相较于儿科医师更多以患者为中心，而非以家庭为中心。对于 CYSHN，青春期与成年早期面临着教育阶段的过渡，所需医疗支持的类型和获取途径往往也随之发生变化。然而，应对该类人群医疗衔接的教育资源和循证指南并不充分，使得成人呼吸科医师在照顾该类人群时往往面临专业性短板。一般建议为应对医疗衔接，医疗团队应在患儿 14 岁时准备一份过渡计划。计划应包含来自患者自身与家庭的观点，预计可能需要的医疗保健服务和相应的财务保障方案。此外，计划中应纳入预防性和疾病特异性治疗以及医疗保险衔接策略，以尽可能减少医疗衔接期间医疗服务的中断。

成功衔接的重要性

10 年前的数据表明，美国每年有超过 50 万名有特殊医疗保健需求的青少年进入成年。伴随着慢性肺

表 10.2　针对不同层面的医疗衔接期治疗建议	
患者层面	尽早开始讨论医疗衔接 制订路线图，以更好地迎接涉及疾病知识、技能、准备程度的评估 创建个人病历摘要，以保障医疗服务的无缝衔接；在儿科与成人医疗团队无法共享电子病历系统的情况下应当尤其注意此点
CF 医疗团队层面	在儿童和成人 CF 团队间建立公开透明的对话 在多学科团队的各个层面（包括患者和家长意见）制订工作衔接方案 建立医疗衔接期患者登记册，定期组织相关讨论 明确项目进展和最终评估指标，对最佳临床实践及儿童-成年医疗团队沟通进行评估
机构层面	寻求机构领导的支持 与其他专注于衔接计划的医疗项目进行合作 建立患者能访问的电子病历系统，内嵌专门的衔接工具

病、技术依赖或其他特殊医疗保健需求者的预期寿命不断增加，社会越来越需要一套系统性、指导性的儿科与成人医疗体系间衔接方案。针对医疗衔接的计划应当在实际衔接前数年开始准备。衔接过程应当涵盖：个人和家庭教育，深化患者对疾病理解（治疗原理、总体预后），针对患者独立就诊和管理治疗的胜任力评估。

有计划的医疗衔接的目标是提高患者生活质量、提升患者独立性、减少患者照护中断。通过设置专门的衔接期协调员可以简化医疗团队间的沟通，确保患者能持续获得药品、操作和医疗设备，直至成人医疗团队接手。虽然不同的医疗保健系统间可能不存在普适的衔接方案，但其原则始终是在系统限制内最大程度地满足患者群体需求（表 10.2）。

医疗保健系统间的衔接是一个复杂过程。其中涉及的方方面面需要多学科团队通力合作，为患者本人和家庭实现顺利过渡（表 10.3）。

成功的医疗衔接在避免慢性疾病恶化的同时，可以让青少年参与并最终接手自我健康管理。反之，医疗衔接不良则容易造成患者错过医疗随访、失访、药物依从性差、疾病发病率升高。上述事件将进一步导致急诊就诊增加和疾病预后不良。研究显示，阻碍医疗衔接顺利进行的因素主要包括：有能力接手的成人医疗团队数量有限，患者自身准备不足、认知障碍、情绪不稳定（焦虑/抑郁），儿童与成人医疗团队沟通不畅。

CF 在慢性呼吸疾病中具有一定代表性。医学界与社会各界在优化 CF 患者的医疗衔接上付出了大量努力。在 CF 基金会的支持下，相关的专业化培训不断推进，成人 CF 患者管理共识指南的颁布进一步明确了管理目标且有利于标准化照护的实施。通过一系列研究

TABLE 10.3 Multidisciplinary Care Team for Transition of Health Care

Multidisciplinary Care Team	Focus for Transition Assessment
Physician/nurse practitioner	Supervising overall transfer and transition process
Registered nurse/care coordinator	Supporting communication of transfer and transition process
Registered dietician	Nutrition and supplementation knowledge, food insecurity risk
Clinic facilitator	Scheduling transfer; meet-and-greet adult team; supplying documents
Pharmacist	Medication knowledge
Behavioral psychologist	Mental/emotional strengths and any barriers to transition
Clinical social worker	Psychosocial strengths and any barriers to transition
Respiratory therapist	Airway clearance knowledge
Physical therapist	Physical activity knowledge as relates to airway clearance
Child life specialist	Age-appropriate disease education and tools for medication adherence

quality improvement projects have identified areas that can make transition a success:

- Make transition to adult care a gradual process.
- Remember that parents and caregivers also are going through a transition.
- Pediatric and adult care teams should work together to improve transition.

Developing a transition program is critically important and does not develop without committed individuals and institutions. Finally, there needs to be pediatric and young adult focused research to better establish guidelines for care that are applicable to this special population.

SUGGESTED READINGS

American Academy of Pediatrics Transition ECHO: https://www.aap.org/en-us/professional-resources/practice-transformation/echo/Pages/Transition.aspx.

CF R.I.S.E. Program materials: https://www.cfrise.com/.

A Consensus Statement on Health Care Transitions for Young Adults With Special Health Care Needs, Pediatrics 110(Suppl 3), 2002.

https://www.aap.org/en-us/Documents/practicesupport_preparing_adolescents_independent_living_webinar.pdf.

The Transition Readiness Assessment Questionnaire (TRAQ): www.rheumatology.org/Portals/0/Files/Transition-Readiness-Assessment-Questionnaire.pdf.

表10.3　医疗衔接中的多学科团队模式	
多学科团队	衔接中评估重点
医师 / 高级执业护师	监督衔接的整体进程
注册护师 / 医疗协调员	参与衔接过程的沟通联系
注册营养师	营养与膳食补充指导、食物风险指导
医疗机构协调员	安排衔接、联系成人医疗团队、提供医疗文件
药剂师	药物指导
行为心理学家	评估心理 / 情感状态及医疗衔接期可能存在的心理障碍
临床社工	评估社会心理状态及医疗衔接期可能存在的社会障碍
呼吸治疗师	气道廓清指导
物理治疗师	与气道廓清相关的体力活动指导
儿童医疗辅导师	根据年龄开展疾病宣教、提供药物依从性工具

和质量改进项目，目前认为有利于推进医疗衔接的因素包括：

- 循序渐进地推进医疗衔接。
- 谨记父母与医疗团队同样需要经历衔接过渡阶段。
- 儿童与成人医疗团队携手推进衔接进程。

制订具体的衔接计划至关重要，而这一过程依赖于个人与机构的积极投入。最后，应当开展以儿童和年轻人为主要对象的研究，为未来针对这一特殊群体制定相应的照护指南提供证据支持。

推荐阅读

American Academy of Pediatrics Transition ECHO: https://www.aap.org/en-us/professional-resources/practice-transformation/echo/Pages/Transition.aspx.

CF R.I.S.E. Program materials: https://www.cfrise.com/.

A Consensus Statement on Health Care Transitions for Young Adults With Special Health Care Needs, Pediatrics 110(Suppl 3), 2002.

https://www.aap.org/en-us/Documents/practicesupport_preparing_adolescents_independent_living_webinar.pdf.

The Transition Readiness Assessment Questionnaire (TRAQ): www.rheumatology.org/Portals/0/Files/Transition-Readiness-Assessment-Questionnaire.pdf.

Preoperative and Postoperative Care

术前和术后照护

11

Preoperative and Postoperative Care

Kim A. Eagle, Kwame Dapaah-Afriyie, Arkadiy Finn

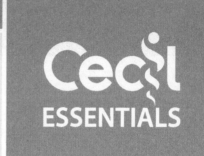

INTRODUCTION

More than 40 million people undergo noncardiac surgical procedures in the United States annually. A general medical and focused cardiovascular preoperative risk assessment involves evaluation of pertinent medical problems with an emphasis on those conditions that may become exacerbated in the perioperative period. Emerging evidence-based practices dictate that the physician should thoughtfully perform an individualized evaluation of the surgical patient to provide an accurate preoperative risk assessment, risk stratification, and modification of risk parameters that can then provide the framework for optimal perioperative risk reduction strategies.

The perioperative period is associated with hemodynamic changes due to surge in sympathetic activity, fluid shifts and their associated effect on the renin-angiotensin system (RAS), and effect of exposure to anesthetic agents.

Assessment of patients' functional status, exercise tolerance, and other preexisting comorbidities are core components of perioperative management. Patients younger than 50 years of age and having no significant medical comorbidities are at very low risk for developing perioperative complications. The increasing prevalence of medical conditions in the surgical patient warrants review of the perioperative approach to those conditions that may pose significant risk. This chapter reviews preoperative and postoperative cardiovascular and medical risk assessment that targets intermediate- to high-risk patients to strategically guide perioperative preventive therapies for optimal outcome.

CARDIAC DISEASE

Preoperative and Postoperative Cardiac Care

It is estimated that the incidence of cardiac complications after noncardiac surgical procedures is between 0.5% and 1%. In other words, 200,000 to 400,000 people will experience perioperative cardiac complications annually. Moreover, more than 25% of these patients will die. Patients who survive a postoperative myocardial infarction (MI) are twice as likely to die in the following 2 years as are patients with uneventful surgical procedures. Emerging evidence-based practices dictate that the physician should thoughtfully perform an individualized evaluation of the surgical patient to provide an accurate preoperative risk assessment, risk stratification, and modification of risk parameters that can then provide the framework for optimal perioperative risk reduction strategies. This section reviews preoperative and postoperative cardiovascular risk assessment that targets intermediate- to high-risk patients to strategically guide perioperative preventive therapies for optimal outcome.

IDENTIFICATION OF PATIENTS WITH ELEVATED RISK

The preoperative evaluation includes an assessment of the risk associated with the planned surgery or procedure. Low-risk procedures (e.g., colonoscopy, cataract surgery) are associated with a less than 1% risk of major adverse cardiovascular events (MACE) of death or MI. Those procedures with a MACE risk of 1% or greater are classified as conferring higher risk. Simple standardized preoperative screening questionnaires have been developed for the purpose of identifying patients at intermediate to high risk who may benefit from a more detailed clinical evaluation (Table 11.1).

TABLE 11.1 Standardized Preoperative Questionnaire[a]

1. Age, weight, and height
2. Are you
   a. Female and 55 years of age or older or male and 45 years of age or older?
   b. If yes, are you also 70 years of age or older?
3. Do you take anticoagulant medications ("blood thinners")?
4. Do you have or have you had any of the following heart-related conditions?
   a. Heart disease
   b. Heart attack within the last 6 months
   c. Angina (chest pain)
   d. Irregular heartbeat
   e. Heart failure
5. Do you have or have you ever had any of the following?
   a. Rheumatoid arthritis
   b. Kidney disease
   c. Liver disease
   d. Diabetes
6. Do you get short of breath when you lie flat?
7. Are you currently on oxygen treatment?
8. Do you have a chronic cough that produces any discharge or fluid?
9. Do you have lung problems or diseases?
10. Have you or any blood member of your family ever had a problem with any anesthesia other than nausea?
    a. If yes, describe
11. If female, is it possible that you could be pregnant?
    a. Perform pregnancy test
    b. Please list date of last menstrual period

[a]University of Michigan Health System patient information report. Patients who answer yes to any of questions 2 through 9 should receive a more detailed clinical evaluation.
From Tremper KK, Benedict P: Paper "preoperative computer," Anesthesiology 92:1212-1213, 2000.

术前和术后照护

王莉芳　刘悦　译　李卫霞　审校　赵晶　通审

引言

在美国，每年有超过 4000 万人接受非心脏手术。必须对全身特别是心血管系统进行术前风险评估，重点关注那些可能在围术期恶化的情况。新近的循证医学实践强调，内科医师需对手术患者进行全面的个体化评估，以提供精确的术前风险评估、风险分层以及风险参数的调整，为优化围术期风险防范策略提供基础框架。

围术期机体会发生血流动力学变化，这些变化是由于交感神经系统兴奋、体液转移、对肾素-血管紧张素系统（RAS）的相关影响以及麻醉药物的使用。

评估患者身体功能状态、活动耐量以及其他并存疾病是围术期管理的核心内容。年龄小于 50 岁且无严重合并症的患者发生围术期并发症的风险很低。现在手术患者伴合并症的比例呈增加趋势，有必要对围术期那些可能造成重大风险的情况予以重点评估。本章回顾了针对中高风险患者的术前和术后心血管系统及其他医疗风险评估，旨在指导制订围术期预防性治疗策略，以获得最佳预后。

心脏病

术前及术后心脏管理

据估计，非心脏手术后心脏并发症发生率大约在 0.5% 至 1% 之间。换言之，每年大约会有 20 万至 40 万人发生围术期心脏并发症，且其中 25% 以上患者会死亡。术后发生心肌梗死（MI）的患者，2 年内死亡的概率是无手术并发症患者的 2 倍。新近的循证医学实践强调，内科医师需对手术患者进行全面的个体化评估，旨在提供精确的术前风险评估、风险分层，以及风险参数的调整，为制订最佳的围术期风险降低策略提供基础框架。本章回顾了针对中高风险患者的术前和术后心血管系统及其他医疗风险评估，旨在指导制订围术期预防性治疗策略，以获得最佳预后。

高风险患者的识别

术前评估内容包括拟行手术或医疗操作相关的风险评估。低危操作（如结肠镜检查、白内障手术）相关的主要不良心血管事件（MACE）如死亡或心肌梗死的发生率低于 1%。MACE 风险大于等于 1% 的手术操作归类于更高危操作。目前已建立简化的标准术前筛查问卷，目的是识别中高危患者，这类患者可能需要进一步详细的临床评估（表 11.1）。

表 11.1　标准术前筛查问卷[a]

1. 年龄、体重和身高
2. 您是否是
   a. 55 岁及以上女性，或 45 岁及以上男性？
   b. 如果是，您是否为 70 岁及以上患者？
3. 您是否使用抗凝药物（"血液稀释剂"）？
4. 您现在或者以前是否有下列任何一种与心脏有关的疾病？
   a. 心脏病
   b. 6 个月内心肌梗死
   c. 心绞痛（胸痛）
   d. 心律不齐
   e. 心力衰竭
5. 您现在或以前是否患过下列任何一种疾病？
   a. 类风湿关节炎
   b. 肾脏病
   c. 肝病
   d. 糖尿病
6. 您躺平时候是否感觉到喘不上气？
7. 您正在接受氧疗吗？
8. 您是否有慢性咳嗽且咳出分泌物或液体？
9. 您有肺部问题或疾病吗？
10. 除恶心以外，您或有血缘关系的亲属是否有过麻醉相关的任何问题？
    a. 如果有，请描述
11. 如果您是女性，您现在有怀孕可能吗？
    a. 做妊娠试验
    b. 请写出末次月经时间

[a] 密歇根大学医疗系统患者信息报告。问题 2 至 9 中任何一项回答"是"的患者须进行进一步临床评估。

引自 Tremper KK, Benedict P: Paper "preoperative computer," Anesthesiology 92: 1212-1213, 2000.

Evaluation of such surgical patients should always begin with a thorough history and physical examination including a 12-lead resting electrocardiogram (ECG) in accordance with the American College of Cardiology/American Heart American (ACC/AHA) guidelines. A determination of the urgency of the surgery should be included in the history because truly emergent procedures are associated with unavoidably higher rates of morbidity and mortality.

Perioperative risk assessment begins with an assessment of the urgency of the noncardiac surgery; emergency surgery should not be delayed but may not allow for in-depth risk stratification. Preoperative testing should be done only for specific clinical conditions based on the history. Healthy patients of any age who are undergoing elective surgical procedures and have no coexisting medical conditions should not need any testing unless the degree of surgical stress could result in unusual changes from the baseline state. The history should focus on symptoms of occult cardiac disease.

PREOPERATIVE CARDIAC RISK ASSESSMENT

During the perioperative risk assessment of patients undergoing noncardiac surgery, there are active cardiac conditions that should be evaluated and treated in accordance with the ACC/AHA guidelines. These conditions include unstable coronary artery disease (CAD), decompensated heart failure, severe arrhythmia, and severe valvular disease (notably severe aortic stenosis and symptomatic mitral stenosis).

Assessment of exercise tolerance in preoperative risk stratification and precise prediction of in-hospital perioperative risk is most applicable in patients who self-report worsening exercise-induced cardiopulmonary symptoms, patients who may benefit from noninvasive or invasive cardiac testing regardless of the scheduled surgical procedure, and patients with known CAD or with multiple risk factors and the ability to exercise. For the prediction of perioperative events, "poor" exercise tolerance has been defined as inability to walk four blocks and climb two flights of stairs or as inability to meet a metabolic equivalent (MET) level of 4 (Table 11.2). Highly functional symptomatic patients (i.e., those who are able to achieve a functional capacity ≥4 METS

without symptoms, as when climbing a flight of stairs or running a short distance) rarely require noninvasive testing or intervention to lower the risk of noncardiac surgery.

If the patient has poor functional capacity or is symptomatic, physicians often use risk indices derived from empirical multivariable predictive models based on clinical assessment of risk factors to identify patients with elevated perioperative cardiac risk. Based on prospective comparison studies, the Revised Cardiac Risk Index (RCRI) is favored by many given its accuracy and simplicity (Table 11.3). A newer predictive model is the National Surgical Quality Improvement Program (NSQIP) risk calculator, which is based on multiple clinical predictors. The RCRI relies on the presence or absence of six identifiable predictive factors: high-risk surgery (suprainguinal vascular, intrathoracic, or intraperitoneal surgery), ischemic heart disease, congestive heart failure (CHF), cerebrovascular disease, diabetes mellitus (requiring insulin therapy), and renal failure (with a serum creatinine concentration >2.0 mg/dL). Each of the RCRI clinical predictors, if present, is assigned 1 point. The risk for cardiac events (i.e., MI, pulmonary edema, ventricular fibrillation or primary cardiac arrest, and complete heart block) can then be predicted. A patient with an RCRI score of 0 has an estimated risk of 0.4% to 0.5% for major cardiac complications; the risk is 0.9% to 1.3% for someone with a score of 1, 4% to 6.6% with a score of 2, and 9% to 11% with a score of 3 (Fig. 11.1). Cardiac risk particularly increases with the presence of two or more predictors and is greatest with three or more. The clinical utility of the RCRI is that it identifies patients who are at higher risk for cardiac complications and helps determine whether they may benefit from further risk stratification with noninvasive cardiac testing or from initiation of preoperative preventive medical management.

TABLE 11.2 Functional Status

Excellent (Activities Requiring >7 METS)
Carry 24 lb up eight steps
Carry objects that weigh 80 lb
Outdoor work (shovel snow, spade soil)
Recreation (ski, basketball, squash, handball, jog or walk 5 mph)

Moderate (Activities Requiring >4 but <7 METS)
Have sexual intercourse without stopping
Walk at 4 mph on level ground
Outdoor work (garden, rake, weed)
Recreation (roller-skate, dance, foxtrot)

Poor (Activities Requiring <4 METS)
Shower/dress without stopping, strip and make bed, dust, wash dishes
Walk at 2.5 mph on level ground
Outdoor work (clean windows)
Recreation (golf, bowl)

MET, Metabolic equivalent.
Modified from Hlatky MA, Boineau RE, Higginbotham MB, et al: A brief self-administered questionnaire to determine functional capacity (the Duke Activity Status Index), Am J Cardiol 64:651-654, 1989.

TABLE 11.3 Revised Cardiac Risk Index: Clinical Markers

1. High-risk surgical procedures
2. Ischemic heart disease
    a. History of myocardial infarction
    b. Current angina considered to be ischemic
    c. Requirement for sublingual nitroglycerin
    d. Positive exercise test
    e. Pathologic Q waves on ECG
    f. History of PTCA and/or CABG with current angina considered to be ischemic
3. Congestive heart failure
    a. Left ventricular failure by physical examination
    b. History of paroxysmal nocturnal dyspnea
    c. History of pulmonary edema
    d. S_3 gallop on cardiac auscultation
    e. Bilateral rales on pulmonary auscultation
    f. Pulmonary edema on chest radiography
4. Cerebrovascular disease
    a. History of transient ischemic attack
    b. History of cerebrovascular accident
5. Diabetes mellitus
    a. Treatment with insulin
6. Chronic renal insufficiency
    a. Serum creatinine concentration >2 mg/dL

CABG, Coronary artery bypass grafting; ECG, electrocardiogram; PTCA, percutaneous transluminal coronary angioplasty.
Modified from Lee TH, Marcantonio ER, Mangione CM, et al: Derivation and prospective validation of a simple index for prediction of cardiac risk of major noncardiac surgery, Circulation 100:1043-1049, 1999.

根据美国心脏病学会 / 美国心脏协会（ACC/AHA）指南，对此类手术患者的评估应从全面的病史采集和体格检查开始，包括 12 导联静息心电图（ECG）检查。手术紧急程度的判断应包括在病史中，因为真正的急诊手术不可避免地会导致更多的合并症和死亡。

围术期风险评估首先要评估非心脏手术的紧急性；因急诊手术不能延误，所以可能出现无法进行深入风险分层的情况。患者的术前检查仅针对有相关疾病病史的情况。对任何年龄拟行择期手术而没有并存疾病的健康患者不需要进行任何检查，除非手术应激的程度可能造成基线状态的异常变化。病史采集须关注隐匿性心脏病的症状。

术前心脏风险评估

对拟行非心脏手术的患者进行围术期风险评估时，应按照 ACC/AHA 指南对活动性心脏病进行评估和治疗，包括不稳定的冠状动脉疾病（CAD），心力衰竭失代偿，严重心律失常，以及严重心脏瓣膜病（尤其是重度主动脉瓣狭窄以及有症状的二尖瓣狭窄）。

通过活动耐量评估进行术前风险分层和精确预测住院期间围术期风险，适用于绝大多数自述运动诱发心肺症状加重的患者，无论拟行何种手术都可能从无创或有创心脏检查中获益的患者，以及已知患有 CAD 或存在多个 CAD 危险因素且有活动能力的患者。在预测围术期事件方面，活动耐量"差"的定义是不能行走 4 个街区的距离，不能爬两层楼梯，或不能达到 4 个代谢当量（MET）（表 11.2）。虽有症状但活动耐量强的患者（也就是在无症状的情况下运动能达到 ≥ 4 METs，例如爬一层楼或短距离跑步）几乎不需要接受其他的无创

检查或干预来降低非心脏手术风险。

当患者活动耐量差或有症状时，医生通常使用基于危险因素临床评估的多变量经验预测模型得出的风险指数，来识别围术期心脏风险较高的患者。基于前瞻性对照研究而得出的改良心脏风险指数（RCRI），因其准确性和便捷性而广受欢迎（表 11.3）。还有一项更新的预测模型，即国家手术质量改进计划（NSQIP）风险计算器，是根据多个临床预测因素建立的。RCRI 基于患者是否具有以下六项可识别的预测因子：高危手术（腹股沟以上的大血管手术、胸内手术或腹腔内的手术），缺血性心脏病，充血性心力衰竭（CHF），脑血管疾病，糖尿病（需胰岛素治疗），以及肾功能衰竭（血肌酐浓度 > 2.0 mg/dl）。当患者存在 RCRI 临床预测因子，每项计 1 分。据此可预测心脏事件（即 MI、肺水肿、心室颤动或原发性心脏停搏及完全性心脏传导阻滞）的风险。RCRI 评分为 0 的患者发生重要心脏并发症的预测风险为 0.4% ～ 0.5%；评分为 1 的患者预测风险为 0.9% ～ 1.3%，评分为 2 的患者预测风险为 4% ～ 6.6%，评分为 3 的患者预测风险为 9% ～ 11%（图 11.1）。有 2 项及以上预测因子的患者，心脏风险大大增加，有 3 项及以上预测因子的患者，心脏风险极高。临床上 RCRI 用于识别心脏并发症风险较高的患者，并帮助医生来决策这些患者是否能从进一步无创心脏检查进行风险分层或从启动术前预防性治疗中获益。

表 11.2　功能状态

良好（需要 > 7 METs 的活动）
提 24 磅重物爬八级台阶
提起 80 磅重物
户外劳动（铲雪、铲土）
娱乐活动（滑雪、篮球、壁球、手球、慢跑或以每小时 5 英里的速度行走）

一般（需要 > 4 METs 但 < 7 METs 的活动）
不中断地完成性生活
在平地上以每小时 4 英里的速度行走
户外劳动（园艺、耙地、播种）
娱乐活动（轮滑、跳舞、狐步舞）

差（需要 < 4 METs 的活动）
不中断地完成洗澡 / 穿衣、整理床铺、打扫灰尘、洗碗
在平地以每小时 2.5 英里的速度行走
户外劳动（擦玻璃）
娱乐活动（高尔夫球、保龄球）

MET，代谢当量。1 磅 ≈ 0.45 kg，1 英里 ≈ 1.61 km。
改编自 Hlatky MA，Boineau RE，Higginbotham MB，et al：A brief self-administered questionnaire to determine functional capacity（the Duke Activity Status Index），Am J Cardiol 64：651-654，1989.

表 11.3　改良心脏风险指数：临床指标

1. 高危手术
2. 缺血性心脏病
   a. 心肌梗死病史
   b. 目前有心绞痛，考虑为心肌缺血所致
   c. 需舌下含服硝酸甘油
   d. 运动试验阳性
   e. ECG 有病理性 Q 波
   f. PTCA 和（或）CABG 术后，目前仍存在心绞痛且考虑为心肌缺血所致
3. 充血性心力衰竭
   a. 查体提示左室功能衰竭
   b. 出现过夜间阵发性呼吸困难
   c. 出现过肺水肿
   d. 听诊心音 S3 奔马律
   e. 听诊双肺啰音
   f. 胸部影像学提示肺水肿
4. 脑血管疾病
   a. 短暂性脑缺血发作史
   b. 脑血管意外史
5. 糖尿病
   a. 胰岛素治疗
6. 慢性肾功能不全
   a. 血肌酐浓度 > 2 mg/dl

CABG，冠状动脉旁路移植术；ECG，心电图；PTCA，经皮冠状动脉血管成形术。
改编自 Lee TH，Marcantonio ER，Mangione CM，et al：Derivation and prospective validation of a simple index for prediction of cardiac risk of major noncardiac surgery，Circulation 100：1043-1049，1999.

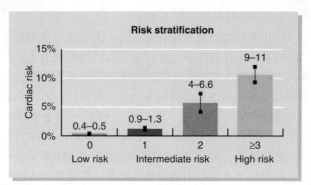

Fig. 11.1 Bar graph shows the predicted risk for cardiac events during surgery according to a patient's Revised Cardiac Risk Index score.

Preoperative Noninvasive Cardiac Testing for Risk Stratification

Evidence discourages widespread application of preoperative noninvasive cardiac testing for all patients. Rather, a selective approach based on clinical risk categorization appears to be both effective and cost-effective. No testing is recommended if it might delay surgical intervention for urgent or emergent conditions.

On a rare occasion, coronary revascularization offers the potential benefit of improving outcomes in high-risk patients—that is, patients with acute coronary syndromes, those with left main CAD, those with two-vessel coronary disease who have significant proximal left anterior descending artery stenosis (and either ischemia on noninvasive testing or reduced left ventricular ejection fraction), and those with three-vessel coronary vessel disease and an ejection fraction of less than 50%. Routine prophylactic coronary revascularization should not be performed in patients with stable CAD before noncardiac surgery. An RCRI score of 3 or higher in a patient with severe myocardial ischemia suggestive of left main or three-vessel disease should lead to consideration of coronary revascularization before noncardiac surgery in appropriate patients.

Noninvasive cardiac testing is most appropriate if it is anticipated that the patient will meet guidelines for initiation of additional medical therapy or coronary angiography and coronary revascularization in the event of a positive test. Noninvasive stress testing of patients with three or more clinical risk factors and poor functional capacity (<4 METS) who require vascular surgery is reasonable, provided that the result might change future management. When feasible, exercise stress testing is the modality of choice and offers the benefit of an objective assessment of functional capacity. Pharmacologic stress tests may be performed instead of exercise tests; they are typically reserved for patients with functional limitations.

Dobutamine echocardiography and nuclear perfusion testing for purposes of identifying patients at risk for perioperative MI or death have excellent negative predictive values (near 100%) but poor positive predictive values (<20%). Therefore, a negative study is reassuring, but a positive study is still only a weak predictor of a "hard" perioperative cardiac event. Which higher-risk patients are most likely to benefit from preoperative noninvasive cardiac testing and treatment strategies to improve outcomes is not well defined.

Preoperative Invasive Cardiac Testing for Risk Stratification

Recommendations for perioperative coronary angiography are similar to those for patients with suspected or known CAD in general and should conform to the ACC/AHA guidelines for coronary angiography. This procedure should be considered for patients who are at high risk for adverse outcomes based on the presence of unstable angina, angina refractory to medical treatment, high-risk results on noninvasive testing, or a nondiagnostic test in a high-risk patient undergoing high-risk noncardiac surgery. It should be considered on an individual basis for those with extensive ischemia revealed during noninvasive testing, for those at intermediate risk undergoing high-risk surgery for whom test results are nondiagnostic, for those convalescing from MI who require urgent noncardiac surgery, and for those with perioperative MI. In patients who have a high clinical risk (RCRI >3) and high-risk features on noninvasive cardiac testing, diagnostic cardiac catheterization should be considered (see Fig. 11.1).

PREOPERATIVE RISK MODIFICATION TO REDUCE PERIOPERATIVE CARDIAC RISK

Coronary Revascularization

Retrospective analyses of the Coronary Artery Surgery Study (CASS) registry and the Bypass Angioplasty Revascularization Investigation (BARI), along with prospective study of patients enrolled in the Coronary Artery Revascularization Prophylaxis (CARP) trial, have shown that prophylactic coronary revascularization with either coronary artery bypass grafting (CABG) or percutaneous coronary intervention (PCI) provides no short-term or mid-term benefit for patients without left main disease or multivessel CAD in the presence of poor left ventricular systolic function. Evidence is lacking to support elective coronary revascularization as a primary strategy for perioperative risk reduction in intermediate-risk patients undergoing major noncardiac surgery.

Recommendations for PCI are similar to those for patients with suspected or known CAD and should conform to the ACC/AHA guidelines. Recommendations by the AHA/ACC Society for Cardiovascular Angiography and Intervention, the American College of Surgeons, and the American Dental Association Science Advisory Committee are for a 30- to 45-day delay of surgery in patients taking thienopyridine dual antiplatelet therapy after bare-metal coronary stent placement and a 365-day wait after placement of a drug-eluting stent. Some studies indicate that the duration of dual antiplatelet therapy may be shortened to less than 1 year in selected patients receiving newer-generation stents (such as everolimus- or zotarolimus-eluting stents).

Currently, studies suggest that optimal medical therapy is the preferred strategy for intermediate- to high-risk patients with RCRI scores of 2 or higher who are without documented severe myocardial ischemia. As stated previously, the CARP trial demonstrated that preoperative coronary revascularization strategies to reduce perioperative cardiovascular risk did not offer significant benefit compared with excellent medical treatment in intermediate- to high-risk patients undergoing vascular surgery. However, high-risk patients with left main coronary stenosis, severe aortic stenosis, left ventricular ejection fraction of 20% or less, or unstable coronary symptoms were excluded from that trial. In many of these patients, coronary or valve surgery may be indicated on its own merit, without factoring in the noncardiac surgery. Therefore, coronary revascularization may be appropriate if diagnostic catheterization reveals left main disease or multivessel disease and depressed ejection fraction.

Using the information obtained from the composite algorithm (Fig. 11.2), a key decision is whether the risk for perioperative cardiac events is sufficiently low to proceed with surgery. For patients identified to be at high cardiac risk who are not candidates for coronary revascularization, the physician may decide to perform an operation that is thought to be less stressful such as a less extensive major plastic reconstruction, laparoscopic versus open procedures or alternative palliative procedures, or attempt to modify cardiac risk by additional intraoperative and perioperative therapies.

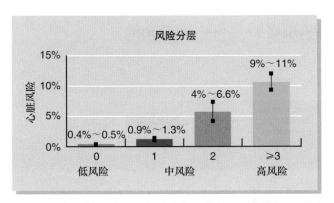

图 11.1　柱状图显示基于患者改良心脏风险指数评分预测术中心脏事件的风险

用于风险分层的术前无创心脏检查

证据显示，不宜对所有患者广泛实施术前无创心脏检查。相反，基于临床风险分类去做选择性检查，似乎更有效且经济。如果心脏检查可能导致紧急或急诊手术推迟，则不推荐。

在一些少见的情况下，冠状动脉血运重建可为下列高危患者改善预后提供潜在获益：急性冠脉综合征的患者，左主干 CAD 的患者，伴左前降支严重狭窄的两支冠脉血管病变患者（无创检查提示缺血改变或左心室射血分数下降），和三支冠脉血管病变以及射血分数低于 50% 的患者。在非心脏手术前不应该对稳定性 CAD 患者进行常规预防性冠状动脉血运重建。而 RCRI 评分 3 分及以上的患者，若存在提示左主干或三支血管病变的严重心肌缺血，应考虑非心脏手术前进行冠状动脉血运重建。

无创心脏检查最适用于下列情况：如果患者检查呈阳性，则会满足指南中开始额外药物治疗或冠状动脉造影及冠状动脉血运重建的情况。具有 3 个及以上临床危险因素和活动耐量差（< 4 METs）且需要进行血管手术的患者，有进行无创负荷试验的适应证，前提是检查结果可能改变后续治疗方案。在可行的情况下，运动负荷试验有利于客观评估运动耐量，是可选方案之一。药物负荷试验可替代运动试验，此检查通常适用于运动功能受限的患者。

多巴酚丁胺负荷超声心动图和核素灌注检查对于识别围术期有 MI 或死亡风险的患者来说具有很好的阴性预测价值（接近 100%），但阳性预测价值较低（< 20%）。因此，上述检查阴性结果让人安心，但阳性结果预测价值低，"很难预测"围术期心脏事件。目前尚不明确哪些高危患者更可能从术前无创心脏检查和治疗策略中获益并改善预后。

用于风险分层的术前有创心脏检查

关于围术期冠状动脉造影的建议，与疑诊或确诊 CAD 的患者建议大致相似，应符合 ACC/AHA 指南中冠状动脉造影的内容。这项检查适用于预期出现不良预后的高风险患者，包括出现不稳定型心绞痛、药物难治性心绞痛、无创检查结果为高危者，或接受高危非心脏手术且仅有非诊断性检查结果的高危患者。对于以下患者应进行个体化医疗决策：无创检查提示广泛心肌缺血的患者，接受高危手术且仅有非诊断性检查结果的中危患者，MI 恢复期需行紧急非心脏手术的患者，以及围术期出现 MI 的患者，应进行个体化医疗决策。对于临床高危（RCRI > 3）及无创心脏检查结果为高危的患者，应考虑诊断性心导管检查（见图 11.1）。

降低围术期心脏风险的术前风险改善策略
冠状动脉血运重建

对冠状动脉手术研究（CASS）注册和旁路血管成形血运重建术研究（BARI）的回顾性分析，以及对冠状动脉血运重建预防（CARP）试验患者的前瞻性研究均提示，在左心室收缩功能差的情况下，通过冠状动脉旁路移植（CABG）或经皮冠状动脉介入治疗（PCI）进行预防性冠脉血运重建治疗，对于不存在左主干病变或不存在多支血管病变 CAD 的患者并不能提供短期或中期获益。以择期冠状动脉血运重建作为接受重大非心脏手术的中危患者降低围术期风险的主要策略，目前仍缺乏证据支持。

推荐行 PCI 的指征与那些疑诊或确诊 CAD 的患者相似，并且应符合 ACC/AHA 指南。AHA/ACC 心血管造影和介入学会、美国外科医师协会以及美国牙科协会科学事务委员会推荐，裸金属冠脉支架放置后服用包括噻吩吡啶类双联抗血小板治疗的患者，外科手术应推迟 30 ～ 45 天，而药物洗脱支架放置后，手术应推迟 365 天。一些研究提示，选择接受新一代支架（如依维莫司或佐他莫司洗脱支架）的患者，双联抗血小板治疗的时间可缩短至 1 年之内。

目前研究建议，对于 RCRI 评分 2 分及以上但无严重心肌缺血病史的中高危患者，进行优化的药物治疗是首选策略。前文已述，CARP 研究提示，对于拟行血管手术的中高危患者，为了降低围术期心血管风险，与完善的药物治疗相比，术前冠脉血运重建策略并不提供足够的获益。然而，有左主干冠脉狭窄、重度主动脉瓣狭窄、左心室射血分数小于等于 20%，或有不稳定型冠脉症状的高危患者被排除在上述研究之外。而往往该类患者中多数人会根据冠脉和瓣膜自身病变选择接受冠脉或瓣膜手术，而非考虑这些危险因素对非心脏手术的影响。因此，若诊断性心导管术提示左主干病变或多支血管病变及射血分数减低，冠脉血运重建可能是适宜的决策。

从下面的流程图（图 11.2）可见，关键的决策在于判断围术期心脏事件的风险是否低至可以进行手术。对于心脏风险高但不适合冠脉血运重建的患者，医生可能会决定实施刺激较小的手术，例如减小大型重建术的范围，以腹腔镜替代开腹手术或选择替代姑息治疗，或努力通过术中及围术期的其他治疗来降低心脏风险。

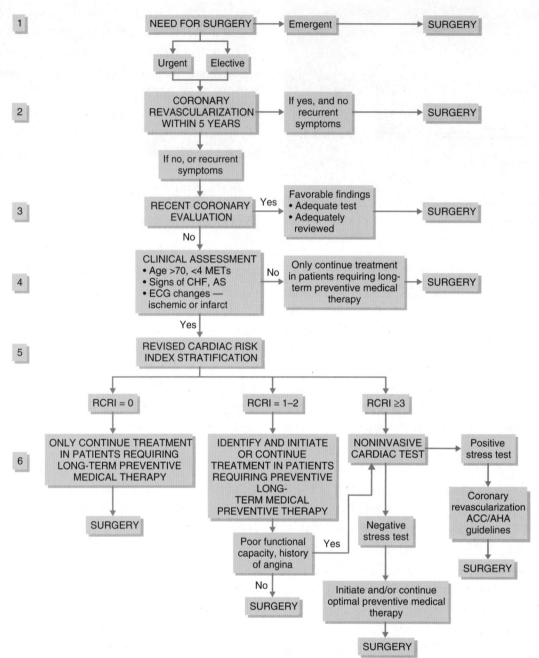

Fig. 11.2 Stepwise clinical evaluation algorithm for diagnostic cardiac catheterization. (1) Emergency surgery; (2) prior coronary revascularization; (3) prior coronary evaluation; (4) clinical assessment; (5) Revised Cardiac Risk Index; (6) risk modification strategies. Preventive medical therapy includes β-blocker and statin therapy. *ACC,* American College of Cardiology; *AHA,* American Heart Association; *AS,* aortic stenosis; *CHF,* congestive heart failure; *ECG,* electrocardiogram; *MET,* metabolic equivalent; *RCRI,* Revised Cardiac Risk Index.

β-Adrenergic Antagonists

There is uncertainty about the effectiveness and safety of perioperative β-blockade in patients undergoing noncardiac surgery. The ACC/AHA guidelines focusing on recommendations for perioperative β-blocker therapy limit class I recommendations to patients undergoing surgery who are already receiving β-blockers to treat angina, symptomatic arrhythmias, or hypertension. Class IIb recommendations are given for the initiation of β-blocker therapy prior to surgery in those with

intermediate- or high-risk myocardial ischemia noted on preoperative noninvasive stress testing (level of evidence C) and patients with three or more RCRI risk factors (level of evidence B).

The Perioperative Ischemic Evaluation (POISE) trial addressed the benefit versus risk of perioperative β-blockade. The POISE trial randomized 8351 intermediate- to high-risk patients older than 45 years of age to receive either a long-acting oral metoprolol succinate (metoprolol CR) or placebo in the perioperative period. The results showed that the

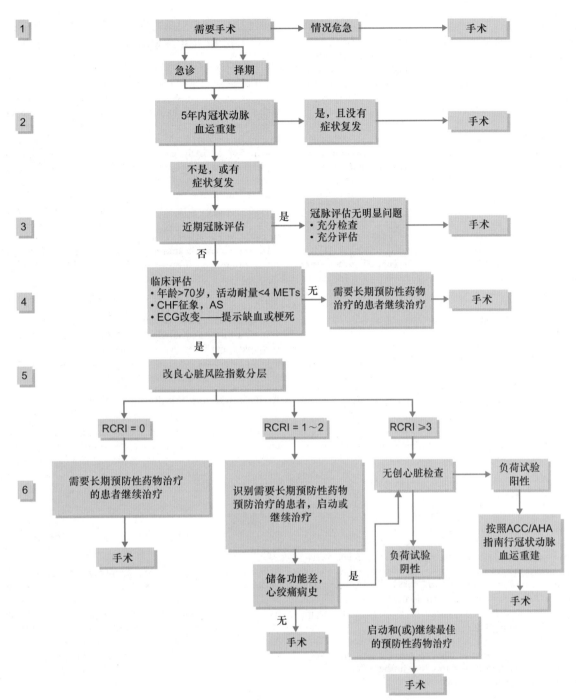

图 11.2　诊断性心导管检查临床分步评估流程。(1) 急诊手术;(2) 既往冠状动脉血运重建;(3) 既往冠脉评估;(4) 临床评估;(5) 改良心脏风险指数;(6) 降低风险的策略。预防性药物治疗包括 β 受体阻滞剂和他汀类药物治疗。ACC,美国心脏病学会;AHA,美国心脏协会;AS,主动脉瓣狭窄;CHF,充血性心力衰竭;ECG,心电图;MET,代谢当量;RCRI,改良心脏风险指数

β 受体阻滞剂

　　非心脏手术的患者围术期使用 β 受体阻滞剂的有效性和安全性目前并不确切。ACC/AHA 指南针对围术期 β 受体阻滞剂治疗的推荐内容中,Ⅰ 类推荐限于已经使用 β 受体阻滞剂治疗心绞痛、有症状的心律失常或高血压的手术患者。术前无创负荷试验提示心肌缺血中危或高危患者(证据等级 C)以及具有 3 项或更多

RCRI 危险因素的患者(证据等级 B),建议术前启动 β 受体阻滞剂治疗,为 Ⅱb 类推荐。

　　围术期缺血评估(POISE)试验探讨了围术期使用 β 受体阻滞剂的获益和风险。POISE 试验纳入 8351 位 45 岁以上中高危患者,随机分为围术期长效口服琥珀酸美托洛尔(美托洛尔 CR)组或安慰剂组。试验结果显示与安慰剂组相比,美托洛尔组心源性死亡、非致死性 MI 或心脏停搏发生率降低。然而,美托洛尔组死亡率和

incidence of cardiac death, nonfatal MI, or cardiac arrest was reduced in the metoprolol group compared with placebo. However, there was an increased incidence of mortality and stroke in the metoprolol group compared with the placebo group. Stroke was associated with perioperative hypotension, bleeding, atrial fibrillation, and a history of stroke or transient ischemic attack. The POISE trialists highlighted the importance of a clear risk and benefit assessment for the initiation of preoperative β-blockers (see Fig. 11.2).

Preexisting β-blockade should be continued because withdrawal might increase perioperative mortality. If β-blockers are newly initiated in appropriately selected higher-risk patients undergoing noncardiac surgery, they should be carefully titrated and not abruptly initiated on a high-dose regimen in order to avoid hypotension or bradycardia.

HMG-CoA Reductase Inhibitors (Statins)

Prospective and retrospective evidence supports the perioperative prophylactic use of 3-hydroxy-3-methylglutaryl–coenzyme A (HMG-CoA) reductase inhibitors (statins) for reduction of perioperative cardiac complications in patients with established atherosclerosis. Statins should be continued in patients who are already on statin therapy and undergoing noncardiac surgery. A class IIa indication is assigned to the use of statins for patients undergoing vascular surgery with or without clinical risk factors.

Angiotensin-Converting Enzyme Inhibitors

Angiotensin-converting enzyme inhibitors (ACEIs) and angiotensin II–receptor blockers (ARBs) are frequently prescribed for the management of hypertension, CHF, chronic renal failure, and ischemic heart disease. Evidence supports the discontinuation of these agents for 24 hours before noncardiac surgery because of adverse circulatory effects after induction of anesthesia in patients on these medications (hypotension) that may result in the need for vasopressin agonists for management of the ensuing refractory hypotension.

Oral Antithrombotic Agents

Evidence-based recommendations regarding perioperative use of aspirin, clopidogrel, other antiplatelet agents, or combination therapy to reduce cardiac risk currently lack clarity. A substantial increase in perioperative bleeding and transfusion requirement in patients receiving dual antiplatelet therapy has been observed. The discontinuation of clopidogrel for 5 days and aspirin for 5 to 7 days before major surgery to minimize the risk of perioperative bleeding and transfusion must be balanced with the potentially increased risk for an acute coronary syndrome, especially in high-risk patients including those with recent coronary stent implantation. If clinicians elect to withhold aspirin before surgery, it should be restarted as soon as possible postoperatively, especially after vascular graft procedures. (See further information on anticoagulants and surgery later in chapter.)

POSTOPERATIVE CARDIAC RISK ASSESSMENT

Monitoring for Myocardial Infarction

Although there are no standard criteria for their diagnosis, most perioperative MIs occur within the first 3 days after noncardiac surgery. Although an ECG is recommended in the setting of signs or symptoms suggestive of myocardial ischemia, MI, or arrhythmia in the postoperative period, the usefulness of postoperative screening with ECGs is uncertain. Measurement of serum cardiac biomarkers should be reserved for patients at high risk and for those who demonstrate ECG changes, symptoms of myocardial ischemia, new arrhythmias, unexplained shortness of breath, or hemodynamic evidence of cardiovascular dysfunction.

NONCARDIAC SURGERY IN PATIENTS WITH SPECIFIC CARDIOVASCULAR CONDITIONS

Valvular Heart Disease

All patients undergoing noncardiac surgery should be assessed especially for aortic stenosis by physical examination and by two-dimensional echocardiography for any suspicious murmur. Symptomatic *severe* stenosis represents an active cardiovascular condition that should be evaluated and managed before elective surgery is undertaken. Appropriately selected patients can be managed with valve replacement or valvuloplasty as a bridge to noncardiac surgery.

Less is known about the perioperative risks associated with mitral stenosis and mitral regurgitation in patients undergoing noncardiac surgery. Usually, a preoperative history and physical examination, chest radiograph, or ECG provides clues to the diagnosis, which can be confirmed by echocardiography. Accurate diagnosis may help optimize intraoperative anesthetic strategies, choice of pharmacologic interventions and invasive monitoring, and postoperative medical management. Patients with severe mitral stenosis are likely to benefit from balloon mitral valvuloplasty or surgical intervention before high-risk surgery.

Patients with aortic or mitral valvular regurgitation benefit from volume control and afterload reduction. In aortic insufficiency, it is thought that faster heart rates are better tolerated than slow ones because slow heart rates lead to increased diastolic filling and can exacerbate left ventricular volume overload.

Arrhythmias and Conduction Defects

Ventricular and atrial arrhythmias historically are recognized as predictors of perioperative cardiac complications. Therefore, identification of a preoperative arrhythmia warrants a careful evaluation for the presence and severity of underlying ischemic heart disease, cardiomyopathy, or other conditions that may contribute to perioperative complications. In general, asymptomatic arrhythmias or conduction defects warrant only observation and maintenance of an optimal metabolic state.

Congestive Heart Failure and Left Ventricular Dysfunction

CHF has been identified as a significant marker of cardiac risk in noncardiac surgery. Every effort should be made to identify the etiology of CHF and optimally control it preoperatively because it is a known risk factor for postoperative cardiac complications. Close monitoring of volume status is needed to avoid perioperative decompensation. Intravenous inotropic agents, vasodilators, or both may be useful for a short duration in the perioperative period to prevent or treat CHF, depending on the situation.

RENAL DISEASE

Renal dysfunction affects critical excretory and synthetic functions required for homeostasis. The major ensuing clinical effects include hypertension, volume overload, and electrolyte derangements.

Hypertension

A well-controlled blood pressure is desirable to reduce perioperative cardiovascular complications. The goal is to have blood pressure within an acceptable range based on current guidelines. Non-urgent procedures should be delayed for adequate BP control to be attained.

The stress response in the perioperative period does increase the incidence of so-called "white coat hypertension." These patients do not require aggressive lowering of blood pressure that can result in

卒中发生率比安慰剂组更高。卒中与围术期低血压、出血、心房颤动以及既往卒中史或短暂性脑缺血发作有关。POISE 研究者强调了在启动术前 β 受体阻滞剂治疗之前，进行明确的风险和获益评估至关重要（见图 11.2）。

由于停药可能增加围术期死亡率，术前已在服用 β 受体阻滞剂的患者应在围术期继续使用。如果拟行非心脏手术的高危患者近期开始非正规服用 β 受体阻滞剂，则需谨慎调整剂量，并且不能以大剂量突然开始使用，以避免低血压或心动过缓的发生。

3- 羟基 -3- 甲基戊二酰辅酶 A（HMG-CoA）还原酶抑制剂（他汀类药物）

前瞻性及回顾性研究证据均支持围术期预防性使用 HMG-CoA 还原酶抑制剂（他汀类药物）以降低动脉粥样硬化患者围术期心脏并发症的发生率。拟行非心脏手术的患者若已经使用他汀类治疗，应继续服用他汀类药物。无论是否有临床危险因素，拟行血管手术的患者服用他汀类药物属于 IIa 类适应证。

血管紧张素转换酶抑制剂

血管紧张素转换酶抑制剂（ACEI）和血管紧张素受体阻滞剂（ARB）常作为高血压、CHF、慢性肾功能衰竭以及缺血性心脏病的治疗用药。有证据支持这些药物在非心脏手术前停药 24 h，因为这些药物在麻醉诱导后对循环有不良影响（低血压），可能导致顽固性低血压，需要使用血管加压素受体激动剂来处理。

口服抗血栓药

关于围术期使用阿司匹林、氯吡格雷、其他抗血小板药物或联合用药方案以降低心脏风险的循证医学建议目前尚不明确。已发现使用双联抗血小板治疗的患者有潜在围术期出血和输血需求增加的风险。在大手术前，尤其是在近期冠脉支架置入的高危患者中，氯吡格雷停药 5 天、阿司匹林停药 5 ~ 7 天可最大程度降低围术期出血和输血的风险，而这一决策必须与潜在的急性冠脉综合征增加的风险进行权衡。若临床医生决定术前停用阿司匹林，则术后应尽快恢复用药，尤其是在血管移植术后。（关于抗凝药与手术更多内容见本章后面内容。）

术后心脏风险评估

心肌梗死监测

尽管缺乏诊断标准，多数围术期 MI 事件一般都发生在非心脏手术后的 3 日之内。尽管术后出现疑似心肌缺血、MI 或心律失常的症状或体征时，推荐行 ECG 检查，但术后进行 ECG 筛查的确切作用尚不明确。高危患者以及出现 ECG 变化、有心肌缺血症状、新发心律失常、难以解释的呼吸困难或血流动力学证据提示心血管功能异常的患者，应行血清心脏生物标志物的测定。

特殊心血管疾病患者的非心脏手术

心脏瓣膜病

所有拟行非心脏手术的患者都需要进行体格检查评估是否存在主动脉瓣狭窄，若出现任何可疑的心脏杂音，须进行二维超声心动图检查。有症状的严重瓣膜狭窄是一种活动性心血管疾病，应在择期手术前评估并治疗。有适应证的患者可通过瓣膜置换或瓣膜成形术作为非心脏手术的桥接治疗。

拟行非心脏手术的患者中，与二尖瓣狭窄和二尖瓣反流相关的围术期风险尚不明确。通常，术前完善病史、体格检查、胸部 X 线片或心电图均能提供诊断线索，超声心动图可予以确诊。准确的诊断有助于优化术中麻醉策略、药物干预和有创监测选择，以及术后治疗方案的制订。对于二尖瓣严重狭窄患者，在高危手术前通过二尖瓣球囊瓣膜成形术或手术干预可能使其获益。

主动脉瓣或二尖瓣反流的患者可通过限制容量和降低后负荷获益。主动脉瓣关闭不全的患者对稍快心率的耐受优于较慢心率，因为心率过慢可造成舒张期充盈增加，加重左心室容量过负荷。

心律失常和传导障碍

室性和房性心律失常历来被认为是围术期心脏并发症的预测因素。因此术前心律失常需要仔细评估是否存在缺血性心脏病、心肌病或其他可能造成围术期并发症的疾病，并评估其严重程度。总体来说，无症状的心律失常或传导障碍只需观察并维持好最佳的代谢状态。

充血性心力衰竭和左心室功能不全

CHF 被认为是非心脏手术心脏风险的一个重要标志。已知 CHF 是术后心脏并发症的危险因素，应尽全力明确 CHF 的病因，并在术前进行最佳的控制。需严密监测容量状态，以防围术期心功能失代偿。静脉使用正性肌力药物、血管扩张剂或两者同时使用，都可以在围术期短时间内有效预防或治疗 CHF，具体视情况而定。

肾病

肾功能不全严重影响机体平衡所需的排泄和合成功能。主要的临床表现包括高血压、容量过负荷和电解质紊乱。

高血压

控制良好的血压是有效降低围术期心血管并发症的必要条件。目标是依据目前的指南将血压维持在可接受范围内。血压控制不佳的非急诊手术应推迟。

围术期应激反应会增加所谓"白大衣高血压"的发生率。这些患者不需要积极降压治疗，因为可能会造成

reduced perfusion to the brain and kidneys, resulting in cerebrovascular accidents and acute kidney injury, respectively.

Antihypertensives (Medications)

- ACEIs, ARBs, and renin antagonists' effect on the RAS have been associated with intraoperative hypotension and should be held on the day of surgery. These can be resumed within 48 hours based on patients' blood pressure, volume status, and renal function
- Diuretics should ideally be held in the perioperative period except in patients with evidence of volume overload. The need for patients to be NPO and associated volume losses during surgery usually result in hypovolemia. Diuretics often need to be adjusted perioperatively to reduce risk of acute kidney injury.
- α-Blockers and β-blockers should not be stopped abruptly except in patients who are hypotensive. These medications are associated with rebound hypertension when stopped abruptly. Doses should rather be reduced and holding parameters instituted in cases of hypotension in order to prevent hypertensive crisis associated with rebound hypertension.
- Calcium-channel blockers and vasodilators can be stopped abruptly if not required for optimization of blood pressure.

Acute Kidney Injury

Refer to the Kidney Disease: Improving Global Outcomes (KDIGO) classification of acute kidney injury (AKI).

Kidney injury can be due to prerenal, intrarenal or postrenal etiologies. Perioperative AKI occurs in about 1% of patients, but risk is much higher in patients having vascular and/or cardiac procedures and in patients with chronic kidney disease, cirrhosis, and heart failure. AKI in the perioperative period is often due to fluid losses, fluid shifts to other body compartments, and/or activation of the RAS. It is essential for the etiology of preoperative AKI to be elucidated and addressed before proceeding with elective surgery. It is critical to maintain euvolemia, while aiming to keep electrolytes—especially serum potassium, magnesium, and sodium—within normal limits.

Management

Prerenal AKI patients typically respond to IVF and measures to ensure adequate renal perfusion by preventing hypotension.

Intrarenal AKI patients require consultation from nephrology colleagues to ensure adequate and timely management to prevent progression of the underlying AKI condition and for initiation of renal replacement therapy if needed.

Postrenal insufficiency is due to obstructive uropathy typically due to BPH, urethral stenosis or calculi. Renal ultrasound or CT of the abdomen and pelvis provides information about the nature and severity of the obstruction. Consultation from urology colleagues is often required.

In all patients with AKI, maintaining adequate renal perfusion by keeping spontaneous bacterial peritonitis (SBP) greater than 110 mm Hg is critical, and avoidance of potential nephrotoxins is essential.

Chronic Kidney Disease (CKD)

Refer to the KDIGO classification for staging.

The majority of the perioperative complications are of cardiac etiology. As much as possible, euvolemic status needs to be attained before surgical procedures are performed. Patients on dialysis need to be dialyzed at least 24 hours before the planned procedure. Patients on peritoneal dialysis who require laparotomy often need temporary conversion to hemodialysis to maintain required volume status and address electrolyte abnormalities.

For non–dialysis dependent patients, adequate renal perfusion needs to be maintained and potential nephrotoxins avoided to prevent worsening of CKD.

Nephrotic Syndrome

Maintenance of adequate volume status and renal perfusion is important. Diuretic doses may need to be adjusted. For patients on corticosteroids (prednisone >5 mg daily) for the management of this condition, it should be assumed that their hypothalamic-pituitary-adrenal (HPA) axis is at least partially compromised. Stress dose corticosteroids given as hydrocortisone 100 mg IV every 8 hours, with a transition to an oral regimen in 24 to 48 hours, and then continuing with the usual dose during the perioperative period is usually an appropriate plan.

Renal Transplant Medicine

Immunosuppressive medications should be continued perioperatively. For patients who are unable to take oral medications such as cyclosporine, IV cyclosporine should be given; the dose required is a third of the oral dose.

Monitoring of drug serum levels is essential in view of potential drug-drug interactions.

HEPATIC DISEASE

Acute and chronic liver diseases (Fig. 11.3) can lead to hepatic dysfunction that may worsen perioperatively because of anesthetic agents and hemodynamic effects of a surgical procedure. The major

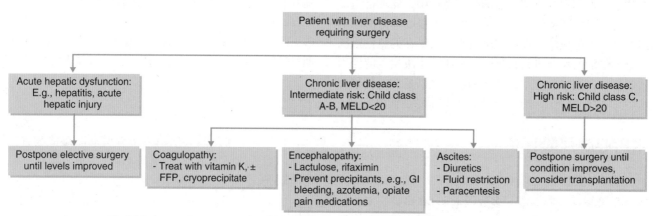

Fig. 11.3 Approach to preoperative risk stratification and interventions in patients with liver disease.

脑和肾脏灌注减少，分别导致脑血管事件和急性肾损伤。

降压（药物）

- ACEI、ARB 及肾素拮抗剂对于 RAS 的作用与术中低血压具有相关性，应在手术当日停用。根据患者的血压、容量状态和肾功能情况在 48 h 内恢复使用。
- 利尿剂最好在围术期暂停使用，除非患者有容量过负荷的证据。术前禁食水（NPO）加上术中的容量丢失常导致低血容量状态。为降低急性肾损伤的发生风险，围术期常需调整利尿剂的使用。
- 不应突然停用 α 受体阻滞剂或 β 受体阻滞剂，除非患者存在低血压。这两类药物的突然停药可能导致反跳性高血压。应该逐渐减少剂量，并在低血压病例中建立停药参数，以防止反跳性高血压相关高血压危象。
- 如果不需要优化血压，钙通道阻滞剂或血管扩张剂可以突然停药。

急性肾损伤

请参考改善全球肾脏预后联盟（KDIGO）中关于急性肾损伤（AKI）的分类。

肾损伤可由肾前性、肾性及肾后性的病因引起。约 1% 的患者发生围术期 AKI，但接受血管和（或）心脏手术的患者以及合并慢性肾病、肝硬化和心力衰竭的患者的发生风险要明显偏高。围术期 AKI 常由于体液丢失、体液向其他部位转移和（或）RAS 的激活造成。对于术前出现的 AKI，在择期手术前查明病因并且进行处理至关重要。维持正常容量状态，同时保持电解质尤其是血钾、镁、钠离子浓度处于正常范围内也十分重要。

处理

肾前性 AKI 患者通常对静脉补液（IVF）和通过预防低血压保证足够肾灌注的措施有治疗反应。

肾性 AKI 需要请肾病科医生会诊，以确保及时充分的治疗，避免潜在的 AKI 病情进展，必要时启动肾脏替代治疗。

肾后性肾功能不全由梗阻性尿路疾病如良性前列腺增生（BPH）、尿道狭窄或结石引起。肾脏超声或腹盆腔 CT 可提供梗阻性质及其严重程度的信息。通常需要请泌尿外科医生会诊。

对于所有 AKI 的患者，关键是通过维持收缩压（SBP）[译者注：原文有误，应为收缩压（systolic blood pressure，SBP）]大于 110mmHg 来保证足够的肾灌注，同时避免使用潜在肾毒性物质也非常重要。

慢性肾脏病（CKD）

请参考 KDIGO 中的分期。

大多数此类患者的围术期并发症是心脏原因引起的。术前应尽可能达到正常的容量状态。透析的患者至少在手术前 24 h 内进行透析。为了维持手术所需容量状态、纠正电解质紊乱，接受开腹手术的腹膜透析患者常需暂时改为血液透析。

为避免非透析依赖患者的 CKD 恶化，应保证足够的肾灌注、避免使用潜在肾毒性物质。

肾病综合征

维持足够容量状态和肾灌注十分重要。利尿剂的剂量可能需要调整。对于接受皮质类固醇（泼尼松＞每天 5 mg）治疗的患者，应考虑到其下丘脑-垂体-肾上腺（HPA）轴至少部分被抑制。合适的围术期方案是：给予应激量的皮质类固醇，如每 8 h 静脉给予氢化可的松 100 mg；然后在第 24 ～ 48 h 内逐步过渡为口服制剂；最后恢复至常规剂量。

肾移植用药

围术期应继续使用免疫抑制剂。对于不能口服环孢素的患者，应静脉给予环孢素，剂量为口服剂量的 1/3。

由于可能存在药物相互作用，监测血药浓度十分必要。

肝脏疾病

急性和慢性肝病（图 11.3）可导致肝功能不全，而麻醉用药及手术造成的血流动力学波动可使围术期肝功能恶化。主要担心的是药物导致的肝脏毒性，可

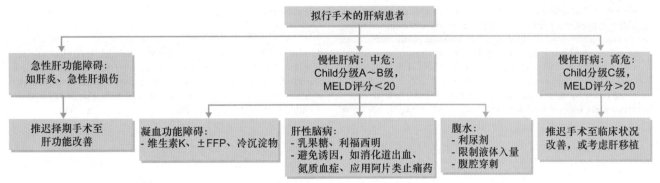

图 11.3 慢性肝病患者的术前风险分层及处理。FFP，新鲜冰冷血浆；MELD，终末期肝病模型

concerns are drug-induced hepatotoxicity, precipitating decompensation of liver cirrhosis and/or development of fulminant liver failure. Perioperative management involves treatment of the complications of liver disease, including coagulopathy, ascites, encephalopathy, and malnutrition.

- Elective procedures in patients with asymptomatic hepatic dysfunction should be postponed pending additional evaluation and reassessment of operative risk.
- Patients with acute hepatic inflammation or hepatocellular and/or cholestatic injury should have elective procedures postponed until there is evidence of recovery.
- Patients with chronic liver disease with preserved hepatic function require close monitoring although their operative risk is minimal.

Cirrhosis is a chronic liver disease, which results in impaired synthetic and metabolic functions.

SBP antibiotic prophylaxis is required for patients with low ascitic fluid protein levels (<1 g/L) for the duration of hospitalization perioperatively. Additional indications for SBP prophylaxis include prior history of SBP and patients with evidence of upper gastrointestinal blood loss.

Patients with ascites due to portal hypertension who may require therapeutic paracentesis will need albumin infusion if more than 5 L is drained to reduce risk for AKI, and the rapid reaccumulation of ascitic fluid.

Diuretic regimens should be adjusted as needed to help maintain required volume status and to keep serum electrolytes within normal limits.

Precipitants of hepatic encephalopathy in patients with cirrhosis need to be avoided as much as possible. Elective procedures in patients who are encephalopathic should be postponed while their clinical condition is managed with the aid of a hepatologist.

Coagulopathy is one of the primary features of chronic advanced liver disease. The etiology is often multifactorial, including hepatic synthetic dysfunction, thrombocytopenia, malnutrition, and the effect of cholestasis on vitamin K absorption. The following measures should be taken to address coagulopathy in the perioperative period.

1. Vitamin K supplementation with or without fresh-frozen plasma (FFP) is often used to correct coagulopathy before surgery. Use of FFP is mainly limited to instances where massive blood transfusion (>4 units) raises concern for dilutional coagulopathy.
2. Cryoprecipitate can address hypofibrinogenemia if serum fibrinogen is less than 100 mg/dL.
3. Platelet transfusion can be used to attain a desired serum platelet level depending on the type of surgical procedure, greater than 50,000 μL for most surgical interventions, but greater than 100,000 μL for neurosurgical procedures.
4. NR values tend to be elevated due to hepatic dysfunction, but this does not confer any antithrombotic properties due to the concept of rebalanced hemostasis. Patients who require deep vein thrombosis (DVT) prophylaxis should still receive subcutaneous heparin or other pharmacologic interventions to reduce DVT risk.

The Model for End-Stage Liver Disease (MELD) and Child-Pugh score/classification (also referred to as Child criteria) have been used for risk assessment of patients with liver disease. The MELD score is calculated using total bilirubin, international normalized ratio (INR), and serum creatinine. This results in four MELD levels, with scores greater than 25 indicating highest mortality risk. Child-Pugh scores are calculated using five clinical measures: total bilirubin, serum albumin, prothrombin time (PT), ascites, and hepatic encephalopathy. The scoring of these clinical measures results in classification of patients in Child class A, B, or C. Patients in class C have the highest mortality risk.

More recently, the integrated MELD score (iMELD), which incorporates serum sodium level for MELD scores less than 12, has been adapted and has been shown to have a better prognostic strength compared with the MELD or Child-Pugh scores.

Surgery is contraindicated in patients with Child-Pugh class C, high MELD/iMELD score (>20), acute hepatitis, severe coagulopathy, or severe extrahepatic manifestations of liver disease (e.g., acute renal failure, hypoxia). Avoid surgery, if possible, in patients with a MELD score of greater than or equal to 18 or Child-Pugh class B unless they have undergone a thorough preoperative evaluation and preparation.

- Use sedatives and neuromuscular blocking agents cautiously.
- Optimize nutrition and medical therapy for cirrhotics:
  - Correct coagulopathy with vitamin K with or without FFP to achieve an INR less than 1.6.
  - The goal platelet count is greater than 50 to 100×10^3/L. This may vary depending on the type of surgical procedure.
  - Address ascitic fluid volume to reduce risk of abdominal wall herniation, wound dehiscence, and compartment syndrome.
- Postoperatively, emphasis should be placed on:
  - Signs of acute liver failure, including worsening jaundice, encephalopathy, and ascites.
  - Monitoring for and correction of renal dysfunction and/or electrolyte abnormalities.
  - Some patients may require IV tranexamic acid to address postoperative bleeding due to the altered fibrinolytic system.

PULMONARY DISEASE

The major components of effective preoperative care are measures to prevent or reduce perioperative complications including pulmonary infections, exacerbation of underlying pulmonary disease, hypoxic hypercarbic respiratory episodes, and avoidance of pulmonary embolism.

For asymptomatic patients there is generally no need for preoperative chest radiographs or pulmonary function tests (PFTs). Preoperative PFTs are, however, essential in patients who are scheduled to have lung resection procedures to help predict postoperative lung function.

Patients with unexplained dyspnea need to be evaluated before having surgical procedures that require general anesthesia.

A combined cardiopulmonary risk index is proposed for risk stratification of pulmonary complications. Pulmonary risk factors have been added to the Goldman Cardiac Risk Index; patients with a combined score of greater than 4 points (of a total of 10) are 17 times more likely to develop complications. These pulmonary risk factors include the following:

- Obesity (i.e., body mass index >27 kg/m^2)
- Cigarette smoking within 8 weeks of surgery
- Productive cough within 5 days of surgery
- Diffuse wheezing within 5 days of surgery
- FEV$_1$/FVC ratio less than 70% and Paco$_2$ greater than 45 mm Hg

In the preoperative history and physical exam, patients should be screened for obstructive sleep apnea (OSA). Adequate management of OSA is critical to prevent cardiopulmonary and neurovascular complications. The commonly used tool is the STOP-BANG score. A formal sleep study is needed in high-risk patients who are scheduled for elective procedures.

COPD/Bronchial Asthma

Patients with these conditions should have their treatment regimen optimized and be instructed to continue with their medications up to the morning of their procedures. Patients with features of exacerbation should be started on systemic corticosteroids. Planned procedures should be rescheduled if possible.

诱发肝硬化失代偿和（或）出现暴发性肝衰竭。围术期管理主要是治疗肝脏疾病的并发症，包括凝血功能障碍、腹水、肝性脑病及营养不良。

- 对于无症状的肝功能异常患者，择期手术应推迟，等待进一步肝功能评估和手术风险评估。
- 对于急性肝脏炎症、肝细胞和（或）胆汁淤积性损伤的患者，应推迟择期手术直至损伤恢复。
- 对于保留肝功能的慢性肝病患者，虽然其手术风险很小，但仍需严密监测。

肝硬化是一种慢性肝病，会导致合成及代谢功能受损。

对于腹水蛋白水平低（＜ 1 g/L）的患者，围术期住院期间应当使用抗生素预防自发性细菌性腹膜炎（spontaneous bacterial peritonitis，SBP）。预防性治疗 SBP 的其他指征包括既往 SBP 病史和有上消化道出血证据的患者。

门静脉高压性腹水的患者可能需要进行治疗性穿刺，如果引流超过 5 L，则应输入白蛋白以降低 AKI 的风险及腹水的快速再蓄积。

为了维持所需容量状态并将电解质维持在正常范围内，应按需调整利尿剂方案。

肝硬化患者应尽可能避免肝性脑病的诱发因素。肝性脑病患者的择期手术应推迟，并请肝脏病专科医生协助治疗其临床状况。

凝血功能障碍是慢性肝病晚期的主要特征表现。其病因是多方面的，包括肝脏合成功能障碍、血小板减少、营养不良及胆汁淤积对维生素 K 吸收的影响。围术期应采取以下措施处理凝血功能障碍。

1. 术前常单用维生素 K 或联合新鲜冰冻血浆（FFP）来纠正凝血功能障碍。FFP 主要限于大量输血（＞ 4 单位）导致的稀释性凝血功能障碍。

2. 若血浆纤维蛋白原低于 100 mg/dl，可使用冷沉淀物纠正低纤维蛋白原血症。

3. 可根据不同手术类型进行血小板输注以达到所需水平，如大部分外科手术需血小板水平大于 50×10^9/L，而神经外科手术需血小板水平大于 100×10^9/L。

4. 肝功能障碍时国际标准化比值（INR）常会升高（译者注：原文有误，应为 INR），但由于止血再平衡的存在，并不会产生抗血栓的特征。因此，深静脉血栓（DVT）高危的患者仍需接受皮下肝素或其他药物干预，以减少 DVT 风险。

终末期肝病模型（MELD）及 Child-Pugh 评分 / 分级（也称 Child 标准）常用于肝病患者的风险评估。MELD 评分通过总胆红素、INR、血肌酐水平计算，共分为 4 级，评分大于 25 表示死亡风险最高。Child-Pugh 评分通过五项临床指标计算：总胆红素、血清白蛋白、凝血酶原时间（PT）、腹水和肝性脑病。根据这些临床指标评分，将患者分为 Child A 级、B 级或 C 级，C 级患者的死亡风险最高。

最近，对于 MELD 评分低于 12 的患者，综合考虑血清钠水平，得到改良的综合 MELD 评分（iMELD），并显示出比 MELD 或 Child-Pugh 评分更强的预后价值。

对于 Child-Pugh C 级、高 MELD/iMELD 评分（＞ 20）、急性肝炎、严重凝血功能障碍或出现肝病的严重肝外表现（如急性肾衰竭、缺氧）的患者，手术是禁忌的。对于 MELD 评分 ≥ 18 或 Child-Pugh 为 B 级的患者，如果可能，应避免手术，除非患者已经进行了充分的术前评估和准备。

- 谨慎使用镇静药和神经肌肉阻滞剂
- 优化肝硬化的营养和药物治疗：
  - 单用维生素 K 或联合 FFP 纠正凝血功能障碍，使 INR 小于 1.6。
  - 根据不同手术类型，血小板的目标需达到（50 ~ 100）$\times 10^9$/L（译者注：原著单位有误）。
  - 控制腹水的量，以减少腹壁疝、伤口裂开及腹腔间隔综合征的风险。
- 术后应重点关注：
  - 急性肝功能衰竭的征象，包括黄疸加重、肝性脑病及腹水。
  - 监测并纠正肾功能不全和（或）电解质紊乱。
  - 一些患者可能需要静脉给予氨甲环酸来控制由于纤溶系统紊乱导致的术后出血。

肺病

有效的术前管理的主要内容是预防或减少围术期并发症（包括肺部感染、基础肺病的加重、低氧高碳酸血症的呼吸事件，及预防肺栓塞）的措施。

对于无症状的患者，术前通常无需进行胸部 X 线检查或肺功能检查（PFT）。但对于拟行肺切除手术的患者，术前 PFT 是必需的，可帮助预测术后的肺功能。

不明原因呼吸困难的患者在进行需要全身麻醉的手术前需要进行评估。

目前提出了一种用于肺部并发症风险分层的联合心肺风险指数。将肺部风险因素加入到 Goldman 心脏风险指数中，综合评分大于 4 分（总分 10 分）的患者其肺部并发症风险增高 17 倍。这些肺风险因素包括以下内容：

- 肥胖（如体重指数 ＞ 27 kg/m²）
- 手术 8 周内吸烟
- 手术 5 天内咳嗽咳痰
- 手术 5 天内肺内存在弥漫性哮鸣音
- FEV_1/FVC 小于 70% 及 $PaCO_2$ 大于 45 mmHg

术前病史询问和体格检查时，应筛查患者是否有阻塞性睡眠呼吸暂停（OSA）。良好的 OSA 管理对于预防心肺和神经血管并发症至关重要。常用的工具是 STOP-BANG 评分。对于安排择期手术的高危患者，应进行正式的睡眠监测。

慢阻肺病 / 支气管哮喘

有上述情况的患者应在术前优化其治疗方案，并持续用药至手术当日早晨。出现加重征象的患者需开始使用全身皮质类固醇治疗；如果可能，应重新安排手术。

HPA axis suppression should be assumed to be present in patients who have received systemic steroids for more than 3 weeks in the past 6 months. These patients should receive stress-dose coverage perioperatively.

There is no role for prophylactic perioperative use of antibiotics. Elective procedures should be cancelled in patients with active infections.

Obstructive Sleep Apnea

Patients require CPAP (continuous positive airway pressure) perioperatively. Blood gas monitoring is required.

Smoking cessation does reduce pulmonary complications and should be encouraged several weeks before planned elective procedures.

Breathing exercises including use of incentive spirometry are worthwhile risk-reduction measures that should be used.

Postoperative management is based on:
- Appropriate use of antibiotics to treat infections
- Use of high-dose steroids of management of flare-up of underlying lung diseases
- Maintenance of adequate oxygenation.

Prevention of Venous Thromboembolism

In patients undergoing major orthopedic surgery such as hip and knee joint replacement, venous thromboembolism (VTE) prophylaxis with low-molecular-weight heparin (LMWH), adjusted dose warfarin, apixaban, rivaroxaban or aspirin should be initiated postoperatively and continued for a period of up to 35 days. Placement of inferior vena cava filters is unlikely to offer added benefit to patients with contraindications to thromboprophylaxis. Patients undergoing nonorthopedic surgeries should be risk stratified for VTE and those at high risk receive prophylaxis with LMWH or low-dose unfractionated heparin. See American College of Chest Physicians guidelines in the suggested readings section.

ENDOCRINE DISEASE

Diabetes Mellitus

Diabetes mellitus is a common condition requiring preoperative management because uncontrolled diabetes is associated with hyperglycemic crises, infection, reduced wound healing, and increased mortality. Optimal perioperative glucose targets vary but generally fall between 80 to 180 mg/dL. Evaluation includes known complications of diabetes including neuropathy, chronic kidney disease, and heart disease. Hemoglobin A_{1C} measurement will correlate with recent (1-3 months) blood glucose levels and may be helpful with assessment of hyperglycemia risk. Oral and noninsulin injectable medications are generally continued until the morning of surgery at which time they are temporarily discontinued. Long-acting basal insulin is continued but may require dose reduction by 20% to 30% if a fasting period is required. Withholding of long-acting insulin in type 1 diabetics may result in onset of ketoacidosis and should be avoided. Short-acting insulin doses may be reduced or temporarily eliminated depending on oral intake restrictions. Intraoperative and postoperative monitoring of blood glucose via fingerstick (every 2-4 hours) will help identify occurrence of hypo- or hyperglycemia. Long- and short-acting insulin should be used to treat and prevent hyperglycemia while being mindful of the patient's insulin sensitivity to avoid hypoglycemia. Transition back to home regimen may begin when the patient is clinically stable, resumes steady oral intake and no further procedures/operations are planned.

Thyroid Disease

Hypo- and hyperthyroidism are each associated with worsening of associated symptoms, morbidity, and even death. Although routine laboratory screening is not recommended, evaluation should be done when symptoms of thyroid dysfunction are noted in patient assessments. Mild to moderate hypothyroidism should be treated with preoperative oral levothyroxine. Treatment of severe hypothyroidism including myxedema coma include IV levothyroxine and IV liothyronine and postponement of elective surgery until thyroid hormone levels are stable. Untreated hyperthyroidism may result in postoperative thyroid storm, which is characterized by tachycardia, confusion, fever, and cardiovascular collapse. Patients with thyrotoxicosis should be treated with β-blockers and antithyroid medications preoperatively (see Chapter 65).

Adrenal Insufficiency and Long-Term Corticosteroid Use

The adrenal glands produce cortisol and various catecholamines in response to stimulation from the HPA axis. Patients receiving long-term exogenous corticosteroids (20 mg daily of prednisone or equivalent for >3 weeks) are considered at risk of adrenal insufficiency due to HPA axis suppression. Because surgery is a state of induced stress, an IV corticosteroid regimen (intravenous hydrocortisone 50-100 mg and up to three times daily) is required with a plan to taper to routine doses based on hemodynamic response.

HEMATOLOGIC DISEASE

Screening for disorders of bleeding hemostasis includes questions identifying episodes of bleeding diathesis, medications posing high bleeding risk, and family history of hemophilia or other inherited bleeding disorders. Patients with liver disease, end-stage renal disease, and collagen vascular disease may have higher perioperative bleeding risk. Commonly obtained laboratory testing includes PT, INR, activated prothrombin time (aPTT), and platelet count.

Management of anticoagulants and antithrombotics in the perioperative setting is a frequent concern given their frequent use in clinical practice. Perioperative risk of bleeding and thromboembolic events should be evaluated because not all surgical procedures require discontinuation of anticoagulation (Table 11.4). In situations of high risk of bleeding, the vitamin K antagonist warfarin is held 5 days prior to the planned procedure. Direct oral anticoagulants such as apixaban, dabigatran, and rivaroxaban may be discontinued within 24 to 48 hours of the procedure depending on overall bleeding risk and renal function. In situations of high risk of thromboembolism due to interruption of therapy, bridging therapy may be provided with heparin infusion or LMWH injection until oral therapy may be safely resumed (Table 11.5). Perioperative management of antithrombotics, such as aspirin, clopidogrel, and other P2Y12 inhibitors should be based upon the indications for antithrombotic use and the type of surgery to be performed as noted in the section on cardiologic disease.

Preoperative anemia is associated with an increase in postoperative transfusion, morbidity, and mortality. A target preoperative hemoglobin is not well established and may depend on the expected blood loss, but most patients will likely tolerate levels as low as 7 g/dL. Screening, work-up, and optimization of anemia should occur with enough lead time to allow for correction and optimization prior to elective surgical procedures.

INFECTIOUS DISEASE

Surgical site infections (SSIs) complicate up to 20% of operations leading to significant morbidity and mortality. SSIs occur within 30 days of surgery and are defined as affecting the superficial, deep or organ/space

对于在 6 个月内使用全身类固醇治疗超过 3 周的患者，应考虑到其 HPA 轴可能受到抑制。此类患者围术期应接受应激剂量的皮质类固醇补充。

围术期无需预防性使用抗生素。若患者存在活动性感染则应取消择期手术。

阻塞性睡眠呼吸暂停

此类患者围术期需要使用持续气道正压通气（CPAP），也需要监测血气。

戒烟可以减少肺部并发症，应在安排择期手术前几周内鼓励患者戒烟。

进行呼吸功能锻炼，包括使用呼吸训练器，是值得使用的降低风险的措施。

术后管理基于：

- 合理使用抗生素治疗感染
- 使用大剂量类固醇治疗基础肺病的突然发作
- 维持足够的氧合

预防静脉血栓栓塞

对于接受髋关节或膝关节置换等骨科大手术的患者，术后应开始使用药物预防静脉血栓栓塞（VTE），包括术后使用低分子量肝素（LMWH），以及对华法林、阿哌沙班、利伐沙班或阿司匹林等药物进行剂量调整，并持续最长 35 天。对于有预防血栓用药禁忌的患者，放置下腔静脉滤器并不太可能带来额外的获益。对于接受非骨科手术的患者，应进行 VTE 风险分层，高危患者应预防性使用 LMWH 或小剂量的普通肝素。参见"推荐阅读"所列美国胸科医师协会指南。

内分泌疾病

糖尿病

糖尿病是一种需要术前管理的常见疾病，因为糖尿病控制不佳与高血糖危象、感染、切口愈合不良和死亡率增加相关。虽然围术期血糖控制的最佳目标并无统一标准，但一般要求控制在 $4.4 \sim 10.0$ mmol/L 之间。评估内容包括已知的糖尿病并发症，包括神经病变、慢性肾病和心脏病。糖化血红蛋白 A_{1C} 与近期（$1 \sim 3$ 个月）血糖水平相关，有助于评估高血糖的风险。口服药或非胰岛素注射药物一般持续用药，手术日早晨暂时停用。长效基础胰岛素继续使用，但若需禁食水，则减量 $20\% \sim 30\%$。1 型糖尿病患者应避免停用长效胰岛素，因为停用会导致酮症酸中毒。短效胰岛素可根据经口进食的限制，适当减量或临时停用。术中及术后（每 $2 \sim 4$ h）指尖血糖监测有助于及时识别低血糖或高血糖的发生。可以使用长效或短效胰岛素治疗或预防高血糖的发生，但同时应考虑患者的胰岛素敏感性以避免低血糖。当患者病情稳定、恢复稳定的经口进食，且没有进一步手术计划时，可以开始过渡到居家治疗方案。

甲状腺疾病

甲状腺功能减退和甲状腺功能亢进均会导致相关症状加重、发病率增加，甚至死亡。尽管不建议常规进行甲状腺功能实验室筛查，但如果评估患者发现甲状腺功能异常的症状时，还是应当进行相关检查。应在术前口服左甲状腺素治疗轻中度的甲状腺功能减退。若出现黏液水肿性昏迷等重度甲状腺功能减退症表现，应静脉补充左甲状腺素及三碘甲状腺原氨酸，并推迟择期手术至甲状腺激素水平稳定。未经治疗的甲状腺功能亢进会导致术后甲状腺危象，表现为心动过速、意识模糊、发热和心血管衰竭。甲状腺功能亢进的患者应在术前给予 β 受体阻滞剂和抗甲状腺药物治疗（见第 65 章）。

肾上腺功能不全和长期使用皮质类固醇

肾上腺受 HPA 轴刺激合成皮质醇和多种儿茶酚胺。长时间接受外源性皮质类固醇（每天 20 mg 泼尼松或等效剂量且持续大于 3 周）的患者，由于 HPA 轴被抑制存在肾上腺功能不全的风险。由于手术会引起应激状态，因此需要静脉注射皮质醇（静脉注射氢化可的松 $50 \sim 100$ mg，每天最多 3 次），并依据血流动力学的反应逐渐减至常规剂量。

血液病

患者出凝血状态的筛查内容包括：询问患者是否有出血倾向、使用高出血风险的药物、血友病家族史或其他遗传性出血疾病。合并肝病、终末期肾病或者结缔组织病（胶原血管病）的患者，围术期出血风险更高。常用的实验室检查包括 PT、INR、活化凝血酶原时间（aPTT）和血小板计数。

由于抗凝药和抗血栓药在临床上频繁使用，相关围术期管理备受关注。并非所有的手术操作都需要停止抗凝治疗（表 11.4），因此应评估围术期出血及血栓栓塞事件的风险。出血风险较高时，维生素 K 拮抗剂华法林应在术前 5 天停用。直接口服抗凝药如阿哌沙班、达比加群和利伐沙班，应根据出血风险和肾功能在术前 $24 \sim 48$ h 内停用。若治疗中断会导致高血栓栓塞风险，则应输注肝素或注射 LMWH 进行桥接治疗，直至可以安全地恢复口服用药（表 11.5）。如"心脏疾病"篇所述，围术期抗血栓药物的管理，如阿司匹林、氯吡格雷和其他 P2Y12 抑制剂，应基于抗血栓药的适应证和手术类型。

术前的贫血与术后输血、发病率及死亡率的升高相关。目前对于术前血红蛋白的目标尚无明确要求，一般与预计出血量相关；大部分患者能够耐受的术前血红蛋白水平为 7 g/dl。应该在择期手术前预留足够的时间筛查和检查贫血，以便及时治疗和优化。

感染性疾病

手术部位感染（SSI）导致多达 20% 的手术复杂化，并显著提高发病率和死亡率。SSI 发生于术后 30 天内，

TABLE 11.4   Risk Factors for Bleeding and Thrombosis in the Anticoagulated Patient

	INDICATIONS FOR ANTICOAGULATION THERAPY[a]		
	Atrial Fibrillation	**Mechanical Heart Valve**	**VTE**
High-risk features for periprocedural bleeding: Consider interruption of therapy	Procedure-related bleeding risk: Consult surgeon or surgical society guidelines for procedure bleeding risk classification. Common high-risk procedures include: vascular surgery, pacemaker lead extraction, kidney biopsy, radical hysterectomy, total hip replacement, and many others. Patient-related bleed risk increased if: Major bleed or intracranial hemorrhage <3 months; thrombocytopenia or abnormal platelet function (uremia and aspirin use); supratherapeutic INR; history of periprocedural bleeding		
High-risk features for perioperative thromboembolism: Consider bridging therapy	• CHADS2-Vasc 7+ • CVA/TIA/VTE <3 months prior • Rheumatic valvular heart disease	• Mitral valve prosthesis • CVA/TIA <6 months prior • Cage-ball or tilting disk aortic valve prosthesis	• VTE <3 months prior • Severe thrombophilia (protein C or S deficiency, antiphospholipid syndrome, history of recurrent thrombosis when off anticoagulation)

CHADS2-VASC, Clinical prediction rule for estimating the risk of stroke in patients with nonrheumatic atrial fibrillation.
[a]Decisions on bridging therapy are clinically based—evaluate thrombotic risk balanced by patient bleeding risk, consider additional information, and use clinical judgement.

TABLE 11.5   Interruption of Therapy and Bridging of Anticoagulation

	Anticoagulant Class	
	Vitamin K Antagonists • Warfarin	**Direct Oral Anticoagulants (DOACs)** • Dabigatran • Apixaban • Rivaroxaban
Interruption of therapy	• INR 2.0-3.0, discontinue 5 days prior to procedure • INR 1.5-1.9, discontinue 3-4 days prior to procedure	• Dependent on creatinine clearance • If renal function is normal, stop 1-2 days prior to surgery
Bridging therapy	• Therapeutic UFH or LMWH • Start UFH when INR <2 • UFH: Stop >4 hours prior to procedure • LMWH: Stop 12-24 hours prior to procedure • LMWH use and dosing must be renally adjusted	• Therapeutic UFH or LMWH • Start UFH when INR <2 • UFH: Stop >4 hours prior to procedure • LMWH: Stop 12-24 hours prior to procedure • LMWH use and dosing must be renally adjusted
Reinitiation of therapy	• Restart at patient's regular dose • Timing is procedure specific: consult with surgeon (most within 24 hours)	• Will render patient therapeutically anticoagulated within hours • Discuss timing of reinitiation with surgeon/proceduralist (most within 24 hours)
Special considerations	• Postprocedure bridging therapy may be considered in patients with moderate or high risk • Discontinue bridging therapy once INR >2.0	• Inability to take PO: may use UFH or LMWH • Obviates need for DVT prophylaxis • Special caution in setting of spinal anesthesia due to risk of hematoma formation

LMWH, Low-molecular-weight heparin; *UFH*, unfractionated heparin.

areas of the wound. Patient risk factors for SSIs include age, nutritional status, and diabetes while operative risk factors include initial contamination of surgical wound, operative technique, and many others. Perioperative care is focused on prevention through the implementation of care bundles (small sets of straightforward evidence-based interventions) including preoperative antibiotics, hair removal, avoidance of hypothermia, and glycemic control. Preoperative antibiotic coverage should include *Staphylococcus aureus* for clean wounds and expand to cover other organisms depending on wound type and risk of contamination. Skin decontamination with topical agents such as chlorhexidine has become routine but may not confer benefit in all patients.

NEUROLOGIC DISEASE

Neurologic conditions that may become exacerbated in the perioperative period include neuromuscular diseases, Parkinson's disease, and stroke.

Neuromuscular Diseases

Conditions such as myasthenia gravis, amyotrophic lateral sclerosis (ALS), and muscular dystrophies predispose patients to a variety of complications. Myasthenia gravis, an autoimmune disease affecting acetylcholine receptors at the neuromuscular junction that leads to skeletal muscle weakness, may worsen acutely in the perioperative period. Respiratory insufficiency or failure due to myasthenic crisis requires assessment of inspiratory function by measuring the negative inspiratory force at the bedside.

Dysphagia, which accompanies many neuromuscular diseases, may lead to aspiration pneumonitis/pneumonia. Swallow evaluation is necessary in the perioperative setting to mitigate this risk in patients with ALS, which is characterized by motor neuron degeneration and may be complicated by postoperative aspiration pneumonia and respiratory failure. Patients with muscular dystrophies are at risk for cardiac arrhythmias and may require cardiac rhythm monitoring. Malignant hyperthermia syndrome is a rare inherited

表 11.4　抗凝治疗的出血及血栓风险

	抗凝治疗的适应证 [a]		
	心房颤动	心脏机械瓣膜	VTE
围术期高出血风险特征：考虑暂停抗凝治疗	操作相关出血风险：可请外科医生会诊或查询外科协会相关指南对不同手术操作出血风险进行分层。常见高出血风险操作包括：血管手术、起搏器导联取出、肾脏活检、根治性子宫切除术、全髋关节置换术等。患者相关出血风险增高的因素有：3 个月内大出血史或颅内出血病史、血小板减少症或血小板功能异常（尿毒症或服用阿司匹林）、超过治疗范围的 INR 值、围术期出血病史		
围术期高血栓栓塞风险特征：考虑桥接抗凝治疗	● CHADS2-Vasc ≥ 7 分 ● 近 3 个月内 CVA/TIA/VTE ● 风湿性心脏瓣膜病	● 二尖瓣假体 ● 近 6 个月内 CVA/TIA ● 主动脉人工瓣为笼球瓣或斜碟瓣	● 近期 3 个月 VTE ● 严重易栓症（蛋白 C 或蛋白 S 缺乏、抗磷脂综合征、停用抗凝治疗后反复栓塞病史）

CHADS2-Vasc，非风湿性心房颤动患者的卒中风险预测评分。CVA，脑血管意外；TIA，短暂性脑缺血发作；VTE，静脉血栓栓塞。
[a] 桥接抗凝治疗决策基于临床：评估患者的血栓风险和出血风险之间的平衡，考虑其他信息并进行临床判断。

表 11.5　抗凝药的暂停和桥接治疗

	抗凝药的分类	
	维生素 K 拮抗剂 ● 华法林	直接口服抗凝药（DOAC） ● 达比加群 ● 阿哌沙班 ● 利伐沙班
暂停抗凝药	● INR 2.0 ~ 3.0 时，术前停用 5 天 ● INR 1.5 ~ 1.9 时，术前停用 3 ~ 4 天	● 根据肌酐清除率决定 ● 如果肾功能正常，术前停用 1 ~ 2 天
桥接治疗	● 治疗量的 UFH 或 LMWH ● 当 INR < 2 时开始使用 UFH ● UFH：术前至少停用 4 h ● LMWH：术前停用 12 ~ 24 h ● LMWH 的使用和剂量须根据肾功能调整	● 治疗量的 UFH 或 LMWH ● 当 INR < 2 时开始使用 UFH ● UFH：术前至少停用 4 h ● LMWH：术前停用 12 ~ 24 h ● LMWH 的使用和剂量须根据肾功能调整
恢复抗凝	● 重启患者的常规剂量 ● 恢复时间根据手术操作决定：与外科医生协商（大部分在 24 h 内）	● 数小时内即可恢复抗凝治疗 ● 与外科医师及操作者协商恢复时间（大部分在 24 h 内）
特殊注意事项	● 中高风险患者需术后考虑继续桥接治疗 ● INR > 2.0 时停止桥接	● 不能经口用药：可考虑使用 UFH 或 LMWH ● 需排除预防 DVT 的必要 ● 椎管内麻醉需特别谨慎，因其有形成血肿的风险

LMWH，低分子量肝素；UFH，普通肝素；DVT，深静脉血栓。

其定义包括浅表、深部或器官 / 间隙的切口感染。患者相关的 SSI 危险因素包括：年龄、营养状况和糖尿病；手术相关危险因素包括：手术切口的初始污染、手术技术等。围术期管理的重点是实施一系列管理措施（小规模循证干预措施）进行预防，包括术前抗生素、备皮、避免低体温和控制血糖。对于洁净切口，术前抗生素应覆盖金黄色葡萄球菌，并根据切口类型及感染风险相应扩大抗菌谱。使用外用药如氯己定去除皮肤污染已成为常规，但不一定能使所有患者获益。

神经系统疾病

多种神经系统疾病会在围术期加重，如神经肌肉疾病、帕金森病及卒中。

神经肌肉疾病

重症肌无力、肌萎缩侧索硬化（ALS）、肌营养不良等情况会导致患者出现多种并发症。重症肌无力是影响神经肌肉接头处乙酰胆碱受体的自身免疫病，会导致骨骼肌无力，可能在围术期急性加重。肌无力危象导致呼吸功能不全或呼吸衰竭时需要评估患者的吸气功能，可在床旁测量最大吸气负压。

吞咽困难见于多种神经肌肉疾病，会导致吸入性肺炎。ALS 以运动神经元退行性变为特征，术后可能出现吸入性肺炎和呼吸功能衰竭，因此应在围术期进行吞咽功能检查以降低此类风险。肌营养不良的患者存在心律失常的风险，可能需要进行心律监测。恶性高热综合征是一种罕见的遗传病，表现为围术期的肌肉强直、发热和心律失常。

condition presenting as perioperative muscle rigidity, fever, and cardiac arrhythmias.

Parkinson's Disease

Parkinson's disease is a common neurodegenerative disorder associated with dyskinesia, dysphagia, dysmetria, and loss of function. Missed doses of levodopa, a common therapy for Parkinson's, may result in fever, dysautonomia, and worsening of Parkinson's disease symptoms. Levodopa therapy should be continued without interruption if possible, depending on the clinical situation. Patients with Parkinson's disease may require longer rehabilitation following surgical procedures.

Stroke

Perioperative stroke incidence is low but carries a high rate of mortality and morbidity. Most perioperative strokes are embolic in mechanism. Risk factors include history of stroke, diabetes mellitus, hypertension, atrial fibrillation, and advanced age. Addressing modifiable risk factors and appropriate management including use of aspirin and statin therapy for known intracranial atheromatous disease should be pursued. In high-risk patients with atrial fibrillation, perioperative bridging of anticoagulation therapy should be considered to minimize risk of stroke.

RHEUMATOLOGIC DISEASE

Autoimmune conditions such as rheumatoid arthritis and lupus are commonly treated with medications aimed at reducing the activity of the immune system. Disease-modifying antirheumatic drugs such as methotrexate, azathioprine, mycophenolate mofetil, which are used in a range of rheumatic conditions, may be continued in the perioperative period. Biologic agents such as adalimumab, infliximab, and other similar agents are thought to raise the risk of perioperative infection and should be held perioperatively. In addition, surgery should ideally be scheduled for the end of the dosing cycle.

SPECIAL NEEDS OF THE GERIATRIC PATIENT

One third of inpatient surgeries in the United States are performed on adults older than age 65. Patients in the geriatric population have a greater risk of perioperative morbidity and mortality. Geriatric preoperative risk assessment should focus on function, cognition, and evaluation of medications, in addition to the systems-based approach in this chapter. Impairment of activities of daily living (ADLs) is directly associated with increased postoperative mortality. Screening for function may be performed with a variety of scales developed for this purpose. Gait speed and the timed Up and Go test are useful objective assessments. Underlying cognitive impairment is an independent risk factor for postoperative delirium. Cognition may be evaluated with the Mini-Cog scale or Montreal Cognitive Assessment. Identification of concerns in the patient's functional status and/or cognition preoperatively may lead to reevaluation of the surgical management plan. Postoperatively, strategies should focus on physical rehabilitation and measures to reduce risk of delirium including minimal use of medications that promote delirium, frequent reorientation, multicomponent interventions, and judicious use of antipsychotic medications.

Review of medications with a view toward postoperative complications should especially include antihypertensives (hypotension), diuretics (volume depletion), diabetes medications (hypo- or hyperglycemia), antithrombotic agents (bleeding or thrombosis), benzodiazepines, opiates, and other sedative hypnotics (sedation and delirium). Indications for each medication should be reviewed and assessment of the risks and benefits should be performed.

SUMMARY

The success of standardized evidence-based preoperative and postoperative risk reduction strategies in patients undergoing noncardiac surgery depends on collaborative teamwork and careful communication among the surgeons, the anesthesiologist, the patient's primary care physician, and the consultant.

The risk for a perioperative cardiac complication varies with the severity of the surgical procedure and with RCRI stratification. A systematic, stepwise approach for preoperative cardiac risk assessment in patients undergoing noncardiac surgery facilitates a decision as to whether the risk for perioperative cardiac events is sufficiently low to proceed with the surgery. The patient's comorbid conditions and risk factors must be assessed for risk of exacerbation and steps taken to reduce risk to the patient in the perioperative period. Postoperatively, close monitoring of the patient's condition is required. Patients who develop complications after the operation will require timely and appropriate interventions by the surgical and medical teams. Finally, cardiac and medical perioperative care are evolving fields and practitioners must strive to keep their knowledge and practices current through literature review and guideline awareness.

For a deeper discussion on this topic, please see Chapters 403, ❖ "Preoperative Evaluation," and 405, "Postoperative Care and Complications," in *Goldman-Cecil Medicine*, 26th Edition.

SUGGESTED READINGS

Auerbach A, Goldman L: Assessing and reducing the cardiac risk of noncardiac surgery, *Circulation* 113:1361–1376, 2006.

Boersma E, Kertai MD, Schouten O, et al.: Perioperative cardiovascular mortality in noncardiac surgery: validation of the Lee cardiac risk index, *Am J Med* 118:1134–1141, 2005.

Doherty JU, Gluckman TJ, Hucker WJ, et al.: 2017 ACC expert consensus decision pathway for periprocedural management of anticoagulation in patients with nonvalvular atrial fibrillation: a report of the American College of Cardiology Clinical Expert Consensus Document Task Force, *J Am Coll Cardiol* 69:871–898, 2017.

Falck-Ytter Y, Francis CW, Johanson NA, Curley C, Dahl OE, Schulman S, et al.: Prevention of VTE in orthopedic surgery patients: Antithrombotic Therapy and Prevention of Thrombosis, 9th ed: American College of Chest Physicians Evidence-Based Clinical Practice Guidelines, *Chest* 141(Suppl 2):e278S–325S, 2012 Feb.

Fleisher LA, Fleischmann KE, Auerbach AD, et al.: 2014 ACC/AHA guideline on perioperative cardiovascular evaluation and management of patients undergoing noncardiac surgery: a report of the American College of Cardiology/American Heart Association task force on practice guidelines, *J Am Coll Cardiol* S0735- 1097(14), 2014, 05536-3.

Hassan SA, Hlatky MA, Boothroyd DB, et al.: Outcomes of noncardiac surgery after coronary bypass surgery or coronary angioplasty in the Bypass Angioplasty Revascularization Investigation (BARI), *Am J Med* 110: 260–266, 2001.

Kristensen SD, Knuuti J, Saraste A, et al.: 2014 ESC/ESA guidelines on non-cardiac surgery: cardiovascular assessment and management: the joint task force on non-cardiac surgery: cardiovascular assessment and management of the European Society of Cardiology (ESC) and the European Society of Anesthesiology (ESA), *Eur Heart J* 35(35):2382–2431, 2014.

McFalls EO, Ward HB, Moritz TE, et al.: Coronary-artery revascularization before elective major vascular surgery, *N Engl J Med* 351:2795–2804, 2004.

POISE Study Group: Effects of extended-release metoprolol succinate in patients undergoing non-cardiac surgery (POISE trial): a randomized controlled trial, *Lancet* 371:1839–1847, 2008.

Rechenmacher SJ, Fang JC: Bridging anticoagulation: primum non nocere, *J Am Coll Cardiol* 66:1392–1403, 2015.

帕金森病

　　帕金森病是一种常见的神经退行性疾病，表现为运动障碍、吞咽困难、辨距不良和生活功能丧失。左旋多巴是治疗帕金森病的常用药，如果漏服会导致发热、自主神经功能紊乱和症状的加重。根据临床情况，左旋多巴的治疗应尽量做到持续无中断。帕金森病患者手术后可能需要更长的恢复时间。

卒中

　　围术期卒中发生率较低，但死亡率和并发症发病率较高。大部分围术期卒中的发生机制是栓塞。危险因素包括：卒中病史、糖尿病、高血压、心房颤动和高龄。应重视处理可改变的风险因素，并采取适当的管理措施，包括对已知患有颅内动脉粥样硬化疾病的患者采用阿司匹林和他汀类药物治疗。对于存在心房颤动的高危患者，应当考虑围术期桥接抗凝治疗，以最大限度降低卒中风险。

风湿性疾病

　　自身免疫性疾病如类风湿关节炎和狼疮，常需使用药物抑制免疫系统功能。很多风湿性疾病患者使用改善病情抗风湿药，如甲氨蝶呤、硫唑嘌呤、吗替麦考酚酯，在围术期可继续使用。生物制剂，如阿达木单抗和英夫利单抗，一般认为会增加围术期感染的风险，应在围术期暂停使用。此外，手术最好安排在每一次给药周期结束时。

老年患者的特殊需求

　　在美国，1/3 的住院手术患者为年龄大于 65 岁的老年人。老年患者的围术期并发症发生率和死亡率的风险明显增高。除了本章涉及的系统性评估外，对于老年患者的术前风险评估应该关注患者的功能状态、认知和用药情况。日常活动能力（ADL）的下降与术后死亡率增加直接相关。功能状态的评估有多种不同的针对性量表。步行速度和起立行走计时是有效的客观评价方法。基础认知功能受损是术后谵妄的独立危险因素。认知功能可以使用 Mini-Cog 量表或蒙特利尔认知评估量表评价。术前对患者的功能状态和（或）认知功能问题的了解和关注可能导致手术方案的重新评估。术后，干预策略应侧重于身体康复和降低谵妄风险的措施，包括尽量减少使用可能引发谵妄的药物、频繁的定向力训练、多维度干预以及合理使用抗精神病药物。

　　应针对可能的术后并发症回顾患者的用药情况，特别是降压药（低血压）、利尿剂（血容量减少）、降糖药（高血糖或低血糖）、抗血栓药（出血或血栓）、苯二氮䓬类、阿片类和其他镇静催眠药（镇静和谵妄）。应审查每种用药的适应证，并评估其风险和获益。

总结

　　在接受非心脏手术的患者中，术前和术后风险降低循证策略的成功实施，依赖于外科医生、麻醉医生、患者的初级保健医生和顾问医师之间的紧密协作和有效沟通。

　　围术期心脏并发症的风险因外科手术的严重程度和 RCRI 分层而异。对接受非心脏手术的患者进行系统的、阶梯的术前心脏风险评估有助于判断围术期心脏事件的风险是否低至可以实施手术。必须评估患者的合并症和危险因素带来的风险，并在围术期采取措施降低风险。术后需要密切关注患者的病情。出现术后并发症的患者需要外科和内科医生及时和适当的干预。最后，心脏和内科围术期管理是一个逐渐发展的领域，医务人员必须努力通过阅读文献和熟悉指南来保持我们知识和实践的与时俱进。

　　有关此专题的深入讨论，请参阅 *Goldman-Cecil* ❖ *Medicine* 第 26 版第 403 章 "术前评估" 和第 405 章 "术后管理与并发症"。

推荐阅读

Auerbach A, Goldman L: Assessing and reducing the cardiac risk of noncardiac surgery, *Circulation* 113:1361–1376, 2006.

Boersma E, Kertai MD, Schouten O, et al.: Perioperative cardiovascular mortality in noncardiac surgery: validation of the Lee cardiac risk index, *Am J Med* 118:1134–1141, 2005.

Doherty JU, Gluckman TJ, Hucker WJ, et al.: 2017 ACC expert consensus decision pathway for periprocedural management of anticoagulation in patients with nonvalvular atrial fibrillation: a report of the American College of Cardiology Clinical Expert Consensus Document Task Force, *J Am Coll Cardiol* 69:871–898, 2017.

Falck-Ytter Y, Francis CW, Johanson NA, Curley C, Dahl OE, Schulman S, et al.: Prevention of VTE in orthopedic surgery patients: Antithrombotic Therapy and Prevention of Thrombosis, 9th ed: American College of Chest Physicians Evidence-Based Clinical Practice Guidelines, *Chest* 141(Suppl 2):e278S–325S, 2012 Feb.

Fleisher LA, Fleischmann KE, Auerbach AD, et al.: 2014 ACC/AHA guideline on perioperative cardiovascular evaluation and management of patients undergoing noncardiac surgery: a report of the American College of Cardiology/American Heart Association task force on practice guidelines, *J Am Coll Cardiol* S0735- 1097(14), 2014, 05536-3.

Hassan SA, Hlatky MA, Boothroyd DB, et al.: Outcomes of noncardiac surgery after coronary bypass surgery or coronary angioplasty in the Bypass Angioplasty Revascularization Investigation (BARI), *Am J Med* 110: 260–266, 2001.

Kristensen SD, Knuuti J, Saraste A, et al.: 2014 ESC/ESA guidelines on non-cardiac surgery: cardiovascular assessment and management: the joint task force on non-cardiac surgery: cardiovascular assessment and management of the European Society of Cardiology (ESC) and the European Society of Anesthesiology (ESA), *Eur Heart J* 35(35):2382–2431, 2014.

McFalls EO, Ward HB, Moritz TE, et al.: Coronary-artery revascularization before elective major vascular surgery, *N Engl J Med* 351:2795–2804, 2004.

POISE Study Group: Effects of extended-release metoprolol succinate in patients undergoing non-cardiac surgery (POISE trial): a randomized controlled trial, *Lancet* 371:1839–1847, 2008.

Rechenmacher SJ, Fang JC: Bridging anticoagulation: primum non nocere, *J Am Coll Cardiol* 66:1392–1403, 2015.

索引 Index

Page numbers followed by "f" indicate figures, "t" indicate tables, and "b" indicate boxes.

页码数字中，"f"代表"图"，"t"代表"表格"，"b"代表"框"。